AF888895

Postoperative Care in Thoracic Surgery

Mert Şentürk • Mukadder Orhan Sungur
Editors

Postoperative Care in Thoracic Surgery

A Comprehensive Guide

Springer

Editors
Mert Şentürk
Department of Anaesthesiology and Intensive Care
Istanbul University, Istanbul Faculty of Medicine
Istanbul
Turkey

Mukadder Orhan Sungur
Department of Anaesthesiology and Intensive Care
Istanbul University, Istanbul Faculty of Medicine
Istanbul
Turkey

ISBN 978-3-319-19907-8 ISBN 978-3-319-19908-5 (eBook)
DOI 10.1007/978-3-319-19908-5

Library of Congress Control Number: 2017933454

© Springer International Publishing Switzerland 2017
This work is subject to copyright. All rights are reserved by the Publisher, whether the whole or part of the material is concerned, specifically the rights of translation, reprinting, reuse of illustrations, recitation, broadcasting, reproduction on microfilms or in any other physical way, and transmission or information storage and retrieval, electronic adaptation, computer software, or by similar or dissimilar methodology now known or hereafter developed.
The use of general descriptive names, registered names, trademarks, service marks, etc. in this publication does not imply, even in the absence of a specific statement, that such names are exempt from the relevant protective laws and regulations and therefore free for general use.
The publisher, the authors and the editors are safe to assume that the advice and information in this book are believed to be true and accurate at the date of publication. Neither the publisher nor the authors or the editors give a warranty, express or implied, with respect to the material contained herein or for any errors or omissions that may have been made.

Printed on acid-free paper

This Springer imprint is published by Springer Nature
The registered company is Springer International Publishing AG
The registered company address is: Gewerbestrasse 11, 6330 Cham, Switzerland

Dedicated to our families and our beloved departed mentor Prof. Dr. Kutay Akpir.

Preface

Postoperative care after thoracic surgery is a multidisciplinary challenge. Obviously, the success of the postoperative care is associated with the success of the surgical process; however, this correlation is probably much stronger in thoracic operations. This "multidisciplinary" character can lead sometimes to some discussions between different disciplines.

This book has several aims: First, and most importantly, it is written to "comprehend" a concrete point of view to the topic. To achieve this, different operations (such as esophagectomy, thymectomy) and different patient populations (such as patients with obstructive pulmonary diseases) have been included. The content of the book limits itself not only to the postoperative period, but covers also preoperative assessment and peroperative management of respiratory and circulatory variables with their relation to a safe and reliable postoperative multidisciplinary planning and management. Second, it is also trying to give the reader some connections of theoretical knowledge and practical approaches. Last but not least, the book is concentrating on a rather "narrow," but challenging area and "claims" to be "reference" in this important topic.

To achieve these aims, the book has some advantages, of which the most important one was that the authors are some of the most "prominent" thoracic anesthesiologists. As a matter of fact, I really believe that it is not easy to find the arguments of so many "experts" of thoracic anesthesia in a book. From this point of view: Yes, the content is not necessarily "evidence-based" and can sometimes be an "expert opinion." But: Yes, these "expert opinions" are also mostly based on the "evidences," which have been introduced, explained, and sometimes debated by these experts. The reader will not only find the "recent knowledge" and the "guidelines" (which she/he can find elsewhere too), but she/he will also face some questions about some routine approaches.

The most important challenge was to prevent the "repetitions." Indeed, the reader will be addressed to some other chapters within the book. Yet, I have intentionally permitted some of the repetitions if I believe that the way of the "expression" was worthy for the reader to understand the argument.

For me, it was a pleasure and honor to edit this book: I just asked my "friends" whether it is a good idea to write a book about this topic and asked them to contribute; and yes, they accepted. Personally, I am very happy with the resulting product. I thank them all, very much. I want to thank also Andrea Ridolfi and other friends from Springer for the encouragement (and also for their patience). And, surely, it would be impossible for me to finish this job by myself. A very hardworking colleague, and a very good friend, Mukadder Orhan Sungur has coedited this book. Without her help, this book would remain as a dream.

We hope that the reader will share similar feelings with us about the book, after reading it.

Istanbul, Turkey Mert Şentürk
2016

Contents

Contributors

Clemens Aigner Department of Thoracic Surgery, Vienna General Hospital, University of Vienna, Vienna, Austria

Catherine Ashes Department of Anaesthetics, St Vincent's Hospital, Fitzroy, NSW, Australia

Lorenzo Ball IRCCS AOU San Martino-IST, Department of Surgical Sciences and Integrated Diagnostics, University of Genoa, Genoa, Italy

Peter Biro Institute of Anesthesiology, University Hospital Zurich, Zurich, Switzerland

Grégoire Blaudszun Department of Anaesthesiology, Pharmacology and Intensive Care, Geneva University Hospitals, Geneva, Switzerland

Pierre-Olivier Bridevaux Division of Pulmonary Medicine, Geneva University Hospitals, Geneva, Switzerland

Jaume Canet Department of Anesthesiology, Hospital Universitari Germans Trias i Pujol, Universitat Autònoma de Barcelona, Badalona, Spain

Tiziano Cassina Division of Anesthesiology, University Hospitals of Geneva, Geneva, Switzerland

Edmond Cohen Departments of Anesthesiology and Thoracic Surgery, The Icahn School of Medicine at Mount Sinai, New York, NY, USA

Maddalena Dameri IRCCS AOU San Martino-IST, Department of Surgical Sciences and Integrated Diagnostics, University of Genoa, Genoa, Italy

Mohamed R. El Tahan Anaesthesiology Department, College of Medicine, University of Dammam, Dammam, Saudi Arabia

Marcelo Gama de Abreu Department of Anesthesiology and Intensive Care Therapy, Pulmonary Engineering Group, University Hospital Carl Gustav Carus, Technische Universität Dresden, Dresden, Germany

Lluis Gallart Department of Anesthesiology, Hospital Universitari Germans Trias i Pujol, Universitat Autònoma de Barcelona, Badalona, Spain

Manuel Granell Department of Anaesthesiology, Critical Care and Pain Relief, General University Hospital of Valencia, Valencia, Spain

University of Valencia, Valencia, Spain

Catholic University of Valencia, Valencia, Spain

Jelena Grusina-Ujumaza Paul Stradins University, Riga, Latvia

Department of Thoracic Surgery, Pauls Stradins Clinical University Hospital, Riga, Latvia

Department of Thoracic Surgery, Group Florence Nightingale Hospitals, Istanbul, Turkey

Thomas Hachenberg Department of Anaesthesiology and Intensive Care Medicine, Otto-von-Guericke University, Magdeburg, Germany

Wilhelm Haverkamp Department of Cardiology, Charite University Medicine, Berlin, Germany

Göran Hedenstierna Hedenstierna Laboratory, Department of Medical Sciences, Clinical Physiology, Uppsala University Hospital, Uppsala, Sweden

Mª José Jiménez Department of Anaesthesiology, Critical Care and Pain Relief, Hospital Clinic of Barcelona, Barcelona, Spain

Thomas Kiss Department of Anesthesiology and Intensive Care Therapy, Pulmonary Engineering Group, University Hospital Carl Gustav Carus, Technische Universität Dresden, Dresden, Germany

Kemalettin Koltka Department of Anesthesiology and Intensive Care Medicine, Istanbul University, Istanbul Faculty of Medicine, Istanbul, Turkey

Lukas Kreienbühl Division of Anesthesiology, University Hospitals of Geneva, Geneva, Switzerland

Marc Joseph Licker Division of Anesthesiology, University Hospitals of Geneva, Geneva, Switzerland

Department of Anaesthesiology, Pharmacology, and Intensive Care, Geneva University Hospitals, Geneva, Switzerland

Juan V. Llau Department of Anaesthesia and Critical Care, Hospital Clínic, Valencia. University of Valencia, Valencia, Spain

Gary H. Mills Sheffield Teaching Hospital and University of Sheffield, Sheffield, UK

Perihan Ergin Özcan Department of Anesthesiology and Intensive Care Medicine, Istanbul University, Istanbul Faculty of Medicine, Istanbul, Turkey

Paolo Pelosi IRCCS AOU San Martino-IST, Department of Surgical Sciences and Integrated Diagnostics, University of Genoa, Genoa, Italy

Giorgio Della Roca Medical University of Udine, Department of Anesthesia and Intensive Care Medicine of the University of Udine, Udine, Italy

Evren Şentürk Department of Anesthesiology and Intensive Care Medicine, Istanbul University, Istanbul Faculty of Medicine, Istanbul, Turkey

Mert Şentürk Department of Anesthesiology and Intensive Care Medicine, Istanbul University, Istanbul Faculty of Medicine, Istanbul, Turkey

Peter Slinger Department of Anesthesia, Toronto General Hospital, Toronto, Canada

Mukadder Orhan Sungur Department of Anesthesiology and Intensive Care Medicine, Istanbul University, Istanbul Faculty of Medicine, Istanbul, Turkey

Zerrin Sungur Department of Anesthesiology and Intensive Care Medicine, Istanbul University, Istanbul Faculty of Medicine, Istanbul, Turkey

Laszlo L. Szegedi, MD, PhD Universitair Ziekenhuis Brussel and Vrije Universiteit Brussel, Brussels, Belgium

Alper Toker Department of Thoracic Surgery, Group Florence Nightingale Hospitals, Istanbul, Turkey

Department of Thoracic Surgery, Istanbul University, Istanbul Faculty of Medicine, Istanbul, Turkey

Frédéric Triponez Service of Thoracic and Endocrine Surgery, Geneva University Hospitals, Geneva, Switzerland

Edda M. Tschernko Department of Cardiothoracic Anesthesia and Intensive Care Medicine, Vienna General Hospital, University of Vienna, Vienna, Austria

Tamás Végh University of Debrecen, Department of Anesthesiology and Intensive Care, Debrecen, Hungary

Outcomes Research Consortium, Cleveland, OH, USA

What Happens to the Lung During Mechanical Ventilation and One-Lung Ventilation?

1

Göran Hedenstierna

1.1 Introduction

Focus of this chapter is on mechanical ventilation of one or both lungs in connection to thoracic surgery. Morphological and functional changes will be discussed as well as possible techniques to minimize any impairment. There is good reason to look for improved ventilator regimes. Despite decades of experience of the caring of the anesthetized patient, several recent multicenter studies show considerable incidence of postoperative lung complications. They may at least in part be attributed to the decreased lung function during anesthesia. However, how to optimize perioperative ventilator regime has not been fully agreed upon. Combinations of low tidal volume, recruitment maneuvers, and positive end-expiratory pressure (PEEP) have been tested, but recommendations differ between studies [1–3]. In a meta-analysis based on 3,365 patients, the total incidence of postoperative lung injury was similar for abdominal and thoracic surgery (3.4 % vs 4.3 %) [4]. Patients who developed postoperative lung injury received ventilation with higher tidal volumes and lower positive end-expiratory pressure levels, or both, than patients who did not. Thus, lung-protective mechanical ventilation strategies, as presently used, may reduce the incidence of postoperative lung injury but uncertainty still remains on what is optimal ventilation, and more can be done.

Functional residual capacity (FRC) is reduced by 0.8–1.0 L by changing the body position from upright to supine, and there is a further decrease by 0.4–0.5 L by the general anesthetic, whether inhaled or given intravenously [5] (except with ketamine that does not lower tone or FRC [6]). Muscle relaxants will presumably have similar effects as the anesthetic. As a result, the end-expiratory lung volume is reduced to close to residual volume.

G. Hedenstierna
Hedenstierna Laboratory, Department of Medical Sciences, Clinical Physiology, Uppsala University Hospital, Uppsala, Sweden
e-mail: goran.hedenstierna@akademiska.se

© Springer International Publishing Switzerland 2017

M. Şentürk, M.O. Sungur (eds.), *Postoperative Care in Thoracic Surgery*,
DOI 10.1007/978-3-319-19908-5_1

The decrease in FRC is a likely explanation to the fall in respiratory compliance and increase in respiratory resistance [7], the former by the reduced ventilated lung volume and the latter by decreased airway dimensions.

1.2 Airway Closure

During anesthesia, airways may close during expiration and reopen during the succeeding inspiration. They may even be continuously closed. The closure occurs because of higher extraluminal than intraluminal airway pressure. Since pleural pressure is higher in lower dependent than upper, nondependent regions, airway closure occurs primarily in the dependent lung. It impedes ventilation and with persisting perfusion causes a ventilation/perfusion mismatch ("low V/Q") [8]. The reduced ventilation in the lower half of the lung, as shown in Fig. 1.1, right panel, is reasonably explained by airway closure. Of similar or perhaps greater importance is that the continuously closed airways cause resorption atelectasis, as will be discussed next.

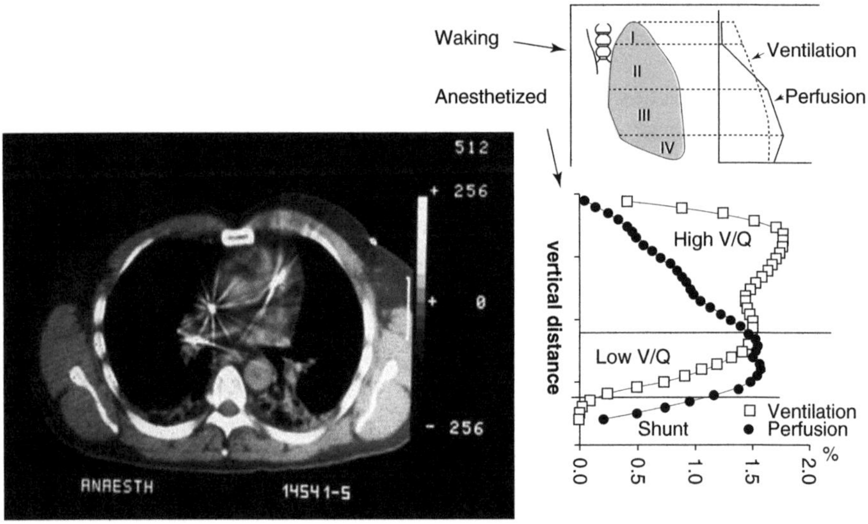

Fig. 1.1 CT scan (*left* panel) and vertical distributions of ventilation (*open squares*) and perfusion (*closed circles*) in an anesthetized subject (*right lower* panel). Ventilation and perfusion distributions in a waking subject are also shown (*right upper* panel). In the anesthetized subject, atelectasis can be seen in the bottom of both lungs. Note also that most of the ventilation is distributed to the upper half of the lung and is decreasing in the lower half until the bottom where the ventilation has ceased. This is different from the distribution in the waking subject. Perfusion on the other hand increases down the lung, similar to the waking situation, except for the lowermost part where a certain decrease can be seen. This causes a considerable ventilation/perfusion mismatch with high V/Q in the upper half of the lung, mimicking dead space ventilation, and low V/Q and shunt in the lowermost regions

1.3 Formation of Atelectasis

In their classic paper, Bendixen and coworkers proposed "a concept of atelectasis" as a cause of impaired oxygenation during anesthesia [9]. However, atelectasis could not be shown on conventional chest X-ray. With the introduction of radiological computed tomography (CT), densities were seen in dependent lung regions in anesthetized pediatric and adult patients [10, 11]. Morphological studies in various animals showed them to be atelectasis (see an example in Fig. 1.1, left panel).

Atelectasis appears in around 90 % of all patients who are anesthetized during spontaneous as well as mechanical ventilation and whether intravenous or inhalational anesthetics are used [11]. The atelectatic area on a CT near the diaphragm is on average 3–4 % of the total lung area but can easily exceed 15–20 %. The amount of tissue that is collapsed is even larger, the atelectatic area comprising mainly lung tissue, whereas the aerated lung consists of tissue and air. Thus, 10–20 % of the lung is regularly collapsed at the base of the lung during uneventful anesthesia before any surgery has been done. Abdominal surgery does not add much to the atelectasis, but the lung collapse can remain for several days in the postoperative period [12]. After thoracic surgery and cardiopulmonary bypass, more than 50 % of the lung can be collapsed still several hours after surgery [13]. The amount of atelectasis decreases toward the apex that is mostly spared (fully aerated). It is likely that the atelectasis is a locus of infection and that it can contribute to pulmonary complications [14, 15].

1.4 Prevention of Atelectasis

The major cause of atelectasis during anesthesia is closure of airways. This is important to remember when considering techniques to prevent atelectasis or reopen collapsed lung tissue. Compression of the lung might be suspected to be a major or additional cause of atelectasis, but this is not likely. Airways will close before alveoli collapse when the lung shrinks. This brings us to the second factor that is needed to cause atelectasis, resorption of the gas that is trapped behind closed airways. The higher the oxygen concentration, the faster is the resorption of gas and atelectasis formation [11] (one may even ask how much of lung collapse in the ARDS patient is caused by compression and how much by gas resorption). Thus, fall in FRC and high oxygen concentration are both needed to produce alveolar collapse, at least when considering the relatively short time of most anesthesias.

Positive end-expiratory pressure PEEP is a simple technique to increase lung volume and airway dimensions. Depending on the magnitude of PEEP, airways may be reopened, but whether the same level of PEEP is high enough to recruit collapsed alveoli is less certain. Airways may close at an airway pressure of 6 cmH_2O in a normal-weight anesthetized subject [16] and, most likely, at higher pressure in an obese subject. Perhaps a rule of thumb (not clearly tested) would be PEEP of 7 cmH_2O when BMI is below 25 kg/m^2, 9 cmH_2O up to 32 kg/m^2, and higher in

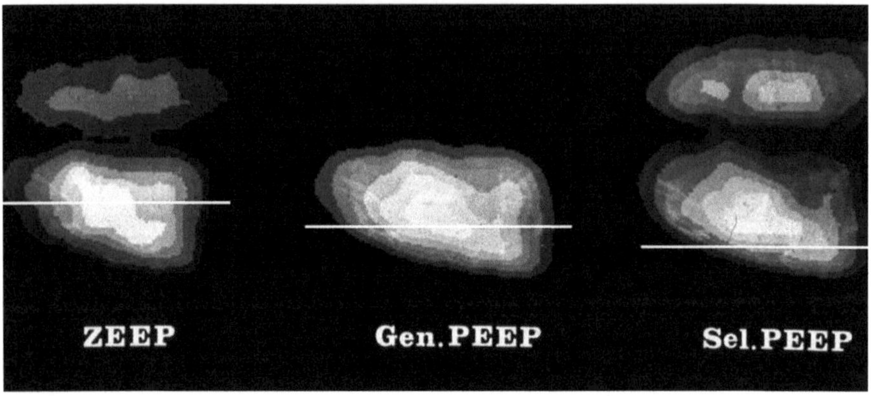

Fig. 1.2 Gamma camera images of lung blood flow in an anesthetized and mechanically ventilated patient in the lateral position. The left panel shows more perfusion to the lower lung, the middle panel shows how perfusion is almost absent in the upper lung with a general PEEP of 10 cmH_2O, and the right panel shows how perfusion is redistributed to the upper lung when a PEEP of 10 cmH_20 has been applied to the dependent lung only. The lung per se cannot be seen but the upper lung is larger than the lower one with no or global PEEP (From Ref. [28], with permission by the publisher)

more obese subjects to keep airways open. If this PEEP is applied before any atelectasis has been produced, it is likely that it can prevent formation of it. To confuse things, it should be mentioned that the application of 10 cmH_2O PEEP consistently reopens collapsed lung tissue. It requires some time, still only minutes, and may rather be an effect of increased inspiratory airway pressure than of PEEP per se [11]. It may not reopen all previously collapsed lung tissue, even if applied during a prolonged period of time. Moreover, arterial oxygenation is not improved in proportion to the decrease in atelectasis because of shift of blood flow to more dependent, still atelectatic lung regions (Fig. 1.2). Also, PEEP higher than 10 cmH_2O may be associated with derangement in hemodynamics [3]. This does not preclude the use of PEEP, but presumably an optimal and individual PEEP is needed to balance the effects of recruitment and circulatory impairment.

Recruitment maneuver: A "sigh," or a double tidal volume, has been suggested to reopen collapsed lung and to improve gas exchange, both for intubated and non-intubated patients [17]. However, the amount of atelectasis does not change during normal tidal breathing or by a "sigh" using an airway pressure of up to 20 cmH_2O [11]. At a sustained inflation of the lungs to an airway pressure of 30 cmH_2O, atelectasis decreases to approximately half the initial size. Additional inflations of the lung to the same airway pressure (30 cmH_2O) only result in minor further opening of lung tissue after the first maneuver. To reopen all collapsed lung tissue in anesthetized adults with healthy lungs, an airway pressure (recruitment pressure) of 40 cmH_2O is required. In morbidly obese patients with increased chest wall elastance, a higher airway pressure is required to reach the same transpulmonary pressure as in normal-weight subjects. A high airway pressure of 55 cmH_2O, kept for 10 s, was also used for lung recruitment in morbidly obese (BMI >45 kg/m^2), anesthetized patient [18].

Recruitment maneuvers also have been used during cardiac surgery [19] (see also below) and in the intensive care setting [20]. As there is a complex interaction between time and pressure, the time frame possibly differs if other recruitment pressures are used [21]. As an alternative, a stepwise increase in PEEP can be used [22].

Oxygen and atelectasis during induction of anesthesia Preoxygenation is provided to prevent hypoxemia in the event of a difficult intubation of the airway and will for the anesthetist be an important procedure to ensure maximum safety. However, the formation of atelectasis should be recalled, and it will by itself shorten the "apnea tolerance time," i.e., the time before hypoxemia develops.

Avoiding the preoxygenation procedure and ventilating with 30 % instead of 100 % O_2 prevents formation of atelectasis during the induction and subsequent anesthesia [23]. In studies atelectasis appeared in all patients who were preoxygenated with 100 % O_2, was much smaller with 80 % O_2, and was almost absent with 60 % O_2. However, the smaller amount of atelectasis with lower oxygen concentration during induction remains only for a limited time. The patients receiving 80 % O_2 during induction had as much atelectasis as those on 100 % O_2 40 min later [24]. This is because the gas trapped behind closed airways consists of 80 % O_2 and will be resorbed during the ensuing period and finally results in airlessness, i.e., atelectasis. Reopening of closed airways by a recruitment maneuver with lower O_2 concentration, e.g., 40 %, even in the absence of atelectasis, will replenish the closed region with lower O_2 gas, and this will slow down resorption atelectasis even more, hopefully for the rest of the anesthesia.

Anesthesia might be induced during ventilation with CPAP that will prevent the fall in FRC and atelectasis formation [25]. Oxygen can be used to full extent, and, moreover, the lung volume is higher compared to no use of CPAP/PEEP, resulting in a larger oxygen reservoir and increased safety time in the event of a complicated intubation of the airway.

Oxygen and atelectasis during anesthesia Ventilation of the lungs with pure oxygen after a vital capacity maneuver that had reopened previously collapsed lung tissue resulted in a rapid reappearance of the atelectasis [11]. If, on the other hand, 40 % O_2 in nitrogen was used for ventilation of the lungs, atelectasis reappeared slowly, and 40 min after the vital capacity maneuver, only 20 % of the initial atelectasis had reappeared. Thus, ventilation during anesthesia should be done with a moderate fraction of inspired oxygen to prevent atelectasis formation, but if higher oxygen is considered necessary, it can be given during PEEP ventilation.

Oxygen and atelectasis during emergence from anesthesia Another situation where a high oxygen concentration is used is at the end of the anesthesia. A post-oxygenation maneuver is regularly performed to reduce the risk of hypoxemia during the wake up. This may be done in combination with airway suctioning to eliminate secretions. However, the combination of oxygenation and airway suctioning will most likely cause atelectasis, and there is indeed no other potential maneuver that can compete with post-oxygenation and airway suctioning in doing so.

The findings of atelectasis during anesthesia and the possibility to recruit lung tissue with an inflation of the lung has prompted studies on the use of recruitment maneuver at the end of the surgery and anesthesia. Again, the influence of inspired oxygen plays an important role. Thus, recruitment at the end of the anesthesia followed by ventilation with 100 % oxygen (the latter again being common in routine anesthesia) caused new atelectasis within the 10 min period before anesthesia was terminated but not if ventilation was with lower FiO_2 [26]. Another approach to prevent atelectasis to persist into the postoperative period is to use PEEP until extubation of the airway and to continue with the CPAP for a limited time, e.g., 15–30 min during which period inspired oxygen concentration is lowered to 30 % in the air. In a small study where this technique was applied, atelectasis was reduced to less than a third compared to control patients with no PEEP/CPAP as assessed by CT one hour after wake up [27].

1.5 Individual Lung Ventilation

An individual lung ventilation technique was developed more than 30 years ago in order to optimize ventilation distribution in proportion to individual lung blood flow. It was successful in improving oxygenation but was considered too complicated to be used in intensive care. Thus, it required that:

1. The patient was in the lateral position
2. A double lumen endobronchial catheter was inserted
3. Two ventilators were used

This made it possible to apply a higher PEEP to the lower lung where most of the atelectasis should be and to ventilate each lung separately so that 50 % of ventilation was given to the upper, nondependent lung and 50 % to the lower, dependent lung. This was assumed to match the distribution of blood flow between the two lungs [28] (Fig. 1.2). Despite its technical complexity, it was also tested in anesthetized patients. Also, during anesthesia, gas exchange could be improved, and CT scanning showed that atelectasis could efficiently be removed from the dependent lung without undue overexpansion of the nondependent lung. The concept has been revived recently, at least experimentally, using better monitoring technique and, more importantly, distributing ventilation in proportion to the lung mechanics of each lung rather than its perfusion. This may not optimize gas exchange but should reduce stress and strain of the lung with possible protective effect on inflammation. Having this as the objective, ventilation will be distributed automatically between the two lungs in proportion to their regional compliances (or, rather, their time constants). Recruitment of collapsed lung tissue with no overexpansion and ventilation of each lung at their optimum PEEP levels can be achieved, as shown in an animal model [29] (see also Fig. 1.3). A simple pneumatic system that allows the use of only one ventilator, still providing different PEEP to the two lungs, does exist [30], and there is today a double lumen tracheal tube that facilitates the insertion and fixation of the tube. The potential value of this in thoracic surgery and in intensive care remains to be studied.

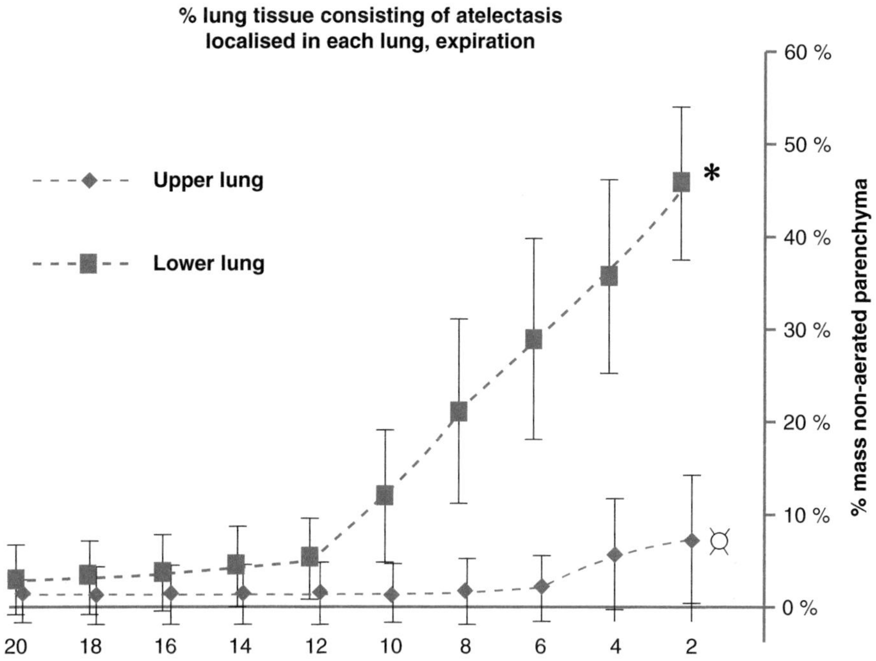

Fig. 1.3 Amount of atelectasis in the nondependent and dependent lung in piglets in the lateral position after creating a ventilator-induced lung injury (repeated lung lavages and vulnerable ventilation). Note that when the end-expiratory pressure decreased from 20 cmH_2O to downward, atelectasis rapidly increased from 12 cmH_2O in the lower dependent lung and not until 6 cmH_2O in the upper nondependent lung (From Ref. [29])

1.6 One-Lung Ventilation

During one-lung ventilation (OLV), one lung is separated from ventilation to enable surgery on that lung, and it does not participate in the pulmonary gas exchange. There is a persisting perfusion that causes shunt and decreased arterial oxygenation. Hypoxic vasoconstriction (HPV) reduces this blood flow, whereas kinking of pulmonary vessels because of compression and distortion of the lung seems to have less effect on blood flow [31].

The other lung is ventilated and perfused. The patient is normally in the lateral position with the non-ventilated lung in the upper position to facilitate surgery and the ventilated lung in the dependent position. Atelectasis is produced in the dependent lung, and pulmonary shunt is regularly larger than 11 % and the PaO_2 reduced by 50 % or more during OLV [32]. A traditional approach to mechanical ventilation during OLV has been high tidal volume (10–12 ml/kg) and zero PEEP to the dependent ventilated lung, high tidal volume to keep the lung open, and no PEEP to preserve the effect of the HPV in the nondependent lung and minimize blood flow to it [33]. However, pulmonary complications are common, both during the anesthesia per se with shunt and hypoxemia (see above) and postoperatively. Pathophysiological

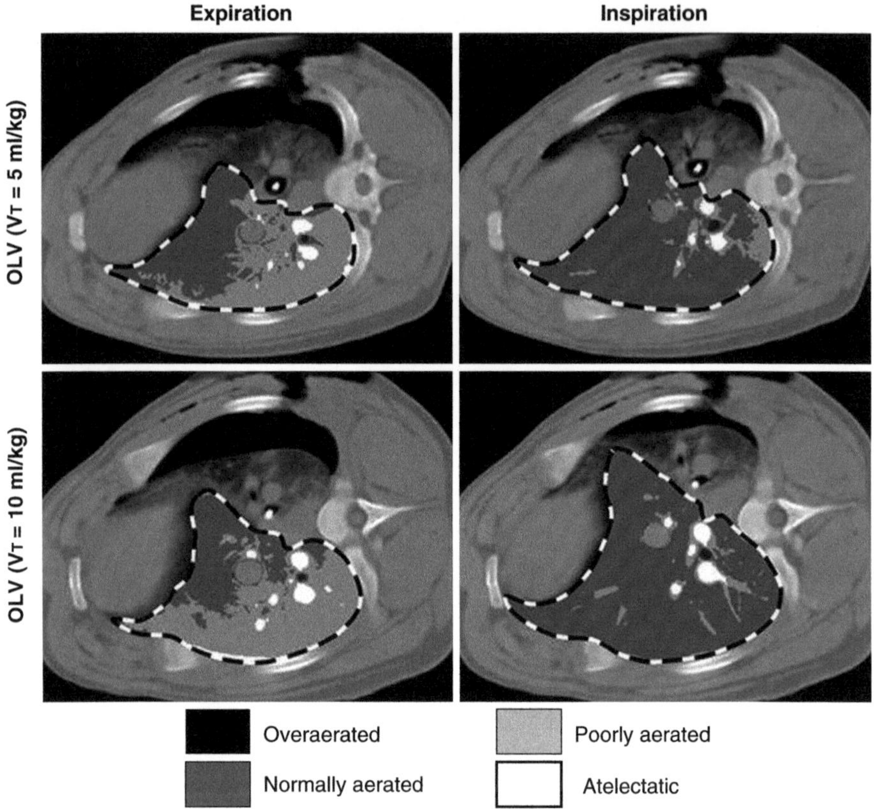

Fig. 1.4 CT images of pig lungs during OLV with VT=5 ml/kg or VT=10 ml/kg in the left lateral position. The left lung has been inscribed. Note the larger amount of atelectasis at end expiration and slightly smaller amount at end inspiration with VT 10 compared to VT 5 ml/kg, thus resulting in larger recruitment/de-recruitment with the large VT (From Ref. [35], with permission by the publisher)

disturbances include high airway pressures, ventilation/perfusion mismatch with shunt, increased pulmonary capillary pressure, and cyclic alveolar collapse. These events may result in alveolar damage followed by pulmonary edema with diffuse alveolar injury, leucocyte sequestration, and alveolar cytokine release, a series of events frequently called mechanotransduction (for a review, see [34]). Moreover, on termination of OLV there can be persisting hyperperfusion in the dependent, ventilated lung, associated with an increased diffuse alveolar damage score, as seen in porcine experiments [35].

Decrease of tidal volume (VT) to 5 ml/kg appears favorable in patients undergoing thoracotomy [36] and, interestingly, reduces cyclic recruitment/de-recruitment of atelectasis and poorly aerated tissue from 65 to 42 % in a porcine model of OLV [37] (Fig. 1.4). This may possibly prevent or reduce an inflammatory reaction. Moreover, the driving pressure, i.e., the difference between end-inspiratory and end-expiratory airway pressure, seems to be an important predictor of outcome in intensive care [38]. It is possible that OLV is another condition where the driving pressure is particularly important.

As with conventional two-lung ventilation, there is no generally accepted standard in determining an optimal level of positive end-expiratory pressure (PEEP) during OLV. One option is to titrate PEEP aiming at best respiratory compliance [39]. However, PEEP has potentially two opposing effects during OLV. On the one hand, it may help to recruit and stabilize collapsed lung units in the ventilated lung, reducing shunt in this lung. On the other hand, PEEP may divert blood flow away from the ventilated lung to the non-ventilated lung, thereby increasing shunt in that lung.

A recruitment maneuver has also been suggested to re-expand collapsed lung during OLV [40]. In addition to an improved oxygenation, due to a reduction in pulmonary shunt, such maneuver may contribute to a more even distribution of ventilation, as suggested by a flattening of the CO_2 curve during a tidal expiration. Using CO_2 washout may also enable detection of excessive airway and alveolar dead spaces and guide in modifying VT and PEEP in OLV [41].

Pressure-controlled ventilation has been suggested to improve gas exchange during OLV, as compared to volume-controlled ventilation. Still, this was not confirmed in a study on patients undergoing thoracic surgery [42]. Indeed, if ventilation was adjusted to reach the same tidal volume, there was no difference in arterial oxygenation, neither was there a difference in end-inspiratory (plateau) airway pressure. The only difference between the two modes was a higher peak pressure in volume-controlled mode, which can be explained by the difference in flow pattern of inspiratory gas between the two modes.

Another line for control of impaired gas exchange during one-lung anesthesia is pharmacological interference with pulmonary blood flow [43]. Inhaled vasodilators such as nitric oxide (NO) and prostaglandins are considered to have a local effect and divert blood away from non-ventilated to well-ventilated lung regions. Interaction with the endothelin system appears to enhance the redistribution of blood flow, as recently demonstrated [44]. Intravenous almitrine has been shown to increase pulmonary artery pressure in a dose-dependent manner and to increase oxygenation in patients with acute respiratory distress syndrome (ARDS) or with sepsis [45]. The effect has been attributed to enhanced HPV and thus a reduction of blood flow in non-ventilated lung regions. Finally, positioning of the patient can alter the degree of shunting [46].

Virtually all anesthetics attenuate HPV [47], but the effect is small as is the difference between anesthetics, e.g., between desflurane and isoflurane during OLV [48]. Intravenous anesthetics blunt HPV even less, but they may trigger inflammatory reactions more than inhaled drugs. Thus, in a study on patients undergoing thoracic surgery during OLV (VT, 7 ml/kg), the effect on inflammatory responses during propofol, desflurane, and sevoflurane anesthesias were compared [49]. The major findings were that OLV increases the concentrations of pro-inflammatory mediators in the ventilated lung and that the inhalational anesthetics, but not propofol, decrease the alveolar inflammatory response.

A special condition of OLV is its execution together with capnothorax, i.e., carbon dioxide insufflation into the pleural cavity. One indication for OLV/

capnothorax is atrial fibrillation surgery. This can be a rather challenging situation with need of rapid decisions regarding ventilatory and circulatory support. In an experimental model using electric impedance tomography (EIT), OLV of the left lung together with right-sided capnothorax caused a decrease in cardiac output, arterial oxygenation, and also mixed venous saturation, whereas changes were less marked in OLV of the right lung and left-sided capnothorax. The model might be useful for further studies [50].

References

1. Futier E, Marret E, Jaber S (2014) Perioperative positive pressure ventilation: an integrated approach to improve pulmonary care. Anesthesiology 121(2):400–408
2. Futier E, Constantin JM, Paugam-Burtz C, Pascal J, Eurin M, Neuschwander A et al (2013) A trial of intraoperative low-tidal-volume ventilation in abdominal surgery. N Engl J Med 369(5):428–437
3. The PNI, for the Clinical Trial Network of the European Society of A (2014) High versus low positive end-expiratory pressure during general anaesthesia for open abdominal surgery (PROVHILO trial): a multicentre randomised controlled trial. Lancet 384(9942):495–503
4. Serpa Neto A, Hemmes SN, Barbas CS, Beiderlinden M, Fernandez-Bustamante A, Futier E et al (2014) Incidence of mortality and morbidity related to postoperative lung injury in patients who have undergone abdominal or thoracic surgery: a systematic review and meta-analysis. Lancet Respir Med 2(12):1007–1015
5. Wahba RW (1991) Perioperative functional residual capacity. Can J Anaesth (Journal canadien d'anesthesie) 38(3):384–400
6. Tokics L, Strandberg A, Brismar B, Lundquist H, Hedenstierna G (1987) Computerized tomography of the chest and gas exchange measurements during ketamine anaesthesia. Acta Anaesthesiol Scand 31(8):684–692
7. Don H (1977) The mechanical properties of the respiratory system during anesthesia. Int Anesthesiol Clin 15(2):113–136
8. Rothen HU, Sporre B, Engberg G, Wegenius G, Hedenstierna G (1998) Airway closure, atelectasis and gas exchange during general anaesthesia. Br J Anaesth 81(5):681–686
9. Bendixen HH, Hedley-Whyte J, Laver MB (1963) Impaired oxygenation in surgical patients during general anesthesia with controlled ventilation. A concept of atelectasis. N Engl J Med 269:991–996
10. Damgaard-Pedersen K, Qvist T (1980) Pediatric pulmonary CT-scanning. Anaesthesia-induced changes. Pediatr Radiol 9(3):145–148
11. Hedenstierna G, Edmark L (2010) Mechanisms of atelectasis in the perioperative period. Best Pract Res Clin Anaesthesiol 24(2):157–169
12. Lindberg P, Gunnarsson L, Tokics L, Secher E, Lundquist H, Brismar B et al (1992) Atelectasis and lung function in the postoperative period. Acta Anaesthesiol Scand 36(6):546–553
13. Tenling A, Hachenberg T, Tyden H, Wegenius G, Hedenstierna G (1998) Atelectasis and gas exchange after cardiac surgery. Anesthesiology 89(2):371–378
14. van Kaam AH, Lachmann RA, Herting E, De Jaegere A, van Iwaarden F, Noorduyn LA et al (2004) Reducing atelectasis attenuates bacterial growth and translocation in experimental pneumonia. Am J Respir Crit Care Med 169(9):1046–1053
15. Nakos G, Tsangaris H, Liokatis S, Kitsiouli E, Lekka ME (2003) Ventilator-associated pneumonia and atelectasis: evaluation through bronchoalveolar lavage fluid analysis. Intensive Care Med 29(4):555–563
16. Hedenstierna G, McCarthy GS (1980) Airway closure and closing pressure during mechanical ventilation. Acta Anaesthesiol Scand 24(4):299–304

17. Scholten DJ, Novak R, Snyder JV (1985) Directed manual recruitment of collapsed lung in intubated and nonintubated patients. Am Surg 51(6):330–335
18. Reinius H, Jonsson L, Gustafsson S, Sundbom M, Duvernoy O, Pelosi P et al (2009) Prevention of atelectasis in morbidly obese patients during general anesthesia and paralysis: a computerized tomography study. Anesthesiology 111(5):979–987
19. Dyhr T, Nygard E, Laursen N, Larsson A (2004) Both lung recruitment maneuver and PEEP are needed to increase oxygenation and lung volume after cardiac surgery. Acta Anaesthesiol Scand 48(2):187–197
20. Gattinoni L, Caironi P, Cressoni M, Chiumello D, Ranieri VM, Quintel M et al (2006) Lung recruitment in patients with the acute respiratory distress syndrome. N Engl J Med 354(17):1775–1786
21. Albert SP, DiRocco J, Allen GB, Bates JH, Lafollette R, Kubiak BD et al (2009) The role of time and pressure on alveolar recruitment. J Appl Physiol (1985) 106(3):757–765
22. Tusman G, Bohm SH, Vazquez de Anda GF, do Campo JL, Lachmann B (1999) 'Alveolar recruitment strategy' improves arterial oxygenation during general anaesthesia. Br J Anaesth 82(1):8–13
23. Rothen HU, Sporre B, Engberg G, Wegenius G, Reber A, Hedenstierna G (1995) Prevention of atelectasis during general anaesthesia. Lancet 345(8962):1387–1391
24. Edmark L, Auner U, Enlund M, Ostberg E, Hedenstierna G (2011) Oxygen concentration and characteristics of progressive atelectasis formation during anaesthesia. Acta Anaesthesiol Scand 55(1):75–81
25. Rusca M, Proietti S, Schnyder P, Frascarolo P, Hedenstierna G, Spahn DR et al (2003) Prevention of atelectasis formation during induction of general anesthesia. Anesth Analg 97(6):1835–1839
26. Benoit Z, Wicky S, Fischer JF, Frascarolo P, Chapuis C, Spahn DR et al (2002) The effect of increased FIO(2) before tracheal extubation on postoperative atelectasis. Anesth Analg 95(6):1777–1781
27. Edmark L, Auner U, Hallen J, Lassinantti-Olowsson L, Hedenstierna G, Enlund M (2014) A ventilation strategy during general anaesthesia to reduce postoperative atelectasis. Ups J Med Sci 119(3):242–250
28. Hedenstierna G, Baehrendtz S, Klingstedt C, Santesson J, Soderborg B, Dahlborn M et al (1984) Ventilation and perfusion of each lung during differential ventilation with selective PEEP. Anesthesiology 61(4):369–376
29. Borges JBAO, Senturk M, Suarez-Sipmann F, Hedenstierna G, Larsson A (2015) Optimum selective PEEP titration during lateral decubitus and differential lung ventilation. Am J Respir Crit Care Med 43(10):e404–e411
30. Darowski M, Hedenstierna G, Baehrendtz S (1985) Development and evaluation of a flow-dividing unit for differential ventilation and selective PEEP. Acta Anaesthesiol Scand 29(1):61–66
31. Miller FL, Chen L, Malmkvist G, Marshall C, Marshall BE (1989) Mechanical factors do not influence blood flow distribution in atelectasis. Anesthesiology 70(3):481–488
32. Lesser T, Schubert H, Klinzing S (2008) Determination of the side-separated pulmonary right-to-left shunt volume. J Med Invest: JMI 55(1–2):44–50
33. Brodsky JB (2005) The evolution of thoracic anesthesia. Thorac Surg Clin 15(1):1–10
34. Karcz M, Vitkus A, Papadakos PJ, Schwaiberger D, Lachmann B (2012) State-of-the-art mechanical ventilation. J Cardiothorac Vasc Anesth 26(3):486–506
35. Kozian A, Schilling T, Freden F, Maripuu E, Rocken C, Strang C et al (2008) One-lung ventilation induces hyperperfusion and alveolar damage in the ventilated lung: an experimental study. Br J Anaesth 100(4):549–559
36. Tugrul M, Camci E, Karadeniz H, Senturk M, Pembeci K, Akpir K (1997) Comparison of volume controlled with pressure controlled ventilation during one-lung anaesthesia. Br J Anaesth 79(3):306–310
37. Kozian A, Schilling T, Schutze H, Senturk M, Hachenberg T, Hedenstierna G (2011) Ventilatory protective strategies during thoracic surgery: effects of alveolar recruitment maneuver and low-tidal volume ventilation on lung density distribution. Anesthesiology 114(5):1025–1035

38. Amato MB, Meade MO, Slutsky AS, Brochard L, Costa EL, Schoenfeld DA et al (2015) Driving pressure and survival in the acute respiratory distress syndrome. N Engl J Med 372(8):747–755
39. Slinger PD, Kruger M, McRae K, Winton T (2001) Relation of the static compliance curve and positive end-expiratory pressure to oxygenation during one-lung ventilation. Anesthesiology 95(5):1096–1102
40. Tusman G, Bohm SH, Sipmann FS, Maisch S (2004) Lung recruitment improves the efficiency of ventilation and gas exchange during one-lung ventilation anesthesia. Anesth Analg 98(6):1604–1609, table of contents
41. Tusman G, Bohm SH, Suarez-Sipmann F (2015) Dead space during one-lung ventilation. Curr Opin Anaesthesiol 28(1):10–17
42. Unzueta MC, Casas JI, Moral MV (2007) Pressure-controlled versus volume-controlled ventilation during one-lung ventilation for thoracic surgery. Anesth Analg 104(5):1029–1033
43. Dembinski R, Henzler D, Rossaint R (2004) Modulating the pulmonary circulation: an update. Minerva Anestesiol 70(4):239–243
44. Trachsel S, Hambraeus-Jonzon K, Bergquist M, Martijn C, Chen L, Hedenstierna G (2015) No redistribution of lung blood flow by inhaled nitric oxide in endotoxemic piglets pretreated with an endothelin receptor antagonist. J Appl Physiol (1985) 118(6):768–775
45. Wysocki M, Delclaux C, Roupie E, Langeron O, Liu N, Herman B et al (1994) Additive effect on gas exchange of inhaled nitric oxide and intravenous almitrine bismesylate in the adult respiratory distress syndrome. Intensive Care Med 20(4):254–259
46. Choi YS, Bang SO, Shim JK, Chung KY, Kwak YL, Hong YW (2007) Effects of head-down tilt on intrapulmonary shunt fraction and oxygenation during one-lung ventilation in the lateral decubitus position. J Thorac Cardiovasc Surg 134(3):613–618
47. Marshall BE (1990) Hypoxic pulmonary vasoconstriction. Acta Anaesthesiol Scand Suppl 94:37–41
48. Schwarzkopf K, Schreiber T, Bauer R, Schubert H, Preussler NP, Gaser E et al (2001) The effects of increasing concentrations of isoflurane and desflurane on pulmonary perfusion and systemic oxygenation during one-lung ventilation in pigs. Anesth Analg 93(6):1434–1438
49. Schilling T, Kozian A, Senturk M, Huth C, Reinhold A, Hedenstierna G et al (2011) Effects of volatile and intravenous anesthesia on the alveolar and systemic inflammatory response in thoracic surgical patients. Anesthesiology 115(1):65–74
50. Reinius H, Borges JB, Freden F, Jideus L, Camargo ED, Amato MB et al (2015) Real-time ventilation and perfusion distributions by electrical impedance tomography during one-lung ventilation with capnothorax. Acta Anaesthesiol Scand 59(3):354–368

Where Should I Send My Patient After the Operation?

2

Lukas Kreienbühl, Tiziano Cassina, and Marc Licker

2.1 Introduction

Thoracic surgery is associated with postoperative mortality rates ranging between 2 and 5 % and cardiopulmonary complications varying between 20 and 40 %, resulting in prolonged hospital stay and increased healthcare costs [1]. Traditionally, a large proportion of thoracic surgical patients were admitted to ICU. In light of growing health costs and budgetary constraints, patients are increasingly admitted in HDU and PACU. In this chapter, we will address the rationale of postoperative care management and selection criteria, guiding the choice to admit the patient in ICU, HDU, or PACU, taking into account available hospital resources, in addition to patient- and procedure-related factors (Fig. 2.1).

A clinician's judgment on postoperative triage is largely based on predicting the occurrence of "avoidable" major complications following surgery. The overall risk profile can be approximated by combining patient- and procedure-related risks. Based on large cohort analysis, several risk scoring systems, including surgical and patient's risk factors, have been developed and validated to estimate postoperative morbidity and mortality in major noncardiac surgery and also more specifically in thoracic surgery.

L. Kreienbühl • T. Cassina • M. Licker (✉)
Division of Anesthesiology, University Hospitals of Geneva, Geneva, Switzerland
e-mail: Marc-Joseph.Licker@hcuge.ch

© Springer International Publishing Switzerland 2017

M. Şentürk, M.O. Sungur (eds.), *Postoperative Care in Thoracic Surgery*,
DOI 10.1007/978-3-319-19908-5_2

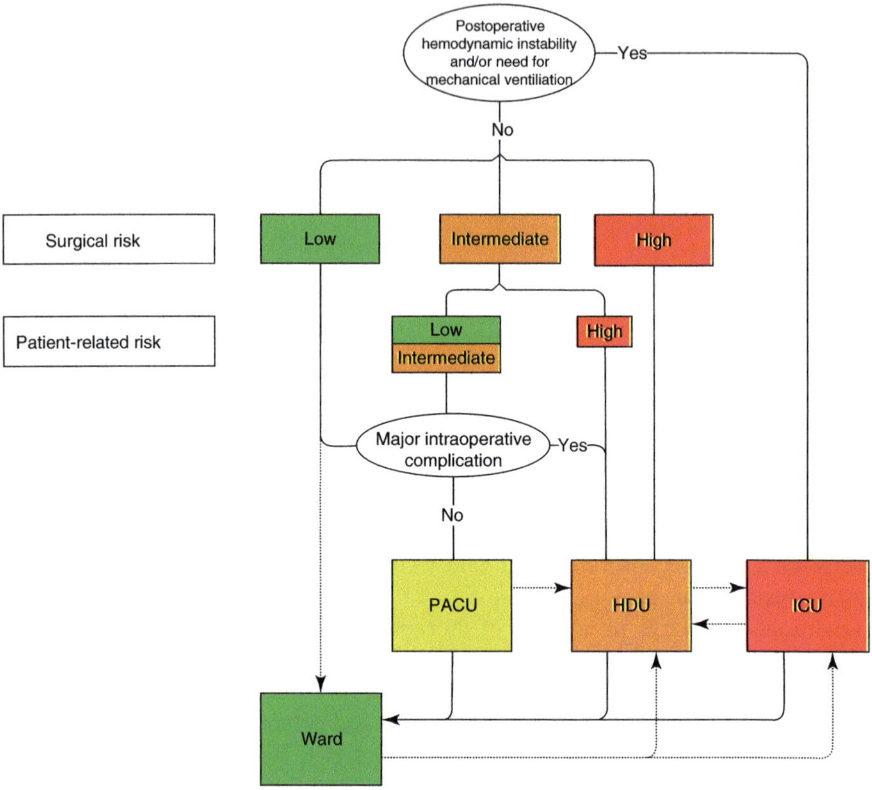

Fig. 2.1 Postoperative patient triage. Abbreviations: *PACU* postanesthesia care unit, *HDU* high dependency unit, *ICU* intensive care unit

2.2 Risk Stratification

2.2.1 Patient-Related Risk Factors

2.2.1.1 General Risk Scores

The American Society of Anesthesiologists' (ASA) classification of physical health (from I to V) is universally applied for assessing preoperative health of patients requiring any surgical, therapeutic, or diagnostic procedure. Although ASA > II is associated with increased risk of postoperative morbidity and mortality, large interobserver variability and poor specificity preclude accurate estimation for individual patient risk [2].

The Charlson Comorbidity Index (CCI), composed of 19 weighted medical diagnoses, is a valid predictor of 1-year mortality in medical patient population, score greater than 5 being associated with 1-year mortality greater than 50 % [3]. In patients undergoing noncardiac surgery, CCI score ≥ 3 was associated with a 16-fold increase of death at one year [4]. Likewise, among lung cancer patients undergoing

Table 2.1 Surgical Mortality Probability Model (S-MPM)

Risk factor	Points
ASA I	0
ASA II	2
ASA III	4
ASA IV	5
ASA V	6
Low surgical risk	0
Intermediate surgical risk	1
High surgical risk	2
Emergency intervention	1
Points	**Mortality %**
0	0.01 %
1	0.02 %
3	0.07 %
4	0.2 %
5	1.5 %
6	4 %
7	10 %
8	25 %
9	50 %

curative resection, a CCI score ≥3 was associated with a tenfold greater incidence of major complications [5].

The National Surgical Quality Improvement Program (NSQIP) was jointly established by the American College of Surgeons (ACS) and the Department of Veterans Affairs (VA) to compare risk-adjusted 30-day mortality between different VA hospitals [6]. Based on 21 variables, the NSQIP is currently available with web-based surgical risk calculator. Derived from the NSQIP database, the Surgical Mortality Probability Model (S-MPM) includes three relevant components – the ASA physical status, surgical risk class, and emergency status – to predict all-cause postoperative mortality at 30 days [7] (Table 2.1).

More specific for thoracic surgery, the Cardiopulmonary Risk Index (CPRI) was developed in 1993 and consists in a combination of a cardiac risk index (congestive heart failure, myocardial infarction during the previous 6 months, greater than five premature ventricular contractions, arrhythmias, age >70 years, important valvular aortic stenosis, poor general medical condition) and a pulmonary risk index (BMI ≥27 kg/m^2, smoking within 8 weeks of surgery, productive cough within 5 days of surgery, diffuse wheezing or rhonchi within 5 days of surgery, FEV1/FVC <70 %, $PaCO_2$ >45 mmHg). Later on, Ferguson et al. have validated a simple scoring system (EVAD) that utilizes pulmonary function test data (forced expiratory volume in one second [FEV1], diffusion capacity of the lung for carbon monoxide [DLCO]) and patient age to predict the likelihood of complications after major lung resection [8].

Table 2.2 Revised Cardiac Risk Index

Risk factor	**Points**
History of coronary artery disease	1
History of heart failure	1
History of cerebrovascular disease	1
High-risk surgery (suprainguinal vascular, intraperitoneal, intrathoracic)	1
Preoperative insuline therapy	1
Serum creatinine > 177 μmol/L	1
Risk of major cardiac event	
Points	**Risk % (95 % CI)**
0	0.4 (0.05 – 1.5)
1	0.9 (0.3 – 2.1)
2	6.6 (3.9 – 10.3)
≥3	≥ 11 (5.8 – 18.4)

CI: Confidence Interval

More recently, the Thoracoscore derived from the French national thoracic database EPITHOR has incorporated eight independent risk factors (age, sex, ASA physical status, performance status, dyspnea, priority of surgery, extent of resection, carcinoma) to predict in-hospital mortality [9].

2.2.1.2 Cardiovascular Risk Scores

The Revised Cardiac Risk Index (RCRI) was developed for prediction of major cardiac complications in non-emergent, noncardiac surgery [10] (Table 2.2). Major cardiac complications include myocardial infarction, pulmonary edema, ventricular fibrillation or primary cardiac arrest, and complete heart block. The RCRI is composed of six variables of approximately equal prognostic importance: high-risk surgery (including intrathoracic surgery), history of ischemic heart disease, history of congestive cardiac failure, history of cerebrovascular disease, insulin therapy for diabetes, and preoperative serum creatinine >177 μmol/L. A RCRI ≥3 is associated with a risk of major postoperative cardiac complications for more than 11 % of patients and may be considered as a cutoff to delineate high-risk patients. Derived from the original RCRI, a thoracic risk score (ThRCRI) for lung resections was established [11] (Table 2.3). The predictive power of both of these scores in patients undergoing lung resections is controversial.

The Myocardial Infarction and Cardiac Arrest (MICA) risk calculator [12] was developed with the intent to improve predictive power for major cardiac adverse events as compared to RCRI. The model was based on analysis of the National Surgical Quality Improvement Program (NSQIP) database with more than 200,000 patients. Five predictors of perioperative risk of MICA at 30 days were identified: type of surgery, age, functional dependency, creatinine >133 umol/L, and ASA class. The MICA risk calculator resulted in a more accurate cardiac risk prediction than RCRI, although no data is available specifically for thoracic surgical patients. The MICA risk calculator is available on the web.

Table 2.3 Thoracic Revised Cardiac Risk Index (ThRCRI)

Risk factor	Points
History of coronary artery disease	1.5
History of cerebrovascular disease	1.5
Pneumonectomy	1.5
Serum creatinine > 177 μmol/L	1
Risk of major cardiac event	
Points	**Risk %**
0	0.9 %
1 – 1.5	4.2 %
2 – 2.5	8 %
> 2.5	18 %

Postoperative pulmonary complications (PPCs) include respiratory failure, reintubation within 48 h, weaning failure, pneumonia, atelectasis, bronchospasm, exacerbation of chronic obstructive pulmonary disease (COPD), pneumothorax, pleural effusion, and various forms of upper airway obstruction. They are a major cause of postoperative morbidity and mortality, possibly accounting for a higher mortality than cardiovascular complications.

2.2.1.3 Pulmonary Risk Scores

The ARISCAT study established a risk score for the development of PPCs in a mixed cohort of surgical patients [13]. Seven independent risk factors emerged: low preoperative SpO2, preoperative anemia, age, lung infection in the previous month, duration of surgery >2 h, upper abdominal or intrathoracic surgery, and emergent surgery (Table 2.4). Both the patient-related and the procedure-related risk factors contributed roughly 50 % to total risk. The score was prospectively and externally validated across many European countries, with a satisfactory predictive power especially for Western European countries [14].

2.2.1.4 Lung Function Tests

The degree of dyspnea is correlated with the risk of postoperative mortality [15]. Standardized symptom-limited stair climbing is a simple cost-effective test to objectively determine cardiorespiratory reserve and may have superior predictive ability than traditional spirometry values [1]. The test involves climbing three flights of stairs without interruption, equivalent to 12 m ascent that corresponds to metabolic equivalents (METs) greater than 4. The inability to climb more than 12 m warrants further lung functional testing. A patient able to climb at least 22 m (5–6 flights of stairs) has a low risk of postoperative complication, regardless of lung function test results [16].

FEV1 is a reliable predictor of perioperative complications in thoracic surgery for patients with FEV1 <70 % [17]. According to the guidelines of European Respiratory Society (ERS) and the European Society of Thoracic Surgery (ESTS) on fitness for lung resection in cancer patients, a predicted postoperative

Table 2.4 ARISCAT score

Age (years)	Score	Preoperative SpO_2, %	Score
51 – 80	3	91 – 95	8
> 80	16	≤ 90	24
Respiratory infection in the last month	17	**Preoperative anemia (≤ 10 g/dL.)**	11
Surgical incision		**Duration of surgery, h**	
Upper abdominal	15	> 2 to 3	16
Intrathoracic	24	> 3	23
Emergency procedure	8		

Risk of PPCs (%)	Score
Low (1.6 % [0.6 – 2.6])	< 26
Intermediate (13.3 % [7.6 – 19])	26 – 45
High (42.1 % [29.3 – 54.9])	>45

PPCs Postoperative pulmonary complications, *SpO_2* pulse oxymetry, *OR* odds ratio

(ppo)-FEV1 <30 % separates patients into normal and high-risk groups. It should be remembered that the calculated ppo-FEV1 may overestimate the actual FEV1 on the first postoperative day by about 30 % and that measured FEV1 on postoperative day one may provide more accurate prediction of cardiopulmonary risk [18–20]. On the other hand, patients with a moderate to severe obstructive pulmonary syndrome may have improved respiratory dynamics after lung resection [21]. The ppo-diffusion capacity of the lung for carbon monoxide (DLCO) is another powerful predictor of perioperative complications. According to the ERS/ESTS guidelines, a ppo-DLCO <30 % delineates a high surgical risk [1].

Peak VO_2 allows further refinement of perioperative risk prediction. Patients with values of peak VO_2 >20 mL/kg/min qualify for resection up to pneumonectomy, whereas values <10 mL/kg/min indicate a high risk for any type of lung resection [22]. A value of ppo-peak VO_2 <10 ml/kg/min is associated with a mortality rate exceeding 50 % [23].

2.2.1.5 Age and Frailty

Given age-related decline in organ function and impairment in physiological reserve, aging is considered a major risk factor for perioperative morbidity and mortality. Sarcopenia affects not only limb skeletal muscles but also respiratory muscles

Table 2.5 Risk classification according to the type of thoracic surgical procedure

Low risk	Intermediate risk	High risk
Pleural drainage Pleurodesis Mediastinoscopy Lung biopsy	Bullectomy Pleural resection Lobectomy Segmentectomy Wedge resection	Pneumonectomy Extended lung resection Tracheal and bronchial resection Mediastinal resections[a] Diaphragmatic resection Lung volume reduction surgery Lung transplantation

[a]Oesophagectomy, mediastinal tumor resection, thymus resection

and those controlling the upper airways. Accordingly, obstructive sleep apnea and occult aspiration occur more frequently particularly in the context of underlying neurological disorders (e.g., previous stroke, dementia, Parkinson disease) [24]. The risk of postoperative hypoxia and hypercapnia is increased because of altered chemosensitivity, respiratory muscle weakness, and increased pulmonary shunting. Impaired thermogenesis favors the occurrence of wound infection, bleeding, and cardiac ischemia events, resulting in prolonged postoperative recovery [25]. The risk of postoperative cognitive disorder (POCD) is increased, especially with benzodiazepine premedication [26].

Frailty is a composite measure of geriatric conditions. It includes measures of cognition, strength, energy, nutrition, physical mobility, mobility, and mood. Patient assessment for frailty may be a valuable aid in determination of operability and planning of postoperative care. A multidimensional frailty score was elaborated for prediction of 1-year postoperative mortality [27]. It represents an adaptation of the comprehensive geriatric assessment (CGA) and comprises a total of nine items, with a maximal score of 15. The authors used a cutoff of a score of 5, to distinguish between a high and a low risk of postoperative mortality (mortality >10 %). Although superior to the ASA score for prediction of 1-year mortality, its computation is complicated and time-consuming and must be performed by a medical consultant familiar with the score.

2.2.2 Procedure-Related Risk Factors (Table 2.5)

2.2.2.1 Lung Resections

The literature on the risk of thoracic surgery primarily focuses on lung resections, particularly in the context of cancer surgery. Broadly, the more extensive the lung resection, the higher is the risk of developing postoperative complications.

The highest risk of postoperative morbidity and mortality is associated with extended pneumonectomy [28]. A study based on the Society for Thoracic Surgeons (STS) General Thoracic Surgery Database (GTSD) examined major morbidity and mortality after pneumonectomy in 1267 patients. The risk factors independently associated with major adverse outcomes were age >65 years, congestive heart failure, FEV1 <60 %, underlying benign lung disease, and extended pneumonectomy. Overall mortality was 5.6 % and the incidence of major morbidity was 30.4 %. A study based on data of the French national database for thoracic surgery (EPITHOR) on 4498 patients with lung cancer reports an overall mortality of 7.8 % for pneumonectomy, with risk factors for mortality identified as age >65 years, ASA physiologic status ≥3, underweight, right-sided pneumonectomy, and extended pneumonectomy [29].

A large study based on the STS GTSD, with 18,800 lung cancer resections performed at 111 participating centers revealed an overall perioperative mortality of 2.2 %. Independent predictors of mortality were pneumonectomy, bilobectomy, ASA rating, functional status, renal dysfunction, induction chemoradiation therapy, steroids, age, urgent procedures, male gender, FEV1, and body mass index [30]. According to an analysis based on data of the American National Cancer Database (NCDB) on almost 120,000 patients, 30-day mortality of lung resections for non-small cell lung carcinoma (NSCLC) was 3.4 % overall, with a mortality of 8.5 % for pneumonectomies, 4 % for extended lobectomies and bilobectomies, and 2.6 % for lobectomies and bilobectomies. Mortality for wedge resections was 4.2 % and slightly higher than for lobectomies, which may be explained by a higher rate of tumor recurrences, and a lower functional preoperative status, indicating a more conservative surgical approach.

Overall, a right-sided lung resection carries a higher risk of complications than a left-sided resection owing to greater propensity to bronchopleural fistula formation, a greater increase in right ventricular afterload, and potential alteration in cardiac sympatho-vagal balance [29, 31].

2.2.2.2 Other Thoracic Surgical Interventions

Thoracic surgical interventions, which require one-lung ventilation (OLV) and a thoracotomy, can be considered high-risk procedures. Similar to lung resections, they expose patients to the risk of cardiovascular complications as well as atelectasis, pneumonia, and ventilator-induced lung injuries (VILI) leading to acute lung injury (ALI) or acute respiratory distress syndrome (ARDS).

For patients undergoing esophagectomies, a nomogram has been developed to predict the occurrence and severity of postoperative complications [32]. Independent risk factors are increasing age, a history of cerebrovascular accident (CVA) or transient ischemic accident (TIA), a history of myocardial infarction, a reduced forced expiratory volume in one second (FEV1), electrocardiographic (ECG) changes, and extensive surgery. The nomogram was validated and proved useful for risk prediction in high-volume hospitals [33].

Lung or pleural biopsies and simple bullectomy with or without pleurodesis under video-assisted thoracic surgery (VATS) are usually short-lasting and minor procedures that require short-term admission in a PACU for monitoring anesthesia emergence, titration of analgesic intravenous regimen, and detection of residual air leakage, lung re-expansion, and atelectasis. Mediastinoscopies can generally be monitored in PACU, with special attention to the risk of occult postoperative hemorrhage.

Uni- or bilateral lung volume reduction surgeries in patients with severe emphysema are considered high-risk procedures given preexisting severe airflow limitations and major impairments in gas exchange. These patients require cautious titration of analgesics (preferably epidural or paravertebral block) and are preferably admitted in ICU or HDU given the risk of life-threatening deterioration in pulmonary function (e.g., bronchopleural fistula, opiate-induced hypercapnic acidosis).

2.2.2.3 Additional Surgical Risk Factors

Little evidence supports the use of a muscle-sparing thoracotomy as opposed to a posterolateral thoracotomy, but incision length may be proportionally related to post-thoracotomy complications [34]. Given limited tissue trauma and consequent reduced neuroendocrine and inflammatory responses, VATS is associated with lower rates of overall perioperative mortality, morbidity (e.g., pneumonia and atrial arrhythmia), as well as length of stay [31]. In the absence of other major risk factors for postoperative complications, patients with a VATS lung resection do not require neuraxial analgesic techniques and are commonly managed in PACU for vital monitoring and anesthesia emergence.

Operative mortality may be lower if board-certified thoracic surgeons perform a minimal case load of procedures [35]. Differences in postoperative mortality rates between hospitals may also be explained by a different quality of postoperative patient management [36]. As a consequence, local experience should be included in the process of postoperative patient triage.

Surgery performed on an emergent basis has repeatedly been associated with worse postoperative outcomes. Various pre- and postoperative scores integrate this factor into risk stratification.

Finally, the occurrence of major intraoperative complications may require a higher level of postoperative monitoring and treatment, than initially planned. Myocardial ischemia, hemodynamically significant arrhythmias, refractory hypotension or hypoxemia, bronchial aspiration, and major bleeding are considered major complications that justify admission in HDU or ICU (Table 2.6).

2.2.2.4 Anesthetic Management

Improving patient outcome can be achieved by implementing perioperative risk-minimizing strategies:

1. Titration of anesthetic agents based on monitoring brain activity
2. Adoption of lung protective ventilatory settings
3. Achievement of optimal oxygen transport to match metabolic demands
4. Control of normothermia and hemostasis
5. Efficient pain control

The type and quality of postoperative pain control influences postoperative triage, since insufficiently controlled postoperative pain increases the risk of postoperative cardiopulmonary complications and length of stay [40]. Thoracic epidural

Table 2.6 Summary of risk factors, indicating a high risk of postoperative complications

Patient-related risk factors	Procedure-related risk factors
ASA physical status ≥4	High-risk procedure (*according to* Table 2.5)
S-MPM ≥6 points	Major intraoperative complication[a]
RCRI ≥2 points	Low level of operator and hospital expertise
ThRCRI >1.5 points	Emergency operation
ARISCAT >45 points	
Preoperative FEV1 <60 %	
ppo-FEV1 <30 %	
ppo-DLCO <30 %	
Peak VO_2 <12 ml/kg/min	
Liver dysfunction[b]	

ASA American Society of Anesthesiologists, *S-MPM* Surgical Mortality Probability Model, *RCRI* Revised Cardiac Risk Index, *ThRCRI* Thoracic Revised Cardiac Risk Index, *FEV1* forced expired volume in one second, *DLCO* diffusion capacity of the lung for carbon monoxide, *VO2* oxygen consumption, *MELD* Model for End-Stage Liver Disease

[a]Refractory hypotension and/or hypoxemia, myocardial ischemia, cardiac arrhythmias requiring treatment, major hemorrhage, and bronchial aspiration

[b]According to [37–39]

analgesia is considered the gold standard for thoracic surgery pain management. Compared to systemic analgesia, it is associated with a lower incidence of postoperative pneumonia and shorter duration of mechanical ventilation [41]. Thoracic paravertebral block (PVB), performed percutaneously by the anesthesiologist or directly placed by the surgeon, may provide similar analgesia, at lower risk of hypotension and urinary retention [42]. In some institutions, refractory hypotension caused by the thoracic epidural pain treatment mandates transfer to HDU or ICU. Over the last decades, the incidence of PPCs and the additional benefit of epidural over systemic analgesia have markedly decreased [41].

2.3 Postoperative Selection of Patients for ICU, HDU, or PACU Admission

For most patients, postoperative triage can be determined and planned preoperatively, based on knowledge of preoperative patient- and procedure-related risk factors, although intraoperative complications may modify the initial assessment. Several risk scores take into account intraoperative complications and can be used at the end of the operation, although none were specifically developed or validated for thoracic surgery.

2.3.1 Scores and Guidelines

The Surgical Apgar Score (SAS) includes three intraoperative parameters – blood loss, lowest mean arterial pressure, and lowest heart rate – that have been shown

Table 2.7 Surgical Apgar score

	0 point	1 point	2 points	3 points	4 points
Estimated blood loss (ml)	>1000	601 – 1000	101 – 600	≤ 100	
Lowest mean arterial pressure (mmHg)	<40	40 – 54	55 – 69	≥ 70	
Lowest hear rate (bpm)	>85[a]	76 – 85	66 – 75	56 – 65	≤ 55

Surgical APGAR score	0 – 4	5	6	7	8	9	10
Complication (%)	32.9	20.5	12.2	9.1	4.8	4	3
Death (%)	7.9	3.4	1.9	1.1	0.5	0.5	0.5

[a]Pathologic bradyarrhythmia, including sinus arrest, atrioventricular block or dissociation, junctional or ventricular escape rhythms, and asystole are also rated 0 points.

useful to predict postoperative major complications or 30-day mortality following noncardiac surgery [43]. So far, thoracic surgical patients have not been included in this exploratory population sample (Table 2.7). The SAS has been successfully validated in single centers and in an international study across eight hospitals of eight different countries [44]. For the purpose of postoperative triage, an Apgar ≤6 may signal a high risk of postoperative complications and prompt the clinician to transfer a patient to HDU or ICU.

The Physiological and Operative Severity Score for the enUmeration of Mortality and morbidity (POSSUM) was developed for audit purposes and is a British equivalent of the NSIQP in the United States. It is based on 12 physiological and 6 operative parameters and allows prediction of in-hospital mortality and morbidity. It proved useful for prediction of postoperative complications in lung resection patients [45]. Subsequently, the POSSUM equation was improved and named Portsmouth-POSSUM (P-POSSUM) [46]. Risk calculation can easily be performed with a web-based risk calculator.

Several ICU scores, such as the Acute Physiology and Chronic Health Evaluation (APACHE) score, the Simplified Acute Physiology Score (SAPS), and the Mortality Probability Model (MPM) may be used for the purpose of risk prediction and stratification in critically ill patients. Nevertheless, they only have limited power to predict individual patient risk and do not take account of surgical parameters.

The American College of Critical Care Medicine (ACCM) has issued guidelines regarding selection criteria of patients admitted to HDU [47] and ICU [48]. Admission in HDU should be considered for "patients who, after major surgery, are hemodynamically stable, but may require fluid resuscitation and transfusion due to major fluid shifts" and "who require close nurse monitoring during the first 24 h." Admission in ICU is restricted for a minority of patients requiring "hemodynamic monitoring/ventilatory support or extensive nursing care."

2.3.2 Local Specificities

The spectrum of postoperative units extends from the day care ward to the surgical ward, to the PACU, to the HDU, and to the ICU. Every hospital has a unique combination of postoperative units, staffing, expertise, and technical equipment, which greatly influence postoperative triage decisions. Triage guidelines must therefore be adjusted to those specificities and developed by a local multidisciplinary team composed of surgeons, anesthetists, pneumologists, and intensivists.

In some institutions, all postsurgical patients are first transferred to PACU before being transferred either to the ward or to HDU. This has the advantage of disposing of more clinical information at the time of the final triage, since the first postoperative hours are a period of major physiological variations with the potential appearance of early pathological processes.

A patient transfer to the ward entails a substantial decrease in the quality and frequency of monitoring. The provision of a medical emergency team, composed of anesthetists and/or intensivists, may be a way to attenuate the risk [49] and may influence postoperative triage decisions.

The triage process is strongly influenced by the ad hoc availability of beds. But in addition, it also depends on aspects such as location of a unit within the hospital (e.g., proximity to imaging facilities and to the operation rooms), administrative barriers, culture of collaboration between staffs, and a unit's level of expertise.

Conclusion

Postoperative preventive and therapeutic management has to be carefully planned in order to limit postoperative morbidity and mortality. The optimal postoperative patient destination depends on the combination of patient-related and procedure-related risk factors and on local specificities. Up-to-date anesthetic management contributes significantly to decrease postoperative risk and to reduce the need for high-level postoperative monitoring. The general trend of thoracic surgery postoperative care moves away from ICU toward HDUs or well-staffed and well-equipped PACUs for many high-risk patients.

References

1. Brunelli A, Charloux A, Bolliger CT et al (2009) ERS/ESTS clinical guidelines on fitness for radical therapy in lung cancer patients (surgery and chemo-radiotherapy). Eur Respir J 34:17–41
2. Wolters U, Wolf T, Stützer H, Schröder T (1996) ASA classification and perioperative variables as predictors of postoperative outcome. Br J Anaesth 77:217–222
3. Charlson ME, Pompei P, Ales KL, MacKenzie CR (1987) A new method of classifying prognostic comorbidity in longitudinal studies: development and validation. J Chronic Dis 40:373–383
4. Monk TG, Saini V, Weldon BC, Sigl JC (2005) Anesthetic management and one-year mortality after noncardiac surgery. Anesth Analg 100:4–10
5. Birim O, Maat APWM, Kappetein AP, van Meerbeeck JP, Damhuis RAM, Bogers AJJC (2003) Validation of the Charlson comorbidity index in patients with operated primary non-small cell lung cancer. Eur J Cardiothorac Surg 23:30–34
6. Khuri SF, Daley J, Henderson W et al (1997) Risk adjustment of the postoperative mortality rate for the comparative assessment of the quality of surgical care: results of the National Veterans Affairs Surgical Risk Study. J Am Coll Surg 185:315–327

7. Glance LG, Lustik SJ, Hannan EL, Osler TM, Mukamel DB, Qian F, Dick AW (2012) The surgical mortality probability model: derivation and validation of a simple risk prediction rule for noncardiac surgery. Ann Surg 255:696–702
8. Ferguson MK, Durkin AE (2003) A comparison of three scoring systems for predicting complications after major lung resection. Eur J Cardiothorac Surg 23:35–42
9. Falcoz PE, Conti M, Brouchet L, Chocron S, Puyraveau M, Mercier M, Etievent JP, Dahan M (2007) The Thoracic Surgery Scoring System (Thoracoscore): risk model for in-hospital death in 15,183 patients requiring thoracic surgery. J Thorac Cardiovasc Surg 133:325–332
10. Lee TH, Marcantonio ER, Mangione CM et al (1999) Derivation and prospective validation of a simple index for prediction of cardiac risk of major noncardiac surgery. Circulation 100:1043–1049
11. Brunelli A, Varela G, Salati M, Jimenez MF, Pompili C, Novoa N, Sabbatini A (2010) Recalibration of the revised cardiac risk index in lung resection candidates. Ann Thorac Surg 90:199–203
12. Gupta PK, Gupta H, Sundaram A et al (2011) Development and validation of a risk calculator for prediction of cardiac risk after surgery. Circulation 124:381–387
13. Canet J, Gallart L, Gomar C et al (2010) Prediction of postoperative pulmonary complications in a population-based surgical cohort. Anesthesiology 113:1338–1350
14. Mazo V, Sabaté S, Canet J, Gallart L, de Abreu MG, Belda J, Langeron O, Hoeft A, Pelosi P (2014) Prospective external validation of a predictive score for postoperative pulmonary complications. Anesthesiology 121:219–231
15. Berrisford R, Brunelli A, Rocco G, Treasure T, Utley M, Audit and guidelines committee of the European Society of Thoracic Surgeons, European Association of Cardiothoracic Surgeons (2005) The European Thoracic Surgery Database project: modelling the risk of in-hospital death following lung resection. Eur J Cardiothorac Surg 28:306–311
16. Brunelli A, Refai M, Xiumé F, Salati M, Sciarra V, Socci L, Sabbatini A (2008) Performance at symptom-limited stair-climbing test is associated with increased cardiopulmonary complications, mortality, and costs after major lung resection. Ann Thorac Surg 86:240–247; discussion 247–248
17. Brunelli A, Al Refai M, Monteverde M, Sabbatini A, Xiumé F, Fianchini A (2002) Predictors of early morbidity after major lung resection in patients with and without airflow limitation. Ann Thorac Surg 74:999–1003
18. Varela G, Brunelli A, Rocco G, Marasco R, Jiménez MF, Sciarra V, Aranda JL, Gatani T (2006) Predicted versus observed FEV1 in the immediate postoperative period after pulmonary lobectomy. Eur J Cardiothorac Surg 30:644–648
19. Varela G, Brunelli A, Rocco G, Novoa N, Refai M, Jiménez MF, Salati M, Gatani T (2007) Measured FEV1 in the first postoperative day, and not ppoFEV1, is the best predictor of cardio-respiratory morbidity after lung resection. Eur J Cardiothorac Surg 31:518–521
20. Varela G, Brunelli A, Rocco G, Jiménez MF, Salati M, Gatani T (2007) Evidence of lower alteration of expiratory volume in patients with airflow limitation in the immediate period after lobectomy. Ann Thorac Surg 84:417–422
21. Brunelli A, Sabbatini A, Xiume' F, Al Refai M, Borri A, Salati M, Marasco RD, Fianchini A (2005) A model to predict the decline of the forced expiratory volume in one second and the carbon monoxide lung diffusion capacity early after major lung resection. Interact Cardiovasc Thorac Surg 4:61–65
22. Licker M, Schnyder J-M, Frey J-G, Diaper J, Cartier V, Inan C, Robert J, Bridevaux P-O, Tschopp J-M (2011) Impact of aerobic exercise capacity and procedure-related factors in lung cancer surgery. Eur Respir J 37:1189–1198
23. Bolliger CT, Wyser C, Roser H, Solèr M, Perruchoud AP (1995) Lung scanning and exercise testing for the prediction of postoperative performance in lung resection candidates at increased risk for complications. Chest 108:341–348
24. Ebihara S, Saito H, Kanda A, Nakajoh M, Takahashi H, Arai H, Sasaki H (2003) Impaired efficacy of cough in patients with Parkinson disease. Chest 124:1009–1015

25. Kozian A, Kretzschmar MA, Schilling T (2015) Thoracic anesthesia in the elderly. Curr Opin Anaesthesiol 28:2–9
26. Dressler I, Fritzsche T, Cortina K, Pragst F, Spies C, Rundshagen I (2007) Psychomotor dysfunction after remifentanil/propofol anaesthesia. Eur J Anaesthesiol 24:347–354
27. Kim S, Han H-S, Jung H, Kim K, Hwang DW, Kang S-B, Kim C-H (2014) Multidimensional frailty score for the prediction of postoperative mortality risk. JAMA Surg 149:633–640
28. Shapiro M, Swanson SJ, Wright CD, Chin C, Sheng S, Wisnivesky J, Weiser TS (2010) Predictors of major morbidity and mortality after pneumonectomy utilizing the Society for Thoracic Surgeons General Thoracic Surgery Database. Ann Thorac Surg 90:927–934; discussion 934–935
29. Thomas PA, Berbis J, Baste J-M, Le Pimpec-Barthes F, Tronc F, Falcoz P-E, Dahan M, Loundou A, EPITHOR group (2015) Pneumonectomy for lung cancer: contemporary national early morbidity and mortality outcomes. J Thorac Cardiovasc Surg 149:73–82
30. Kozower BD, Sheng S, O'Brien SM, Liptay MJ, Lau CL, Jones DR, Shahian DM, Wright CD (2010) STS database risk models: predictors of mortality and major morbidity for lung cancer resection. Ann Thorac Surg 90:875–881; discussion 881–883
31. Rosen JE, Hancock JG, Kim AW, Detterbeck FC, Boffa DJ (2014) Predictors of mortality after surgical management of lung cancer in the National Cancer Database. Ann Thorac Surg 98:1953–1960
32. Lagarde SM, Reitsma JB, Maris A-KD, van Berge Henegouwen MI, Busch ORC, Obertop H, Zwinderman AH, van Lanschot JJB (2008) Preoperative prediction of the occurrence and severity of complications after esophagectomy for cancer with use of a nomogram. Ann Thorac Surg 85:1938–1945
33. Grotenhuis BA, van Hagen P, Reitsma JB, Lagarde SM, Wijnhoven BPL, van Berge Henegouwen MI, Tilanus HW, van Lanschot JJB (2010) Validation of a nomogram predicting complications after esophagectomy for cancer. Ann Thorac Surg 90:920–925
34. Elshiekh MAF, Lo TTH, Shipolini AR, McCormack DJ (2013) Does muscle-sparing thoracotomy as opposed to posterolateral thoracotomy result in better recovery? Interact Cardiovasc Thorac Surg 16:60–67
35. Chowdhury MM, Dagash H, Pierro A (2007) A systematic review of the impact of volume of surgery and specialization on patient outcome. Br J Surg 94:145–161
36. Ghaferi AA, Birkmeyer JD, Dimick JB (2009) Variation in hospital mortality associated with inpatient surgery. N Engl J Med 361:1368–1375
37. Ziser A, Plevak DJ, Wiesner RH, Rakela J, Offord KP, Brown DL (1999) Morbidity and mortality in cirrhotic patients undergoing anesthesia and surgery. Anesthesiology 90:42–53
38. Hanje AJ, Patel T (2007) Preoperative evaluation of patients with liver disease. Nat Clin Pract Gastroenterol Hepatol 4:266–276
39. Canet J, Sabaté S, Mazo V, Gallart L, de Abreu MG, Belda J, Langeron O, Hoeft A, Pelosi P (2015) Development and validation of a score to predict postoperative respiratory failure in a multicentre European cohort. Eur J Anaesthesiol 32:1–13
40. Ganter MT, Blumenthal S, Dübendorfer S, Brunnschweiler S, Hofer T, Klaghofer R, Zollinger A, Hofer CK (2014) The length of stay in the post-anaesthesia care unit correlates with pain intensity, nausea and vomiting on arrival. Perioper Med Lond Engl 3:10
41. Pöpping DM, Elia N, Marret E, Remy C, Tramèr MR (2008) Protective effects of epidural analgesia on pulmonary complications after abdominal and thoracic surgery: a meta-analysis. Arch Surg Chic Ill 1960 143:990–999; discussion 1000
42. Powell ES, Cook D, Pearce AC, Davies P, Bowler GMR, Naidu B, Gao F, UKPOS Investigators (2011) A prospective, multicentre, observational cohort study of analgesia and outcome after pneumonectomy. Br J Anaesth 106:364–370
43. Gawande AA, Kwaan MR, Regenbogen SE, Lipsitz SA, Zinner MJ (2007) An Apgar score for surgery. J Am Coll Surg 204:201–208
44. Haynes AB, Regenbogen SE, Weiser TG, Lipsitz SR, Dziekan G, Berry WR, Gawande AA (2011) Surgical outcome measurement for a global patient population: validation of the Surgical Apgar Score in 8 countries. Surgery 149:519–524

45. Brunelli A, Fianchini A, Gesuita R, Carle F (1999) POSSUM scoring system as an instrument of audit in lung resection surgery. Physiological and operative severity score for the enumeration of mortality and morbidity. Ann Thorac Surg 67:329–331
46. Prytherch DR, Whiteley MS, Higgins B, Weaver PC, Prout WG, Powell SJ (1998) POSSUM and Portsmouth POSSUM for predicting mortality. Physiological and Operative Severity Score for the enUmeration of Mortality and morbidity. Br J Surg 85:1217–1220
47. Nasraway SA, Cohen IL, Dennis RC, Howenstein MA, Nikas DK, Warren J, Wedel SK (1998) Guidelines on admission and discharge for adult intermediate care units. American College of Critical Care Medicine of the Society of Critical Care Medicine. Crit Care Med 26:607–610
48. (1999) Guidelines for intensive care unit admission, discharge, and triage. Task Force of the American College of Critical Care Medicine, Society of Critical Care Medicine. Crit Care Med 27:633–638
49. Bellomo R, Goldsmith D, Uchino S, Buckmaster J, Hart G, Opdam H, Silvester W, Doolan L, Gutteridge G (2004) Prospective controlled trial of effect of medical emergency team on postoperative morbidity and mortality rates. Crit Care Med 32:916–921

Does It Matter How I Ventilate the Patient During the Operation?

3

Laszlo L. Szegedi

3.1 Introduction

With better surgical techniques and better and safer anesthesia drugs, monitoring, and training, there is possibility to schedule patients for operations and one-lung ventilation with more and more comorbidities, while the planned surgery is more and more complex. Although the number of operable patients for lung cancer surgery remains limited, the number of patients presenting for surgery requiring one-lung ventilation (OLV) is increasing, because of the broader indications for this technique. From the classical "absolute and relative" indications for OLV, we moved to rather indications for facilitating surgery (the majority of the indications for OLV), preventing cross-contamination of the contralateral lung and controlling the distribution of ventilation to one lung. These last years, the use of OLV increased not only for lung cancer surgery but also for other newer surgical procedures or diagnostic procedures, like pleura surgery, thoracic aorta surgery, esophagus surgery, thoracic spine surgery, thoracic sympathicolysis, minimally invasive cardiac surgery, cardiac electrophysiological surgery, whole-lung lavage, radiofrequency ablation of hepatic tumors, and so on, without forgetting the increased number of lung transplant procedures.

In the previous decades, because of its complexity, OLV was managed almost exclusively by specialists in academic settings. Nowadays there is increased necessity for all anesthesia staff members to master OLV techniques and trying to obtain the best postoperative outcome for the patients.

Studies on how to one-lung ventilate the patients correctly are lacking, and most of the recommendations for OLV are derived from two-lung ventilation (TLV). Unfortunately, for the *OLV addicts*, most of the published studies were done in intensive care unit (ICU) settings, during TLV of patients with either acute

L.L. Szegedi, MD, PhD
Universitair Ziekenhuis Brussel and Vrije Universiteit Brussel, Brussels, Belgium
e-mail: Laszlo.Szegedi@uzbrussel.be

© Springer International Publishing Switzerland 2017

M. Şentürk, M.O. Sungur (eds.), *Postoperative Care in Thoracic Surgery*,
DOI 10.1007/978-3-319-19908-5_3

respiratory distress syndrome (ARDS) or acute lung injury (ALI), and just a few studied TLV during general anesthesia (GA) and even less OLV.

Khuri et al. [1] identified some of the determinants of 30-day postoperative mortality and long-term survival after major surgery. While patient-dependent risk and surgical factors are difficult to control by the anesthesiologists, the anesthesia-dependent factors are under our responsibility – the type of anesthesia, the pain management, the amount of administered fluids, and last, but surely not least, the ventilatory management of the operated patients.

Postoperative pulmonary complications are the main cause of overall perioperative morbidity and mortality in patients following GA. The incidence of postoperative pulmonary complications may vary dramatically, ranging from 2 to 40 %, depending on the clinical treatment setting, the kind of surgery studied, and the definition of postoperative pulmonary complications used [2].

The above mentioned facts are not really new, but they still remain a common clinical problem. One should not forget that mechanical ventilation, even if done in the best manner, is not a physiological process, because of positive pressure, shear stress of the lungs, secretion of inflammatory mediators, the gas mixtures used to ventilate, and the drugs and anesthetic gases which are also potential independent variables in producing variable degrees of injuries to the lung tissues.

3.2 The Protective Ventilation Was Born with ARDS

It's worth to go back in history and see the evolution of proposed ventilator strategies for anesthesia and mechanical ventilation. There are two interesting studies, which should be mentioned here. More than 50 years ago, at the beginning of modern mechanical ventilation, in 1963, Bendixen et al. found a relation between the degree of ventilation and the magnitude of fall in arterial oxygen tension [3]. Large tidal volumes (VTs) appeared to protect against falls in oxygen tension, presumably by providing continuous hyperinflation, while shallow VTs lead to atelectasis and increased shunting, with impaired oxygenation. The second study [4], at the beginning of this century, a multicenter, randomized study, compared two methods of mechanical ventilation in patients with ALI and ARDS. Traditional ventilation method with VT of 12 ml/kg of predicted body weight (PBW) and an end-inspiratory airway pressure (plateau pressure) of 50 cmH_2O or less was compared with ventilation with an initial VT of 6 ml/kg of PBW and a plateau pressure of 30 cmH_2O or less. In patients with ALI and ARDS, mechanical ventilation with a lower VT than was traditionally used at that time resulted in decreased mortality and increased the number of postoperative days without a need for mechanical ventilation. Interesting to mention, too, is that the trial was stopped before the initially proposed number of patients was reached, because the results were very satisfactory.

Better understanding of the pathophysiology of ARDS has led to the proposal that airway pressures and tidal volumes should be limited in ventilator management of these patients [5]. This means that sometimes a rise in the arterial partial pressure of carbon dioxide ($PaCO_2$) should be accepted. Severe hypercapnia and acidosis can have adverse effects, including increased intracranial pressure, depressed myocardial contractility, pulmonary hypertension, and depressed renal blood flow. The view that these risks are preferable to the higher plateau pressure required to achieve normocapnia has represented a substantial shift in ventilatory management. Cyclic inflation-deflation of injured lung units or alveoli can exacerbate lung injury, and medium to high levels of positive end-expiration pressure (PEEP) should be used to keep alveoli open throughout the ventilatory cycle. Overall, this type of approach has been termed lung-protective ventilation strategy. Ventilation with lower VT was also associated with lower levels of systemic inflammatory mediators [6].

3.3 Is There a Rationale to Use Lung-Protective Ventilation in Patients with Normal Lungs?

In a retrospective cohort study of patients with normal lungs at the onset of mechanical ventilation in ICU, three different VTs were used for mechanical ventilation (either <9, 9–12, or >12 ml/kg PBW). The study showed the occurrence of ventilator-associated lung injury in these patients; however, their incidence was significantly lower in those who were ventilated with lower VT [7].

A preventive, randomized controlled trial, also in ICU settings, compared 6 vs 10 ml/kg PBW VTs in mechanically ventilated patients without ALI at the start of mechanical ventilation. The percentage of occurrence of ALI/ARDS in the group ventilated with 6 ml/kg was 2.6 % as compared to 13.5 % in the second group [8].

These presented studies have identified the use of large VTs as a major risk factor for development of lung injury in mechanically ventilated patients without acute lung injury.

3.4 What About Patients Ventilated During General Anesthesia?

A multicenter observational study of intraoperative ventilatory management during GA and TLV showed that according to ideal body weight, approximately 30 % of patients are still ventilated with VTs higher than 10 ml/kg [9].

A recent meta-analysis [10] assessed whether incidence, morbidity, and in-hospital mortality associated with postoperative lung injury are affected by type of surgery and whether outcomes are dependent on type of ventilation. The total incidence of postoperative lung injury was similar for abdominal and thoracic surgery. Patients who developed postoperative lung injury were older, with higher ASA scores and prevalence of sepsis or pneumonia, more frequently received blood transfusions during surgery, and were ventilated with higher tidal volumes, lower PEEP, or both, than patients who did not. ICU and hospital stay were longer, and in-hospital mortality was higher in the patients with lung injury than in those without injury and also higher in the patients who underwent thoracic interventions as compared to abdominal surgery. Lung-protective ventilatory strategies reduced the incidence of postoperative lung injury but did not improve mortality.

The main differences between mechanical ventilation in ICU patients and patients in OR settings are the duration of ventilation (short term, rarely exceeding 6–8 h in OR, with in most cases an easy weaning, while in ICU ventilation is most of times lasting for more than 24 h, with sometimes difficult weaning). However, even short-term ventilation can produce lung damage, and injurious mechanical ventilation may lead to epithelial cell apoptosis (far from the lungs, including kidneys and the small intestine) [11].

As anesthesiologists and physicians first of all, we are striving to improve quality of care in medicine and of course in mechanical ventilation too. There is enough evidence in the literature with physiological rationale, meta-analyses, or just small studies which suggest the low-VT option as a valuable one.

3.5 The Role of PEEP

The main determinants of ventilator-induced lung injury were proposed to be the end-inspiratory transpulmonary pressure and the regional overdistension – mainly determined by the high VT – which would not occur during "normal" spontaneous breathing. There are other causes which even during very short-term mechanical ventilation may cause injury to the lungs, surfactant deactivation by mechanical ventilation causing problems in surfactant adsorption and desorption, or elevated tissue stress between lung structures with different mechanical properties. The second main mechanism is the low end-expiratory lung volume injury, in other words the atelectasis-induced lung injury, the so-called silent killer of peripheral airways [12].

Normally, in a healthy, erect subject, ventilation occurs above closing capacity (CC) (the resting volume in the lungs at which peripheral airway closure occurs, with inhomogeneity of distribution of ventilation and impaired gas exchange and consequent risk of peripheral airway injury). Airway closure, which can occur when the CC exceeds the end-expiratory lung volume (FRC), is commonly observed in diseases characterized by increased CC (e.g., chronic obstructive pulmonary disease, asthma, aging) and/or decreased FRC (e.g., obesity, chronic heart failure). Airway closure is a commonly observed phenomenon during GA and not only in obese patients, where FRC is already decreased.

Applying high VT with high inspiratory pressures, during mechanical ventilation, will lead to barotrauma or volutrauma, with release of inflammatory cytokines interleukin (IL)-1 beta, IL-6, IL-8, tumor necrosis factor (TNF)-alpha leading to biotrauma. On the other hand, if low VT is used without PEEP, atelectrauma will occur with the same consequences [13].

Atelectasis and pulmonary gas exchange were studied in supine patients without lung disease. Positive end-expiratory pressure reduced the atelectasis in all patients but did not change the degree of shunt. It was concluded that the development of atelectasis in dependent lung regions is a major cause of gas exchange impairment during GA, during both spontaneous breathing and mechanical ventilation, and that

PEEP diminishes the atelectasis, but not necessarily the shunt [14]. Even if a PEEP is associated with low-VT ventilation, prolonged impaired lung function after major surgery is not ameliorated [15].

3.6 The Role of Oxygen

Some minutes after induction of general anesthesia, in healthy patients, FRC decreases by almost 20 % [16]. All anesthetic drugs (but ketamine), even with spontaneous breathing, decrease FRC after induction of anesthesia. During sleep, FRC is reduced during rapid eye movement (REM) sleep at the same level as after induction of GA. Reduced respiratory muscle tone and airway closure are likely causative factors. However, during sleep, atelectasis does not develop, because the FiO_2 is low [17]. At the induction of GA, preoxygenation with FiO_2 of 80 % instead of 100 % may be sufficient in most patients with no anticipated difficulty in managing the airway, but time to hypoxemia during apnea decreases. Continuous positive airway pressure (CPAP)/PEEP was proposed to prevent fall in FRC. Inspired oxygen concentration of 30–40 %, or even less, should suffice if the lung is kept open [18].

3.7 Alveolar Recruitment Maneuver

Alveolar recruitment maneuvers (ARMs) were proposed to ameliorate oxygenation before applying a PEEP [19]. Different methods of ARM were described. But very simply explained, it consists of inflation to an airway pressure of 40 cmH_2O for 10 s and to higher airway pressures in patients with reduced abdominal compliance (obese and patients with abdominal disorders), while respecting a driving pressure of maximum 15 cmH_2O and increasing PEEP. A low and constant driving pressure during all the procedure allows an increased safety margin when a higher PEEP is employed during ARM. Alveolar recruitment maneuvers followed by PEEP reduce atelectasis and improve oxygenation in morbidly obese patients, whereas either PEEP or ARM alone does not [20]. The effect of ARMs on patient outcome in the postoperative period is, however, not yet known.

There is large evidence that during GA, lung-protective ventilation should be used. Ideally it should be a combination of low VT (how low is low?) and ARM (early and repeated) before applying PEEP. A study comparing standard mechanical ventilation lasting more than 2 h (VT 9 ml/kg, without PEEP or ARM) versus lung-protective ventilation (VT 7 ml/kg with PEEP 10 cmH_2O and ARM) obtained better inflammatory responses and better chest X-ray postoperatively in the group with protective ventilation [21]. The IMPROVE study ($n = 400$) [22] compared ventilation with VTs of 10–12 ml/kg, without PEEP or ARM, to ventilation with VT of 8 ml/kg, with PEEP 6–8 cmH_2O and ARM after intubation and repeated every 30–40 min. As compared with a practice of non-protective mechanical ventilation, the use of a lung-protective ventilation strategy in intermediate-risk and high-risk patients undergoing major abdominal surgery was associated with improved clinical outcomes.

The PROVHILO international study ($n=900$) [23] compared two groups during abdominal surgery too, using the same VT of 8 ml/kg for both groups, but in the conventional ventilation group with a PEEP <2 cmH_2O and in the protective ventilation group with a PEEP of 12 cmH_2O and ARM after intubation, after any disconnection of ventilator, and before extubation. Compared with patients in the lower PEEP group, those in the higher PEEP group developed intraoperative hypotension and needed more vasoactive drugs. The high level of PEEP and ARM during open abdominal surgery did not protect against postoperative pulmonary complications. Their recommendations were that an intraoperative protective ventilation strategy should include a low tidal volume and low PEEP (not the 12 cmH_2O used), without ARM.

After all these large, international studies, with different and sometimes contradictory findings, the question, if they are of real help or more confusing, may be justified [24].

3.8 Pressure- or Volume-Controlled Two-Lung Ventilation

There are benefits for both of them; however, the incidence of perioperative complications is not different. The best mode depends on the patient and the anesthesiologists should apply the mode that they best know and master. Even in obese patients, no real benefits could be demonstrated when using these two types of mechanical ventilation, which remains rather physician dependent, than really goal oriented.

Mechanical ventilation should no longer be considered only as a way to supply gas exchange during GA. Inadequate ventilatory settings can produce lung damage even in patients with healthy lungs, even for short periods of mechanical ventilation, not only in ICU, but in OR too. Lung-protective ventilation is the standard of care in most ARDS patients and it should become in OR too.

The relative contribution of low VT, low pressures, and PEEP in prevention of ventilator-induced lung injury is uncertain. Driving pressure (VT/compliance of respiratory system (CRS)), in which VT is intrinsically normalized to functional lung size (instead of predicted lung size in healthy persons), was suggested to be a better parameter associated with survival than VT or PEEP in patients who are not actively breathing [25].

3.9 The "Baby Lung" During OLV

The "baby lung" concept was described by Gattinoni et al., to characterize the normally aerated lung tissue in ARDS/ALI patients, which was comparable to the lung dimensions of a young child. They suggested that in these patients, the CRS is linearly related to the dimensions of the aerated lung regions, which is not at all stiff, but with normal elasticity; thus, for ventilator-induced lung injury, what is important is the ratio of VT to aerated lung volume and to body weight; the smaller the "baby lung," the greater is the potential for unsafe mechanical ventilation [26]. This principle may be extrapolated for OLV also.

3.10 One-Lung Ventilation with Lessons from Two-Lung Ventilation?

One-lung ventilation is a technique that adds supplementary difficulties to the complexity of anesthesia management per se (generally combined sometimes with epidural technique) and to the management of patients which present in most of cases with compromised pulmonary (and other organ system) functions.

During OLV, one lung is ventilated, while the other is excluded from ventilation and remains perfused, adding an extra intrapulmonary shunting, to the physiologic and general anesthesia-induced one. It is normal that at the start of OLV, if keeping the same inspired oxygen concentration and the same hemodynamic and metabolic status for the patient, the arterial oxygen partial pressure will decrease, and the alveolar-to-arterial oxygen partial pressure difference will increase. Fortunately, there are some mechanisms which to divert blood flow from the non-ventilated lung toward the ventilated one, trying to diminish shunt. These are active, like the hypoxic pulmonary vasoconstriction, and passive, like gravitational redistribution of blood flow from the upper, non-ventilated lung toward the lower, ventilated one, surgical manipulation of lung tissue (this may be beneficial through mechanical manipulation; however, in the same time, it may lead to secretion of vasodilatory and proinflammatory **mediators**), preexisting lung pathology, and ventilatory methods. It is obvious that in clinical situations it is impossible to determine the individual contribution of each of these factors.

In the last few decades, there is a significant decrease of reported intraoperative hypoxemia during OLV, from 20 to 25 % reported in the 1970s to less than 5 % nowadays (some are saying even less).

This decrease is multifactorial: better surgical techniques, new anesthetic drugs, better lung-separating devices, better training with hands-on workshops at congresses, and the routine use of the fiber-optic bronchoscope for positioning of lung-separating devices and better ventilatory techniques.

In the textbooks of thoracic anesthesia (unfortunately most of them available are more than 10 years old!), the recommendations for ventilatory management during thoracic surgery are as follows: maintain TLV until the pleura is opened; manage OLV by increasing the FiO_2 if necessary to 100 %; use VTs of 10–12 ml/kg; adjust respiratory rate in order to maintain normocapnia; even if an auto-PEEP is present, try to eliminate it; and use total intravenous anesthesia instead of inhaled anesthetics. If hypoxemia occurs, check the position of the double-lumen tube, apply a CPAP to the nondependent lung, use low levels of PEEP to the dependent lung, resume TLV, or ask the surgeon to clamp the pulmonary artery for pneumectomy. These criteria, which are focusing almost only on oxygenation, are relatively inadequate for modern OLV. A couple of years ago, the author of this chapter has published a study on COPD patients during OLV, in which high VT was used with variable respiratory rate and constant minute volume, in order to diminish intrinsic PEEP. Fortunately, all the patients were evaluated without postoperative complications, but such studies are nowadays, for obvious reasons, no more possible [27].

Even with a decrease in the incidence of hypoxemia during OLV, anesthesiologists are aware that not only hypoxemia is the problem during OLV, but the possibility of lung injury too.

In an observational study including patients undergoing lung surgery, two clinical forms of ALI were described: a delayed-onset form triggered by intercurrent complications and an early form associated with preoperative alcohol consumption, pneumectomy, high intraoperative pressures, and excessive fluid intake over the first 24 h [28].

One-lung ventilation with VT as used during TLV is a suggested algorithm but may impose mechanical stress of the dependent lung and potentially aggravate alveolar mediator release. A study comparing ventilation with different VTs assessed if there were changes in pulmonary immune function, hemodynamics, and gas exchange. Patients undergoing open thoracic surgery were randomized to receive either minute volume with a VT of either 10 ml/kg or 5 ml/kg, and respiratory rate was adjusted to obtain normal $PaCO_2$ during and after OLV. Fiber-optic bronchoalveolar lavage (BAL) of the ventilated lung was performed, and cells, protein, TNF-alpha, IL-8, soluble intercellular adhesion molecule (sICAM)-1, IL-10, and elastase were determined in the BAL. In all patients, an increase of pro-inflammatory variables was found. The time courses of intra-alveolar cells, protein, albumin, IL-8, elastase, and IL-10 did not differ between the groups after OLV and postoperatively. TNF-alpha and sICAM-1 concentrations were significantly smaller after OLV with the lower VTs. These results indicate that OLV too may induce epithelial damage and a pro-inflammatory response in the ventilated lung, just like TLV. Reduction of VT during OLV may reduce alveolar concentrations of TNF-alpha and of sICAM-1 [29].

Most of clinical studies using BAL fluid analysis have demonstrated pulmonary inflammatory reactions in the ventilated, dependent lung. However, few clinical studies have investigated such inflammatory reactions in the dependent lung compared with the collapsed nondependent lung. A study comparing the inflammatory reactions in the dependent lung and the nondependent lung during thoracic surgery was performed on patients during OLV, under total intravenous anesthesia with propofol and remifentanil. Levels of inflammatory mediators, TNF-alpha, IL-1 beta, IL-6, IL-8, IL-10, and IL-12, were measured before and after OLV. All inflammatory mediators were elevated at the end of surgery compared with their baseline levels; however IL-6 was significantly higher in the dependent lung than in the nondependent lung [30]. One-lung ventilation can damage the ventilated lung just like TLV.

Nevertheless, using protective approach OLV to prevent lung injury, by reduction of VT and application of PEEP, did not completely inhibit thromboxane B2 formation in isolated rabbit lungs [10, 31] or the enhanced alveolar pro-inflammatory response in laboratory animals.

During esophagus surgery, protective ventilatory strategy decreased the pro-inflammatory systemic response, improved lung function, and resulted in earlier extubation [32].

In a survey on the habitudes of thoracic anesthesiologists, done by the thoracic subcommittee and endorsed by the European Association of Cardiothoracic Anesthesiology (EACTA), the good news for the management of OLV is that 100 %

of the respondent anesthesiologists were using fiber-optic bronchoscopy to position and check the position of lung-separating devices during OLV, which is an enormous help to avoid hypoxemia due to malposition of these devices. Concerning the modes of one-lung ventilation, 60 % of the anesthesiologists were using volume-controlled modes, while 40 % pressure-controlled modes for OLV. The inspiratory airway pressures used during PCV ranged from 15 to 40, which may be considered as high. During VCV, the acceptable plateau pressures varied from 15 to 35. There are studies investigating the VCV vs. PCV during OLV. In one study [33], it was found that oxygenation was better when using PCV as compared to VCV. Ten years later, another study assessed the same modes and did not find any differences [34]. This difference in the outcome of the studies might be due to the patients included in the studies: differences were found in favor of PCV for OLV of patients with altered lung functions, the other study included only healthy lung patients.

A study evaluated the use of ARM to decrease the VT used during OLV in piglets. It was found that ARM improves aeration and respiratory mechanics. Moreover, in contrast to OLV with high VT, OLV with reduced VT did not reinforce tidal recruitment, indicating decreased mechanical stress [35]. Alveolar recruitment maneuvers during OLV, applied to the ventilated lung, improve oxygenation significantly, to PaO_2 values comparable of those during TLV [36].

Unfortunately, there are no data on the effects of OLV on postoperative ventilation/perfusion matching. An animal study in a pig model evaluated the influence of OLV on ventilation /perfusion mismatch using a single-photon emission computed tomography technique and related these findings to lung histopathology after OLV. One-lung ventilation resulted in significant ventilation/perfusion mismatch, hypoperfusion, and alveolar damage in the dependent lung, contributing to gas exchange impairment after OLV [37].

Data suggest that pro-inflammatory reactions during OLV are influenced by the type of general anesthesia. Several prospective, randomized studies suggest an immunomodulatory role for the volatile anesthetic sevoflurane during OLV for thoracic surgery with significant reduction of pro-inflammatory mediators and a significantly better clinical outcome (defined by postoperative adverse events), as compared to intravenous propofol [38].

When BAL was done in the nondependent lung too, less increase in inflammatory mediators was found with sevoflurane as compared with propofol anesthesia, which suggest decreased postoperative adverse events when using sevoflurane. Better effects were found for desflurane too, as compared to propofol anesthesia [39]. It seems that the old recommendations of using total intravenous anesthesia for OLV had become obsolete by the introduction of new halogenated agents. Volatile anesthetics inhibit the local alveolar, but not the systemic inflammatory response [40].

Before, we tried to maintain normocapnia, but a recent study showed that normocapnia is not mandatory for OLV. At the contrary, under intravenous anesthesia, therapeutic hypercapnia inhibited local and systematic inflammation and improved respiratory function after OLV in lobectomy patients without severe complications [11].

Some surgeons advocate that a high fraction of inspired oxygen (FiO_2) is needed for wound healing. However, this theory remains controversial. Indeed a higher arterial oxygen partial pressure (PaO_2) is needed to force oxygen into injured and healing tissues, particularly in the subcutaneous tissue, fascia, tendon, and bone, the tissues most at risk for healing.

In order to use a lower FiO_2, the effects of low VT with limited plateau pressure to try to establish ideal ventilatory parameters were studied, using a crossover design; however, just low VT combined with PEEP resulted in reduced oxygenation [41].

In a healthy porcine lung model of OLV, moderate PEEP can improve oxygenation. This effect implies both expiratory and inspiratory pulmonary recruitment. Co-administration of inspired nitric oxide was ineffective [42].

Positive end-expiratory pressure is commonly applied to the ventilated lung to try to improve oxygenation during OLV, but it is an unreliable therapy and occasionally causes PaO_2 to decrease further. The effects of PEEP on oxygenation depend on the static compliance curve of the lung to which it is applied. The effects of the application of 5 cmH_2O PEEP on oxygenation during OLV correspond to individual changes in the relation between the plateau end-expiratory pressure and the inflection point of the static compliance curve. When the application of PEEP causes the end-expiratory pressure to increase from a low level toward the inflection point, oxygenation is likely to improve, but, if the addition of PEEP causes an increased inflation of the ventilated lung that raises the equilibrium end-expiratory pressure beyond the inflection point, oxygenation is likely to deteriorate. Unfortunately, there is yet no possibility for the use of a device that could establish the inflection point in the current clinical practice [43].

Applying CPAP to the non-ventilated lung can have beneficial effects. Results suggest that increased IL-1 or TNF-alpha production by alveolar macrophages may be responsible for fever caused by atelectasis. By applying CPAP to the non-ventilated, atelectatic lung, this may be prevented. In the same time, it is beneficial for reducing FiO_2 during OLV [44].

Re-expansion pulmonary edema is a rare complication caused by rapid re-expansion of a collapsed lung. Elevated levels of pro-inflammatory cytokines in pulmonary edema fluid are suggested to play important roles in its development. Pro-inflammatory cytokines are upregulated upon re-expansion and ventilation after short-period lung collapse, though no changes are observed in pulmonary capillary permeability [45].

Because of the regular use of fiber-optic bronchoscope, the positioning of lung-separating devices became safer; thus, very high FiO_2 is most of times not necessary. High FiO_2 may induce atelectasis, and it was shown that during OLV inflammatory and oxidative responses were more favorable when using lower (under 50 %) FiO_2 [46].

Conclusions

The practice of OLV practice has changed over the past few decades, with VT decreasing significantly. However, patients during OLV are still ventilated with large, and perhaps too large, VT. Even if there is increasing evidence for the use of protective settings for OLV, however, what are the optimal settings? According to the EACTA thoracic subcommission's survey, still less than 60 % of anesthesiologists who are regularly performing OLV are using higher VT than 6 ml/kg, less than 50 % are doing no ARM at all, just a few of the rest are doing ARM before applying a PEEP, and just a very few use FiO_2 less than 100 % for induction of GA, and a lot 100 % for OLV. What is the low VT that we may use during OLV to keep the balance between oxygen delivery and prevention of lung injury, and how much is the optimal PEEP that we should use during OLV? The ventilatory method for OLV (pressure vs volume controlled) seems to be not an issue, given that the differences are not really relevant. As an alternative for conventional ventilatory methods, high-frequency jet ventilation was proposed too; however, studies are lacking. Unfortunately, even if it remains evidence based, the use of ARM, low VT, low driving pressure, PEEP, and low FiO_2 is not yet generally accepted by thoracic anesthesiologists. Prospective studies to evaluate optimal settings for OLV (while keeping the balance between oxygenation and lung injury) are needed; the more and more sophisticated monitoring devices that are available for clinical use, like electrical impedance tomography or volumetric capnography, could help assess these uncertainties.

References

1. Khuri SF, Henderson WG, DePalma RG, Mosca C, Healey NA, Kumbhani DJ et al (2005) Determinants of long-term survival after major surgery and the adverse effect of postoperative complications. Ann Surg 242(3):326–341; discussion 41–43
2. Rock P, Rich PB (2003) Postoperative pulmonary complications. Curr Opin Anaesthesiol 16(2):123–131
3. Bendixen HH, Hedley-Whyte J, Laver MB (1963) Impaired oxygenation in surgical patients during general anesthesia with controlled ventilation. A concept of atelectasis. N Engl J Med 269:991–996
4. (2000) Ventilation with lower tidal volumes as compared with traditional tidal volumes for acute lung injury and the acute respiratory distress syndrome. The Acute Respiratory Distress Syndrome Network. N Engl J Med 342(18):1301–1308
5. Artigas A, Bernard GR, Carlet J, Dreyfuss D, Gattinoni L, Hudson L et al (1998) The American-European Consensus Conference on ARDS, part 2: ventilatory, pharmacologic, supportive therapy, study design strategies, and issues related to recovery and remodeling. Acute respiratory distress syndrome. Am J Respir Crit Care Med 157(4 Pt 1):1332–1347
6. Ranieri VM, Suter PM, Tortorella C, De Tullio R, Dayer JM, Brienza A et al (1999) Effect of mechanical ventilation on inflammatory mediators in patients with acute respiratory distress syndrome: a randomized controlled trial. JAMA 282(1):54–61
7. Gajic O, Dara SI, Mendez JL, Adesanya AO, Festic E, Caples SM et al (2004) Ventilator-associated lung injury in patients without acute lung injury at the onset of mechanical ventilation. Crit Care Med 32(9):1817–1824
8. Determann RM, Royakkers A, Wolthuis EK, Vlaar AP, Choi G, Paulus F et al (2010) Ventilation with lower tidal volumes as compared with conventional tidal volumes for patients without acute lung injury: a preventive randomized controlled trial. Crit Care (Lond, Engl) 14(1):R1
9. Jaber S, Coisel Y, Chanques G, Futier E, Constantin JM, Michelet P et al (2012) A multicentre observational study of intra-operative ventilatory management during general anaesthesia: tidal volumes and relation to body weight. Anaesthesia 67(9):999–1008
10. Serpa Neto A, Hemmes SN, Barbas CS, Beiderlinden M, Fernandez-Bustamante A, Futier E et al (2014) Incidence of mortality and morbidity related to postoperative lung injury in

patients who have undergone abdominal or thoracic surgery: a systematic review and meta-analysis. Lancet Respir Med 2(12):1007–1015
11. Gao W, Liu DD, Li D, Cui GX (2015) Effect of therapeutic hypercapnia on inflammatory responses to one-lung ventilation in lobectomy patients. Anesthesiology 122(6):1235–1252
12. Pelosi P, Rocco PR (2007) Airway closure: the silent killer of peripheral airways. Crit Care (Lond, Engl) 11(1):114
13. Tusman G, Bohm SH, Warner DO, Sprung J (2012) Atelectasis and perioperative pulmonary complications in high-risk patients. Curr Opin Anaesthesiol 25(1):1–10
14. Tokics L, Hedenstierna G, Strandberg A, Brismar B, Lundquist H (1987) Lung collapse and gas exchange during general anesthesia: effects of spontaneous breathing, muscle paralysis, and positive end-expiratory pressure. Anesthesiology 66(2):157–167
15. Treschan TA, Kaisers W, Schaefer MS, Bastin B, Schmalz U, Wania V et al (2012) Ventilation with low tidal volumes during upper abdominal surgery does not improve postoperative lung function. Br J Anaesth 109(2):263–271
16. Hedenstierna G, Strandberg A, Brismar B, Lundquist H, Svensson L, Tokics L (1985) Functional residual capacity, thoracoabdominal dimensions, and central blood volume during general anesthesia with muscle paralysis and mechanical ventilation. Anesthesiology 62(3): 247–254
17. Appelberg J, Pavlenko T, Bergman H, Rothen HU, Hedenstierna G (2007) Lung aeration during sleep. Chest 131(1):122–129
18. Hedenstierna G (2012) Oxygen and anesthesia: what lung do we deliver to the post-operative ward? Acta Anaesthesiol Scand 56(6):675–685
19. Tusman G, Bohm SH, Suarez-Sipmann F, Turchetto E (2004) Alveolar recruitment improves ventilatory efficiency of the lungs during anesthesia. Can J Anaesth 51(7):723–727
20. Reinius H, Jonsson L, Gustafsson S, Sundbom M, Duvernoy O, Pelosi P et al (2009) Prevention of atelectasis in morbidly obese patients during general anesthesia and paralysis: a computerized tomography study. Anesthesiology 111(5):979–987
21. Severgnini P, Selmo G, Lanza C, Chiesa A, Frigerio A, Bacuzzi A et al (2013) Protective mechanical ventilation during general anesthesia for open abdominal surgery improves postoperative pulmonary function. Anesthesiology 118(6):1307–1321
22. Futier E, Constantin JM, Paugam-Burtz C, Pascal J, Eurin M, Neuschwander A et al (2013) A trial of intraoperative low-tidal-volume ventilation in abdominal surgery. N Engl J Med 369(5):428–437
23. Anaesthesiology PNIftCTNotESo, Hemmes SN, Gama de Abreu M, Pelosi P, Schultz MJ (2014) High versus low positive end-expiratory pressure during general anaesthesia for open abdominal surgery (PROVHILO trial): a multicentre randomised controlled trial. Lancet 384(9942):495–503
24. Hedenstierna G, Edmark L, Perchiazzi G (2015) Postoperative lung complications: have multicentre studies been of any help? Br J Anaesth 114(4):541–543
25. Amato MB, Meade MO, Slutsky AS, Brochard L, Costa EL, Schoenfeld DA et al (2015) Driving pressure and survival in the acute respiratory distress syndrome. N Engl J Med 372(8):747–755
26. Gattinoni L, Pesenti A (2005) The concept of "baby lung". Intensive Care Med 31(6): 776–784
27. Szegedi LL, Barvais L, Sokolow Y, Yernault JC, d'Hollander AA (2002) Intrinsic positive end-expiratory pressure during one-lung ventilation of patients with pulmonary hyperinflation. Influence of low respiratory rate with unchanged minute volume. Br J Anaesth 88(1):56–60
28. Licker M, de Perrot M, Spiliopoulos A, Robert J, Diaper J, Chevalley C et al (2003) Risk factors for acute lung injury after thoracic surgery for lung cancer. Anesth Analg 97(6): 1558–1565
29. Schilling T, Kozian A, Huth C, Buhling F, Kretzschmar M, Welte T et al (2005) The pulmonary immune effects of mechanical ventilation in patients undergoing thoracic surgery. Anesth Analg 101(4):957–965, table of contents

30. Sugasawa Y, Yamaguchi K, Kumakura S, Murakami T, Kugimiya T, Suzuki K et al (2011) The effect of one-lung ventilation upon pulmonary inflammatory responses during lung resection. J Anesth 25(2):170–177
31. Gama de Abreu M, Heintz M, Heller A, Szechenyi R, Albrecht DM, Koch T (2003) One-lung ventilation with high tidal volumes and zero positive end-expiratory pressure is injurious in the isolated rabbit lung model. Anesth Analg 96(1):220–228
32. Michelet P, D'Journo XB, Roch A, Doddoli C, Marin V, Papazian L et al (2006) Protective ventilation influences systemic inflammation after esophagectomy: a randomized controlled study. Anesthesiology 105(5):911–919
33. Tugrul M, Camci E, Karadeniz H, Senturk M, Pembeci K, Akpir K (1997) Comparison of volume controlled with pressure controlled ventilation during one-lung anaesthesia. Br J Anaesth 79(3):306–310
34. Unzueta MC, Casas JI, Moral MV (2007) Pressure-controlled versus volume-controlled ventilation during one-lung ventilation for thoracic surgery. Anesth Analg 104(5):1029–1033, tables of contents
35. Kozian A, Schilling T, Schutze H, Senturk M, Hachenberg T, Hedenstierna G (2011) Ventilatory protective strategies during thoracic surgery: effects of alveolar recruitment maneuver and low-tidal volume ventilation on lung density distribution. Anesthesiology 114(5):1025–1035
36. Tusman G, Bohm SH, Sipmann FS, Maisch S (2004) Lung recruitment improves the efficiency of ventilation and gas exchange during one-lung ventilation anesthesia. Anesth Analg 98(6):1604–1609, table of contents
37. Kozian A, Schilling T, Freden F, Maripuu E, Rocken C, Strang C et al (2008) One-lung ventilation induces hyperperfusion and alveolar damage in the ventilated lung: an experimental study. Br J Anaesth 100(4):549–559
38. De Conno E, Steurer MP, Wittlinger M, Zalunardo MP, Weder W, Schneiter D et al (2009) Anesthetic-induced improvement of the inflammatory response to one-lung ventilation. Anesthesiology 110(6):1316–1326
39. Schilling T, Kozian A, Kretzschmar M, Huth C, Welte T, Buhling F et al (2007) Effects of propofol and desflurane anaesthesia on the alveolar inflammatory response to one-lung ventilation. Br J Anaesth 99(3):368–375
40. Schilling T, Kozian A, Senturk M, Huth C, Reinhold A, Hedenstierna G et al (2011) Effects of volatile and intravenous anesthesia on the alveolar and systemic inflammatory response in thoracic surgical patients. Anesthesiology 115(1):65–74
41. Roze H, Lafargue M, Perez P, Tafer N, Batoz H, Germain C et al (2012) Reducing tidal volume and increasing positive end-expiratory pressure with constant plateau pressure during one-lung ventilation: effect on oxygenation. Br J Anaesth 108(6):1022–1027
42. Michelet P, Roch A, Brousse D, D'Journo XB, Bregeon F, Lambert D et al (2005) Effects of PEEP on oxygenation and respiratory mechanics during one-lung ventilation. Br J Anaesth 95(2):267–273
43. Slinger PD, Kruger M, McRae K, Winton T (2001) Relation of the static compliance curve and positive end-expiratory pressure to oxygenation during one-lung ventilation. Anesthesiology 95(5):1096–1102
44. Hughes SA, Benumof JL (1990) Operative lung continuous positive airway pressure to minimize FIO2 during one-lung ventilation. Anesth Analg 71(1):92–95
45. Funakoshi T, Ishibe Y, Okazaki N, Miura K, Liu R, Nagai S et al (2004) Effect of re-expansion after short-period lung collapse on pulmonary capillary permeability and pro-inflammatory cytokine gene expression in isolated rabbit lungs. Br J Anaesth 92(4):558–563
46. Olivant Fisher A, Husain K, Wolfson MR, Hubert TL, Rodriguez E, Shaffer TH et al (2012) Hyperoxia during one lung ventilation: inflammatory and oxidative responses. Pediatr Pulmonol 47(10):979–986

4 Can Postoperative Pulmonary Complications Be Objectively Evaluated?

Marcelo Gama de Abreu, Thomas Kiss, Lluis Gallart, and Jaume Canet

4.1 Introduction

It has been estimated that more than 230 million major surgical procedures are conducted every year across the world and that more than 1 % of those procedures, i.e., approximately 2.6 million, carry a high risk of complications [1]. Again, roughly half of the patients who are submitted to high-risk interventions experience complications, and more than 300,000 die during the hospital stay. Among those complications, pulmonary adverse events, or postoperative pulmonary complications (PPCs), occur as often as cardiac and circulatory adverse events [2]. Observational studies have shown that PPCs occur in up to 10 % of patients who undergo surgery under general anesthesia [3]. In patients with low preoperative peripheral oxygen saturation, upper airway infection up to 1 month before surgery, and anemia and in the elderly, the risk of PPCs increases importantly. Also the type of surgery, emergency procedures, and the duration of surgery itself are associated with a higher risk of developing adverse pulmonary events [3]. Following upper abdominal and thoracic surgery, the incidence of PPCs can be as high as 19–59 % [4].

There are different reasons for assessing the risk of PPCs. The stratification of patients according to the likelihood of such complications allows preventive measurements to be taken, such as planned admission in units better equipped for monitoring and treating those patients, thereby decreasing the risk of further complications that might develop. It has been shown that postoperative lung failure dramatically increases the risk of death following abdominal and thoracic surgery [5].

M.G. de Abreu (✉) • T. Kiss
Department of Anesthesiology and Intensive Care Therapy, Pulmonary Engineering Group, University Hospital Carl Gustav Carus, Technische Universität Dresden, Dresden, Germany
e-mail: mgabreau@uniklinikum-dresden.de

L. Gallart • J. Canet
Department of Anesthesiology, Hospital Universitari Germans Trias i Pujol, Universitat Autònoma de Barcelona, Badalona, Spain

© Springer International Publishing Switzerland 2017

M. Şentürk, M.O. Sungur (eds.), *Postoperative Care in Thoracic Surgery*,
DOI 10.1007/978-3-319-19908-5_4

Furthermore, when groups of patients with a similar probability of developing PPCs are identified, specific interventions to prevent them can be designed and trials may be better planned. Last but not the least, allocation of financial resources can be conducted in a more objective and efficient way, given that such complications have marked economic impact on health systems.

In the present chapter, we will present the state of the art of the evaluation of PPCs. We will critically review the most commonly used definitions of PPCs and provide a thorough appraisal of the current tools for stratifying patients at higher risk. We will present a comprehensive state of the art in prediction of PPCs, focusing on patients undergoing thoracic surgery procedures, and the particularities of this type of intervention.

4.2 Definitions of Postoperative Pulmonary Complications

In clinical practice, any postoperative pulmonary adverse event can be seen as a PPC, independent of the degree of severity or further consequences it may cause. Among the most common events considered as PPC are [2, 6–8] (a) respiratory failure from pulmonary or cardiac origin, (b) pneumonia and respiratory infection, (c) pleural effusion and atelectasis, (d) pneumothorax, (e) bronchospasm, and (f) need for noninvasive respiratory support or reintubation. Although apparently less harmful, and occurring more frequently than other events, peripheral oxygen desaturation requiring supplemental oxygen has been considered also a PPC by different authors [9–12]. It is worth noting that once a PPC occur, the average hospital stay is prolonged and the risk of in-hospital death increases despite the subjectively attributable severity of the specific event [3–13]. Obviously, the incidence of PPCs varies considerably depending on the definition used, and this may impact on the interpretation of studies and use of risk scores.

Recently, the joint task force of the European Society of Anaesthesiology (ESA) and the European Society of Intensive Care Medicine (ESICM) on perioperative outcome measures proposed specific definitions for PPCs based on a consensus among experts and more common used terms across different studies [12]:

- Acute respiratory failure – Postoperative PaO_2 <60 mmHg on room air, a PaO_2/FIO_2 ratio <300 mmHg, or arterial oxyhemoglobin saturation measured with pulse oximetry <90% and requiring oxygen therapy. Although not directly addressed by the ESA-ESICM task force [12], respiratory failure may be subdivided into mild, moderate, and severe forms. The mild form refers to adequate response to supplemental oxygen, the moderate form corresponds to inadequate response to supplemental oxygen requiring noninvasive or invasive mechanical ventilation, and the severe form is the development of the acute respiratory distress syndrome [14].
- Atelectasis – Lung opacification with a shift of the mediastinum, hilum, or hemidiaphragm toward the affected area and compensatory overinflation in the adjacent non-atelectatic lung.

- Respiratory infection – The patient has received antibiotics for a suspected respiratory infection and met one or more of the following criteria: new or changed sputum, new or changed lung opacities, fever, and white blood cell count $>12\times10^9\ L^{-1}$.
- Pleural effusion – Chest radiograph demonstrating blunting of the costophrenic angle, loss of sharp silhouette of the ipsilateral hemidiaphragm in upright position, evidence of displacement of adjacent anatomical structures, or (in supine position) a hazy opacity in one hemithorax with preserved vascular shadows.
- Pneumothorax – Air in the pleural space with no vascular bed surrounding the visceral pleura.
- Bronchospasm – Newly detected expiratory wheezing treated with bronchodilators.
- Aspiration pneumonitis – Acute lung injury after the inhalation of regurgitated gastric contents.

Usually, these adverse events are grouped together to build a so-called collapsed composite. When one component variable of the composite outcome is fulfilled, the patient is considered to have a PPC. One of the major advantages of using collapsed PPC composites is that they may increase the power of studies addressing interventions. Since the incidence of a particular event can be relatively low, accounting for a group of events that can be influenced by a specific intervention seems reasonable. On the other hand, it has been suggested that differences in the frequency of component variables of a collapsed composite, as well as their severity, should be ideally comparable, or at least their relative weighs taken into account [15].

4.3 Postoperative Pulmonary Complications After Thoracic Surgery

One of the particularities of surgical interventions in the thorax, mainly those involving lung procedures, is that one or more of the adverse events previously mentioned represent an otherwise common consequence of surgery. For example, partial atelectasis of the operated lung, pleural effusion, and ipsilateral pneumothorax are more likely related to the surgical procedure and/or the preoperative condition than to the intraoperative respiratory or circulatory management. On the other hand, the presence of prolonged air leaks, acute lung edema, pulmonary embolism, purulent pleuritis, and even hemorrhage [16] may be partly related to the modulation of the immune, pro-inflammatory, and pro-coagulatory responses, which are influenced, at least in part, by the management of hemodynamics and ventilation during thoracic surgery.

Given that mild forms of acute respiratory failure likely represent the most common adverse event following thoracic surgery, and aiming at delivering a comprehensive, but also specific list of adverse pulmonary events that is summarized in Table 4.1.

Table 4.1 Most frequent and relevant postoperative pulmonary complications after thoracic surgery

Adverse pulmonary event	Definition	Observation
Acute respiratory failure	Postoperative PaO_2 <60 mmHg on room air, a PaO_2/FIO_2 ratio <300 mmHg, or arterial oxyhemoglobin saturation measured with pulse oximetry <90 % and requiring oxygen therapy [12]	It may present as mild, moderate, or severe form Mild, adequate response to supplemental oxygen; moderate, inadequate response to supplemental oxygen requiring noninvasive or invasive mechanical ventilation; severe, acute respiratory distress syndrome [14]
Prolonged air leak	Air leak requiring >7 days of postoperative chest tube drainage [16]	After acute respiratory failure, possibly the most common pulmonary complication following thoracic surgery
Respiratory infection	Receiving antibiotics for a suspected respiratory infection and met one or more of the following criteria: new or changed sputum, new or changed lung opacities, fever, white blood cell count>12 × 10^9 L^{-1} [12]	
Postoperative hemorrhage	Bleeding through the chest tubes requiring reoperation or three or more red blood cell packs [16]	
Atelectasis	Lung opacification with a shift of the mediastinum, hilum, or hemidiaphragm toward the affected area and compensatory overinflation in the adjacent non-atelectatic lung [12]	
Pneumothorax	Air in the pleural space with no vascular bed surrounding the visceral pleura [12]	As far as not related to the surgical procedure alone
Bronchospasm	Newly detected expiratory wheezing treated with bronchodilators [12]	In mechanically ventilated patients, increased airway pressure during positive-pressure ventilation or prolonged expiratory phase [16]
Pulmonary embolism	As documented by pulmonary arteriogram or autopsy or supported by a ventilation/perfusion radioisotope scans [16]	
Aspiration pneumonitis	Acute lung injury after the inhalation of regurgitated gastric contents	

Table 4.1 (continued)

Adverse pulmonary event	Definition	Observation
Pleural effusion	Chest radiograph demonstrating blunting of the costophrenic angle, loss of sharp silhouette of the ipsilateral hemidiaphragm in upright position, evidence of displacement of adjacent anatomical structures, or (in supine position) a hazy opacity in one hemithorax with preserved vascular shadows	As far as not related explained by the preoperative patient condition alone
Acute pulmonary edema	Evidence of fluid accumulation in the alveoli as documented by lung imaging	Not explained by poor cardiac function
Purulent pleuritis	Receiving antibiotics for a suspected infection	As far as not related explained by the preoperative patient condition alone

4.4 Risk of Developing Postoperative Pulmonary Complications

Along the last 16 years, more than 50 risk factors for PPCs have been identified and discussed in the literature [9, 10, 17]. Factors related to development of PPCs can be seen also as "predictors" and addressed in terms of relative contribution to the odds of developing such complications. They may be combined by means of statistical models into scores that will ultimately reflect the probability of patients to develop PPCs.

The milestone of a structured presentation of factors related to the development of pulmonary adverse events in surgery patients has been established by the American College of Physicians (ACP) in the year 2006 [17]. Those are factors related to the patient's preoperative condition, the surgical procedure itself, as well as the type of anesthesia delivered and have been expanded and improved in subsequent studies.

4.4.1 Risk Factors Related to the Patient's Condition

4.4.1.1 Age

Advanced age has been recognized as a major risk for different adverse postoperative events [18] and represents the most frequent factor related to PPCs [17]. Aging may increase the vulnerability of organ systems to a major surgical stress, or decrease the capability of organ systems to respond to a combination of multiple minor stressors, which may ultimately compromise their ability to respond to such challenges [19]. Although such phenomenon, usually known as frailty, is not exclusive of the elderly patient, it is more often observed in higher age groups. In fact, advanced age seems to be only a surrogate of frailty, which is accompanied by an increased pro-inflammatory response in both nonsurgical [20] and surgical patients [21]. Nevertheless, age still properly stratifies the risk of PPCs.

4.4.1.2 Functional Dependence

Functional dependence reflects perhaps a relevant degree of disability of a patient, and as such it is closely related to age and frailty. It has been shown that this patient-related risk factor and its severity are associated with increased serum levels of pro-inflammatory markers [22]. Particularly, patients with advanced age frequently present frailty and some degree of disability with functional dependence, which further increases the risk for postoperative complications [23].

4.4.1.3 Classification of the American Society of Anesthesiologists (ASA)

The ASA classification for general risk evaluation is popular among anesthesiologists, even if considerable variability among assessors has been reported in different studies [24, 25]. As a score derived from the degree of impairment of several organ systems, the ASA classification is unspecific but has the advantage of integrating possible single factors that may have higher sensibility for PPCs [9]. However, when taken into account for computing risk of PPCs, the ASA classification may jeopardize the contribution of relevant risk factors. Thus, its use as part of risk assessment must be judiciously considered.

4.4.1.4 Smoking

It has been claimed that in lung cancer surgery, the odds of smoking as a risk factor for PPCs is increased [26]. However, the impact of smoking on the development of PPCs after thoracotomy [27], even in patients undergoing lung cancer resection, has been questioned [28]. Therefore, compared to other factors, smoking seems to play a less important role for PPCs.

4.4.1.5 Respiratory Symptoms

The presence of respiratory symptoms is associated with advanced impairment of the pulmonary function in obstructive disease [29]. Among those symptoms, cough, sputum, dyspnea, and wheezing seem to play an important role [30].

4.4.1.6 Peripheral Oxygen Saturation and Pulmonary Function Tests (PFTs)

Low peripheral oxygen saturation adds importantly to the risk of PPCs following different types of surgical interventions, including thoracic surgery [11]. Despite its almost intuitive rationale, this risk factor has been recognized only recently [9].

In the context of thoracic surgery, PFTs comprehend spirometry and diffusing capacity of the lung for carbon monoxide (DLCO). According to the American College of Chest Physicians, impairment of the forced expiratory volume in one second (FEV1) and DLCO are useful in stratifying the risk of disability and even mortality following lung resectional surgery [31]. In patients with lung cancer undergoing surgery, FEV1 represented the PFT parameter that was better associated with PPCs and better contributed to the risk evaluation [32]. The predictive value of PFTs holds useful regardless of the surgical approach, i.e., also for minimally invasive lobectomy [33].

4.4.1.7 Respiratory Infection Prior to Surgery

Infection of the respiratory system in the last month preceding surgery has been linked to an increased the risk of PPCs [3, 11], but its contribution to predict these complications has been challenged recently [34].

4.4.1.8 Preoperative Hypoalbuminemia, Weight Loss, and Body Mass Index (BMI)

These factors are closely related to the nutritional status. Low serum albumin concentrations seem to increase the risk of PPCs in the general population [17], possibly to increased incidence of anastomose leakage. In patients undergoing pneumonectomy, hypoalbuminemia was associated with bronchopleural fistula formation [35]. Also, weight loss exceeding 10 % in the past 6 months preceding surgery increases the risk of postoperative pneumonia [36]. Whereas a BMI <18.5 kg/m^2 increases the risk of death after lobectomy for cancer [37], a BMI >18.5 kg/m^2 increases the risk of PPCs after thoracotomy.

4.4.1.9 Preoperative Anemia

Patients with preoperative hemoglobin concentrations <10 g/dL who undergo lung resection surgery are at increased risk for PPCs [38]. Also in the general surgical population, anemia adds to the risk of PPCs [3].

4.4.1.10 Chronic Obstructive and Other Pulmonary Diseases

Chronic obstructive pulmonary disease (COPD) is a comparatively high prevalent disease [39] that carries a considerable risk for patients to develop both non-pulmonary and pulmonary postoperative adverse events [40]. This disease has been incorporated into numerous scores for prediction of risk of PPCs [7, 41–47]. In thoracic surgery patients, COPD is a common comorbidity that underlies many of the indications for such interventions, for example, lung volume reduction surgery, bullectomy, and lung transplantation [48], as well as lung cancer resection and spontaneous pneumothorax surgery [49]. In addition, the degree of severity of COPD plays a relevant role for prognosis prediction, since it is associated with increased need for ICU admission following pulmonary resection [50]. Importantly, the attributable risk of COPD may be decreased upon pulmonary rehabilitation measures [29]. In the general population, chronic pulmonary diseases have been implicated in the need for postoperative reintubation [45].

4.4.1.11 Congestive Heart Failure (CHF)

Congestive heart failure (CHF), even if adequately compensated, adds considerably to the risk of PPCs in the general surgery population [17, 51]. In older patients undergoing lung cancer surgery, CHF increased the risk of death [52].

4.4.1.12 Renal Disease

Patients with renal disease may be at higher risk to develop PPCs [17]. In surgical patients, acute renal failure increases the need for reintubation and ventilatory failure [53].

4.4.1.13 Liver Disease

Preoperative liver disease adds to the odds of developing PPCs [11]. In the general surgical population, cirrhosis is associated with higher risk of death following surgery [51].

4.4.1.14 Obstructive Sleep Apnea (OSA)

Surgical patients with OSA have an increased risk for postoperative complications, especially circulatory and pulmonary, also following thoracic surgery [54, 55].

4.4.1.15 Current Alcohol Use

Alcohol impairs the immune response [56] and causes neurologic impairment, which may facilitate aspiration and the development of pneumonia postoperatively. Alcohol use has been identified as a risk factor for development of PPCs in the general surgical population [17], as is associated with higher risk of death following pneumonectomy [57].

4.4.1.16 Diabetes Mellitus

Diabetes mellitus has been associated with an increased risk of ARDS following surgery [44], but it is comparatively less relevant than of other factors. In patients undergoing lung cancer resection, diabetes mellitus did not increase the risk of postoperative pneumonia [58].

4.4.2 Procedure-Related and Intraoperative Risk Factors

Thoracic surgery, as compared to other types of surgical interventions, has been associated with relatively high risk for PPCs in different investigations [3, 17, 44]. This figure is explained by the fact that the intervention itself causes direct injury to the lungs, the airways, and also the respiratory muscles, likely interfering with the capability to ventilate, mobilize secretions, and cough. Also, the presence of atelectasis may impair the gas exchange and lead to hypoxemia. Certainly, the surgical approach contributes to determine the impact on the risk of PPCs.

4.4.2.1 Thoracotomy Versus Median Sternotomy

During thoracotomy, the intercostal muscles are likely more injured than during sternotomy, which could be associated with more severe pain and ventilatory impairment. In patients undergoing lung cancer resection, median sternotomy was associated with shorter length of hospital stay, but did not improve survival [59].

4.4.2.2 Video-Assisted Thoracoscopic Versus Open Thoracic Surgery

Laparoscopy compared to open surgery has been found to decrease mortality in the general surgical population [51]. A recent meta-analysis showed that in lung cancer patients with compromised lung function, lobectomy with video-assisted thoracoscopy (VATS) is associated with lower risk for pulmonary morbidity than open surgery [60]. In fact, compared to most open surgical approaches, VATS has been classified as low risk for postoperative ARDS [44].

4.4.2.3 Extent of Lung Resection

Extensive lung resection may be associated with a shift of the pulmonary perfusion to the remaining capillary bed, increasing the shear stress to those areas and consequent failure [61]. In patients undergoing thoracic surgery for lung cancer, the incidence of acute lung injury was more than three times higher after pneumonectomy than lobectomy or lesser resections [62].

4.4.2.4 Duration of Surgery

The duration of surgery has been shown to increase the risk of PPCs in different studies [3, 17, 44, 51]. Particularly, interventions lasting more than 2 h in the general surgical population [3, 11], or requiring more than 2 h of anesthetic time for pneumonectomy [63], have been independently associated with an increased probability of developing adverse pulmonary events.

4.4.2.5 Volatile Versus Intravenous Anesthetics

The anesthesia regimen has the potential to modulate the incidence of PPCs, given that certain anesthetics promote organ protection. In rats [64], but also in patients [65], volatile agents compared to intravenous anesthetics reduced lung injury and/or inflammation. However, up to this date, no randomized controlled trial demonstrated an advantage of volatile anesthetics in terms of outcome.

4.4.2.6 Muscle Paralysis

The use of neuromuscular blocking agents (NMBAs) for intubation of the trachea with devices that enable lung separation is almost mandatory, since such devices are comparatively larger than conventional endotracheal tubes and optimal conditions more difficult to obtain. Also, NMBAs are used to achieve optimal thoracic surgical conditions. In the general surgical population, intermediate-acting NMBAs have been implicated in an increased incidence of PPCs, especially if reversal of muscle paralysis is not appropriately performed [66].

4.4.2.7 Restrictive Versus Liberal Fluid Strategy

Liberal fluid strategies have been shown to increase the risk for lung injury after thoracic procedures. Fluid overload, impairment of lung lymphatic outflow, and damage of the pulmonary endothelium have been implicated as possible causes for such complication [67]. A retrospective study in patients undergoing anatomic lung resections showed that infusion rates exceeding 6 mL/kg/h increased the risk of PPCs [68].

4.4.2.8 Transfusion of Blood and Blood Products

Transfusion-related acute lung injury (TRALI) is a leading cause of transfusion-related death. This syndrome is related to the passive infusion of human leukocyte antigen and human neutrophil antigen, which may elicit an antibody-mediated [69] inflammatory response, but a non-antibody mediated due to aged cellular blood products has been also identified [70]. Neutrophils seem to play a key role in TRALI. Those cells are activated by different insults, for example, hypotension, mechanical ventilation, or ischemia-reperfusion, which are usually present in thoracic surgery and serve as a first hit. The transfusion of blood and blood products leads then to a second hit, with resulting inflammatory response.

4.4.2.9 Mechanical Ventilation

Mechanical stress inflicted by the ventilator to the lung parenchyma has the potential to cause harm. In patients undergoing esophagectomy, a protective ventilation with low tidal volume (5 mL/kg, predicted body weight – PBW) with positive end-expiratory pressure (PEEP) of 5 cmH2O was associated with less lung inflammation than a non-protective mechanical ventilation with high tidal volume (10 mL/kg PBW) with PEEP of 0 cmH2O [71]. In a retrospective study in lung cancer patients, intraoperative ventilation with lower plateau inspiratory pressure was associated with a decreased incidence of acute lung injury [62]. In addition, a recent meta-analysis showed that protective compared to non-protective ventilation reduced the incidence of postoperative lung injury following abdominal and thoracic surgery. Since the term "protective ventilation" is not well defined and mostly seen as a bundle of measures (low tidal volume, PEEP, recruitment maneuvers, low inspiratory oxygen fraction), it is not clear which of those elements are responsible for lung protection. Apparently, low tidal volumes play an important role in lung protection, whereas the relevance of PEEP has not been demonstrated [72].

4.5 Predictive Models of Postoperative Pulmonary Complications in Thoracic Surgery

Several predictive models of postoperative complications have been developed, but only a few of them are specific for the thoracic surgery population and pulmonary complications. Those scores usually are limited by one or more of the following factors: (1) use of preoperative variables only; (2) lack of clearness of the model's development as listed in the STROBE guidelines and defined according by the "Transparent Reporting of a Multivariable Prediction Model for Individual Prognosis or Diagnosis (TRIPOD)" statement [73]; (3) lack of external validation in independent studies; (4) lack of generalizability to other patient populations; and (5) lack of capability of predicting the outcome of individual patients, rather than groups. However, they still build the fundament for stratification of patients for testing interventions, allocation of resources, benchmarking, and also professional audits. Moreover, for the treating physician, they may be helpful to justify and obtain informed consent for certain procedures on a more objective risk/benefit analysis basis. Also, they might contribute to improve a patient's condition depending whether potentially modifiable risk factors are involved in a poor prognosis. In this subsection, we will briefly describe a few relevant scoring systems for prediction of PPCs, with emphasis in the application in noncardiac thoracic surgery.

4.5.1 The Physiological and Operative Severity Score for the Enumeration of Mortality and Morbidity (POSSUM)

The POSSUM score, which is based on 12 preoperative factors, was originally developed for predicting adverse outcome in the general population [74]. In patients undergoing lung resection, the POSSUM scoring system showed acceptable performance for predicting PPCs [75].

4.5.2 The Cardiopulmonary Risk Index (CPRI)

The CPRI combines cardiopulmonary variables into one single score ranging from 1 to 10, where 10 represents the worst value. In patients undergoing pneumonectomy, but not other types of thoracic surgery, a CPRI $\geq$4 was associated with increased incidence of PPCs [76].

4.5.3 The Expiratory Volume Age Diffusion (EVÁD) Capacity Score

The EVÁD score uses three main covariates to assess the risk of complications after lung resection, namely, age, spirometry, and diffusing capacity [77]. Compared to the CPRI and POSSUM scoring systems, EVÁD showed a better predictive value for PPCs after major lung resection.

4.5.4 The Postoperative Respiratory Failure (PRF) and the Postoperative Pneumonia Risk (PPR) Index

The PRF index has been developed within a retrospective analysis of patients admitted to the National Veterans Affairs Surgical Quality Improvement Program (NSQIP) [7] and is able to identify high-risk patients with a 30 % likelihood of developing respiratory failure. Later on, a score to predict pneumonia was proposed by the same group and using NSQIP data, which applies also to patients undergoing thoracic surgery [36]. Both the PRF and PPR indices, with 7 and 14 predictors, respectively, have not been validated externally.

4.5.5 The Assess Respiratory Risk in Surgical Patients in Catalonia (ARISCAT) Score

The ARISCAT score is a specific predicting tool for PPCs [3]. It has been developed in a European region only (Catalonia, Spain) but undergone extensive recalibration and external validation in a large cohort from different countries, the so-called Prospective Evaluation of a RIsk Score for postoperative pulmonary COmPlications in Europe (PERISCOPE) study [11]. Furthermore, the PERISCOPE study identified also a group of preoperative variables that allow the prediction of postoperative respiratory failure (PERISCOPE-PRF score) [34]. To date, the ARISCAT score, as recalibrated in the PERISCOPE study, represents one of the most valuable tools for prediction of PPCs. However, it has not been specifically developed for thoracic surgery and therefore does not address some particular complications that may occur in such population, for example, persistent leakage of the operated lung. Furthermore, it is not clear how some of the elements of the collapsed composite PPC, for example, pneumothorax and lung edema, should be dealt with if they occur in the operated hemithorax. Also, intraoperative variables other than duration of surgery are not taken into account.

4.5.6 Preoperative and Intraoperative Predictors of Postoperative Acute Respiratory Distress Syndrome

Postoperative ARDS probably represents the most severe form of PPC. Using data from a single US center, investigators developed a score for predicting ARDS in the general surgical population, which may find application also in thoracic surgery [41]. One important advantage of that score is that preoperative and intraoperative predictors have been identified. However, the lack of external validation still poses doubt about its generalizability.

4.5.7 Further Scoring Systems Developed from Single-Center Databases

A number of prediction scoring systems have been developed, which could be useful in the field of thoracic surgery. They addressed the need for unplanned postoperative tracheal intubation [43, 45], as well as the development of postoperative acute lung injury [44]. Recently, a prediction rule for estimating PPCs has been proposed [47], but patients undergoing pulmonary surgery have been excluded a priori.

4.6 Summary

PPCs are common after thoracic surgery. Usually, the term PPC is defined not as a single complication, but rather a collapsed composite that consists of mild, moderate, and severe complications. Despite differences in severity, they increase the length of stay in hospital and even mortality, especially when two or more complications are present. Preoperative but also intraoperative factors have been identified that are associated with an increased risk for PPCs after thoracic surgery. Those factors, which have been drawn from retrospective, observational prospective, single- and multiple-center studies, have combined by multivariable analyses into scores that might be useful to predict the risk of developing PPCs. Some of those scores addressing general surgical populations have undergone extensive external evaluation in separate studies, whereas others have focused on thoracic surgical patients, but not been validated so far. Albeit the ideal score for predicting PPCs after thoracic surgery has not been developed and validated yet, the available tools already allow the estimation of the risk of pulmonary adverse advents in this surgical population.

References

1. Weiser TG, Makary MA, Haynes AB, Dziekan G, Berry WR, Gawande AA (2009) Standardised metrics for global surgical surveillance. Lancet 374:1113–1117
2. Smetana GW (2009) Postoperative pulmonary complications: an update on risk assessment and reduction. Cleve Clin J Med 76(Suppl 4):S60–S65
3. Canet J, Gallart L, Gomar C, Paluzie G, Valles J, Castillo J, Sabate S, Mazo V, Briones Z, Sanchis J (2010) Prediction of postoperative pulmonary complications in a population-based surgical cohort. Anesthesiology 113:1338–1350
4. Garcia-Miguel FJ, Serrano-Aguilar PG, Lopez-Bastida J (2003) Preoperative assessment. Lancet 362:1749–1757
5. Serpa Neto A, Hemmes SN, Barbas CS, Beiderlinden M, Fernandez-Bustamante A, Futier E, Hollmann MW, Jaber S, Kozian A, Licker M, Lin WQ, Moine P, Scavonetto F, Schilling T, Selmo G, Severgnini P, Sprung J, Treschan T, Unzueta C, Weingarten TN, Wolthuis EK, Wrigge H, Gama de Abreu M, Pelosi P, Schultz MJ, PN investigators (2014) Incidence of mortality and morbidity related to postoperative lung injury in patients who have undergone abdominal or thoracic surgery: a systematic review and meta-analysis. Lancet Respir Med 2:1007–1015
6. Smetana GW (1999) Preoperative pulmonary evaluation. N Engl J Med 340:937–944
7. Arozullah AM, Daley J, Henderson WG, Khuri SF (2000) Multifactorial risk index for predicting postoperative respiratory failure in men after major noncardiac surgery. The National Veterans Administration Surgical Quality Improvement Program. Ann Surg 232:242–253
8. Qaseem A, Snow V, Fitterman N, Hornbake ER, Lawrence VA, Smetana GW, Weiss K, Owens DK, Aronson M, Barry P, Casey DE Jr, Cross JT Jr, Sherif KD, Weiss KB (2006) Risk assessment for and strategies to reduce perioperative pulmonary complications for patients undergoing noncardiothoracic surgery: a guideline from the American College of Physicians. Ann Intern Med 144:575–580
9. Canet J, Gallart L (2013) Predicting postoperative pulmonary complications in the general population. Curr Opin Anaesthesiol 26:107–115
10. Canet J, Gallart L (2014) Postoperative respiratory failure: pathogenesis, prediction, and prevention. Curr Opin Crit Care 20:56–62
11. Mazo V, Sabate S, Canet J, Gallart L, de Abreu MG, Belda J, Langeron O, Hoeft A, Pelosi P (2014) Prospective external validation of a predictive score for postoperative pulmonary complications. Anesthesiology 121:219–231
12. Jammer I, Wickboldt N, Sander M, Smith A, Schultz MJ, Pelosi P, Leva B, Rhodes A, Hoeft A, Walder B, Chew MS, Pearse RM (2015) Standards for definitions and use of outcome measures for clinical effectiveness research in perioperative medicine: European Perioperative

Clinical Outcome (EPCO) definitions: a statement from the ESA-ESICM joint taskforce on perioperative outcome measures. Eur J Anaesthesiol 32(2):88–105
13. Fernandez-Perez ER, Keegan MT, Brown DR, Hubmayr RD, Gajic O (2006) Intraoperative tidal volume as a risk factor for respiratory failure after pneumonectomy. Anesthesiology 105:14–18
14. Force ADT, Ranieri VM, Rubenfeld GD, Thompson BT, Ferguson ND, Caldwell E, Fan E, Camporota L, Slutsky AS (2012) Acute respiratory distress syndrome: the Berlin Definition. JAMA 307:2526–2533
15. Mascha EJ, Sessler DI (2011) Statistical grand rounds: design and analysis of studies with binary- event composite endpoints: guidelines for anesthesia research. Anesth Analg 112:1461–1471
16. Stephan F, Boucheseiche S, Hollande J, Flahault A, Cheffi A, Bazelly B, Bonnet F (2000) Pulmonary complications following lung resection: a comprehensive analysis of incidence and possible risk factors. Chest 118:1263–1270
17. Smetana GW, Lawrence VA, Cornell JE (2006) Preoperative pulmonary risk stratification for noncardiothoracic surgery: systematic review for the American College of Physicians. Ann Intern Med 144:581–595
18. Griffiths R, Beech F, Brown A, Dhesi J, Foo I, Goodall J, Harrop-Griffiths W, Jameson J, Love N, Pappenheim K, White S, Association of Anesthetists of Great B, Ireland (2014) Peri-operative care of the elderly 2014: Association of Anaesthetists of Great Britain and Ireland. Anaesthesia 69(Suppl 1):81–98
19. Hubbard RE, Story DA (2014) Patient frailty: the elephant in the operating room. Anaesthesia 69(Suppl 1):26–34
20. Compte N, Boudjeltia KZ, Vanhaeverbeek M, De Breucker S, Pepersack T, Tassignon J, Trelcat A, Goriely S (2013) Increased basal and alum-induced interleukin-6 levels in geriatric patients are associated with cardiovascular morbidity. PLoS One 8:e81911
21. Hubbard RE, O'Mahony MS, Savva GM, Calver BL, Woodhouse KW (2009) Inflammation and frailty measures in older people. J Cell Mol Med 13:3103–3109
22. Adriaensen W, Mathei C, Vaes B, van Pottelbergh G, Wallemacq P, Degryse JM (2014) Interleukin-6 predicts short-term global functional decline in the oldest old: results from the BELFRAIL study. Age 36:9723
23. Robinson TN, Eiseman B, Wallace JI, Church SD, McFann KK, Pfister SM, Sharp TJ, Moss M (2009) Redefining geriatric preoperative assessment using frailty, disability and co-morbidity. Ann Surg 250:449–455
24. Mak PH, Campbell RC, Irwin MG, American Society of Anesthesiologists (2002) The ASA Physical Status Classification: inter-observer consistency. American Society of Anesthesiologists. Anaesth Intensive Care 30:633–640
25. Castillo J, Canet J, Gomar C, Hervas C (2007) Imprecise status allocation by users of the American Society of Anesthesiologists classification system: survey of Catalan anesthesiologists. Rev Esp Anestesiol Reanim 54:394–398
26. Shiono S, Katahira M, Abiko M, Sato T (2015) Smoking is a perioperative risk factor and prognostic factor for lung cancer surgery. Gen Thorac Cardiovasc Surg 63:93–98
27. Barrera R, Shi W, Amar D, Thaler HT, Gabovich N, Bains MS, White DA (2005) Smoking and timing of cessation: impact on pulmonary complications after thoracotomy. Chest 127:1977–1983
28. Seok Y, Hong N, Lee E (2014) Impact of smoking history on postoperative pulmonary complications: a review of recent lung cancer patients. Ann Thorac Cardiovasc Surg Off J Assoc Thorac Cardiovasc Surg Asia 20:123–128
29. Niewoehner DE (2010) Clinical practice. Outpatient management of severe COPD. N Engl J Med 362:1407–1416
30. Cotes JE (1987) Medical Research Council Questionnaire on Respiratory Symptoms (1986). Lancet 2:1028
31. Brunelli A, Kim AW, Berger KI, Addrizzo-Harris DJ (2013) Physiologic evaluation of the patient with lung cancer being considered for resectional surgery: Diagnosis and management

of lung cancer, 3rd ed: American College of Chest Physicians evidence-based clinical practice guidelines. Chest 143:e166S–e190S
32. Stanzani F, Paisani Dde M, Oliveira A, Souza RC, Perfeito JA, Faresin SM (2014) Morbidity, mortality, and categorization of the risk of perioperative complications in lung cancer patients. Jornal brasileiro de pneumologia publicacao oficial da Sociedade Brasileira de Pneumologia e Tisilogia 40:21–29
33. Zhang R, Lee SM, Wigfield C, Vigneswaran WT, Ferguson MK (2015) Lung function predicts pulmonary complications regardless of the surgical approach. Ann Thorac Surg 99:1761–1767
34. Canet J, Sabate S, Mazo V, Gallart L, de Abreu MG, Belda J, Langeron O, Hoeft A, Pelosi P, PERISCOPE group (2015) Development and validation of a score to predict postoperative respiratory failure in a multicentre European cohort: A prospective, observational study. Eur J Anaesthesiol 32(7):458–470
35. Matsuoka K, Misaki N, Sumitomo S (2010) Preoperative hypoalbuminemia is a risk factor for late bronchopleural fistula after pneumonectomy. Ann Thorac Cardiovas Surg Off J Assoc Thorac Cardiovas Surg Asia 16:401–405
36. Arozullah AM, Khuri SF, Henderson WG, Daley J (2001) Development and validation of a multifactorial risk index for predicting postoperative pneumonia after major noncardiac surgery. Ann Intern Med 135:847–857
37. Tewari N, Martin-Ucar AE, Black E, Beggs L, Beggs FD, Duffy JP, Morgan WE (2007) Nutritional status affects long term survival after lobectomy for lung cancer. Lung Cancer 57:389–394
38. Fernandes EO, Teixeira C, Silva LC (2011) Thoracic surgery: risk factors for postoperative complications of lung resection. Rev Assoc Med Bras 57:292–298
39. May SM, Li JT (2015) Burden of chronic obstructive pulmonary disease: healthcare costs and beyond. Allergy Asthma Proc Off J Reg State Allergy Soc 36:4–10
40. Hausman MS Jr, Jewell ES, Engoren M (2015) Regional versus general anesthesia in surgical patients with chronic obstructive pulmonary disease: does avoiding general anesthesia reduce the risk of postoperative complications? Anesth Analg 120:1405–1412
41. Blum JM, Stentz MJ, Dechert R, Jewell E, Engoren M, Rosenberg AL, Park PK (2013) Preoperative and intraoperative predictors of postoperative acute respiratory distress syndrome in a general surgical population. Anesthesiology 118:19–29
42. Gupta H, Gupta PK, Fang X, Miller WJ, Cemaj S, Forse RA, Morrow LE (2011) Development and validation of a risk calculator predicting postoperative respiratory failure. Chest 140:1207–1215
43. Hua M, Brady JE, Li G (2012) A scoring system to predict unplanned intubation in patients having undergone major surgical procedures. Anesth Analg 115:88–94
44. Kor DJ, Warner DO, Alsara A, Fernandez-Perez ER, Malinchoc M, Kashyap R, Li G, Gajic O (2011) Derivation and diagnostic accuracy of the surgical lung injury prediction model. Anesthesiology 115:117–128
45. Brueckmann B, Villa-Uribe JL, Bateman BT, Grosse-Sundrup M, Hess DR, Schlett CL, Eikermann M (2013) Development and validation of a score for prediction of postoperative respiratory complications. Anesthesiology 118:1276–1285
46. Gupta H, Gupta PK, Schuller D, Fang X, Miller WJ, Modrykamien A, Wichman TO, Morrow LE (2013) Development and validation of a risk calculator for predicting postoperative pneumonia. Mayo Clin Proc 88:1241–1249
47. Jeong BH, Shin B, Eom JS, Yoo H, Song W, Han S, Lee KJ, Jeon K, Um SW, Koh WJ, Suh GY, Chung MP, Kim H, Kwon OJ, Woo S, Park HY (2014) Development of a prediction rule for estimating postoperative pulmonary complications. PLoS One 9:e113656
48. Marchetti N, Criner GJ (2015) Surgical approaches to treating emphysema: lung volume reduction surgery, bullectomy, and lung transplantation. Semin Respir Crit Care Med 36:592–608
49. Ichinose J, Nagayama K, Hino H, Nitadori JI, Anraku M, Murakawa T, Nakajima J (2016) Results of surgical treatment for secondary spontaneous pneumothorax according to underlying diseases. Eur J Cardiothorac Surg 49(4):1132–1136

50. Pinheiro L, Santoro IL, Perfeito JA, Izbicki M, Ramos RP, Faresin SM (2015) Preoperative predictive factors for intensive care unit admission after pulmonary resection. Jornal brasileiro de pneumologia publicacao oficial da Sociedade Brasileira de Pneumologia e Tisilogia 41:31–38
51. Pearse RM, Moreno RP, Bauer P, Pelosi P, Metnitz P, Spies C, Vallet B, Vincent JL, Hoeft A, Rhodes A (2012) Mortality after surgery in Europe: a 7 day cohort study. Lancet 380:1059–1065
52. Miura N, Kohno M, Ito K, Senba M, Kajiwara K, Hamaguchi N, Makino H, Kanematsu T, Okamoto T, Yokoyama H (2015) Lung cancer surgery in patients aged 80 years or older: an analysis of risk factors, morbidity, and mortality. Gen Thorac Cardiovasc Surg 63:401–405
53. Wakeam E, Hyder JA, Jiang W, Lipsitz SA, Finlayson S (2015) Risk and patterns of secondary complications in surgical inpatients. JAMA Surg 150:65–73
54. Mador MJ, Goplani S, Gottumukkala VA, El-Solh AA, Akashdeep K, Khadka G, Abo-Khamis M (2013) Postoperative complications in obstructive sleep apnea. Sleep Breath 17:727–734
55. Hai F, Porhomayon J, Vermont L, Frydrych L, Jaoude P, El-Solh AA (2014) Postoperative complications in patients with obstructive sleep apnea: a meta-analysis. J Clin Anesth 26:591–600
56. Liang Y, Harris FL, Brown LA (2014) Alcohol induced mitochondrial oxidative stress and alveolar macrophage dysfunction. Biomed Res Int 2014:371593
57. Safi S, Benner A, Walloschek J, Renner M, op den Winkel J, Muley T, Storz K, Dienemann H, Hoffmann H, Schneider T (2015) Development and validation of a risk score for predicting death after pneumonectomy. PLoS One 10:e0121295
58. Wang Z, Cai XJ, Shi L, Li FY, Lin NM (2014) Risk factors of postoperative nosocomial pneumonia in stage I-IIIa lung cancer patients. Asian P J Cancer Prev APJCP 15:3071–3074
59. Asaph JW, Handy JR Jr, Grunkemeier GL, Douville EC, Tsen AC, Rogers RC, Keppel JF (2000) Median sternotomy versus thoracotomy to resect primary lung cancer: analysis of 815 cases. Ann Thorac Surg 70:373–379
60. Zhang R, Ferguson MK (2015) Video-assisted versus open lobectomy in patients with compromised lung function: a literature review and meta-analysis. PLoS One 10:e0124512
61. Zeldin RA, Normandin D, Landtwing D, Peters RM (1984) Postpneumonectomy pulmonary edema. J Thorac Cardiovasc Surg 87:359–365
62. Licker M, de Perrot M, Spiliopoulos A, Robert J, Diaper J, Chevalley C, Tschopp JM (2003) Risk factors for acute lung injury after thoracic surgery for lung cancer. Anesth Analg 97:1558–1565
63. Algar FJ, Alvarez A, Salvatierra A, Baamonde C, Aranda JL, Lopez-Pujol FJ (2003) Predicting pulmonary complications after pneumonectomy for lung cancer. Eur J Cardiothorac Surg 23:201–208
64. Fortis S, Spieth PM, Lu WY, Parotto M, Haitsma JJ, Slutsky AS, Zhong N, Mazer CD, Zhang H (2012) Effects of anesthetic regimes on inflammatory responses in a rat model of acute lung injury. Intensive Care Med 38:1548–1555
65. Schilling T, Kozian A, Kretzschmar M, Huth C, Welte T, Buhling F, Hedenstierna G, Hachenberg T (2007) Effects of propofol and desflurane anaesthesia on the alveolar inflammatory response to one-lung ventilation. Br J Anaesth 99:368–375
66. McLean DJ, Diaz-Gil D, Farhan HN, Ladha KS, Kurth T, Eikermann M (2015) Dose-dependent association between intermediate-acting neuromuscular-blocking agents and postoperative respiratory complications. Anesthesiology 122:1201–1213
67. Chau EH, Slinger P (2014) Perioperative fluid management for pulmonary resection surgery and esophagectomy. Semin Cardiothorac Vasc Anesth 18:36–44
68. Arslantas MK, Kara HV, Tuncer BB, Yildizeli B, Yuksel M, Bostanci K, Bekiroglu N, Kararmaz A, Cinel I, Batirel HF (2015) Effect of the amount of intraoperative fluid administration on postoperative pulmonary complications following anatomic lung resections. J Thorac Cardiovasc Surg 149:314–320, 21 e1
69. Peters AL, Van Stein D, Vlaar AP (2015) Antibody-mediated transfusion-related acute lung injury; from discovery to prevention. Br J Haematol 170:597–614

70. Peters AL, van Hezel ME, Juffermans NP, Vlaar AP (2015) Pathogenesis of non-antibody mediated transfusion-related acute lung injury from bench to bedside. Blood Rev 29:51–61
71. Michelet P, D'Journo XB, Roch A, Doddoli C, Marin V, Papazian L, Decamps I, Bregeon F, Thomas P, Auffray JP (2006) Protective ventilation influences systemic inflammation after esophagectomy: a randomized controlled study. Anesthesiology 105:911–919
72. Serpa Neto A, Hemmes SN, Barbas CS, Beiderlinden M, Biehl M, Binnekade JM, Canet J, Fernandez-Bustamante A, Futier E, Gajic O, Hedenstierna G, Hollmann MW, Jaber S, Kozian A, Licker M, Lin WQ, Maslow AD, Memtsoudis SG, Reis Miranda D, Moine P, Ng T, Paparella D, Putensen C, Ranieri M, Scavonetto F, Schilling T, Schmid W, Selmo G, Severgnini P, Sprung J, Sundar S, Talmor D, Treschan T, Unzueta C, Weingarten TN, Wolthuis EK, Wrigge H, Gama de Abreu M, Pelosi P, Schultz MJ (2015) Protective versus conventional ventilation for surgery: a systematic review and individual patient data meta-analysis. Anesthesiology 123:66–78
73. Guglielminotti J, Dechartres A, Mentre F, Montravers P, Longrois D, Laouenan C (2014) Reporting and methodology of multivariable analyses in prognostic observational studies published in 4 anesthesiology journals: a methodological descriptive review. Anesth Analg 121(4):1011–1029
74. Copeland GP, Jones D, Walters M (1991) POSSUM: a scoring system for surgical audit. Br J Surg 78:355–360
75. Brunelli A, Fianchini A, Gesuita R, Carle F (1999) POSSUM scoring system as an instrument of audit in lung resection surgery. Physiological and operative severity score for the enumeration of mortality and morbidity. Ann Thorac Surg 67:329–331
76. Melendez JA, Carlon VA (1998) Cardiopulmonary risk index does not predict complications after thoracic surgery. Chest 114:69–75
77. Ferguson MK, Durkin AE (2003) A comparison of three scoring systems for predicting complications after major lung resection. Eur J Cardiothorac Surg 23:35–42

Fluid Management During and After the Operation: Less Is More or More Is Less?

5

Catherine Ashes and Peter Slinger

5.1 Introduction

Acute lung injury is a major cause of mortality after lung resection surgery [1], and a principle focus of the thoracic anesthesiologist is prevention of this devastating complication. Fluid therapy is an integral component of the perioperative management of these complex patients [2], and the risks of fluid overload and tissue edema must be balanced against the risk of hypovolemia and end-organ ischemia [3].

5.2 Epidemiology and Impact of ALI/ARDS After Lung Resection Surgery

Post-pneumonectomy pulmonary edema (PPPE) was first described in 1984 by Zeldin et al. [4], where ten cases of lung injury following pneumonectomy were described. It has since been recognized that the syndrome may occur after lesser degrees of resection and surgery requiring one-lung ventilation (OLV) without lung resection [5, 6]. PPPE has been found to share histological features with acute respiratory distress syndrome (ARDS) [7], is not of cardiogenic origin [3], and the most severe form of PPPE follows a course indistinguishable from ARDS [5]. Accordingly, the condition may be described as post-thoracotomy acute lung injury (ALI) or ARDS. Post-thoracotomy ALI is generally classified by the American-European Consensus on ARDS criteria [8].

C. Ashes
Department of Anaesthetics, St Vincent's Hospital, Fitzroy, Darlinghurst, NSW, Australia

P. Slinger (✉)
Department of Anesthesia, Toronto General Hospital, Toronto, Canada
e-mail: Peter.Slinger@uhn.ca

© Springer International Publishing Switzerland 2017

M. Şentürk, M.O. Sungur (eds.), *Postoperative Care in Thoracic Surgery*,
DOI 10.1007/978-3-319-19908-5_5

While the incidence of lung injury after lung resection is fairly consistent, between 2 and 4 % [9–11], the mortality rate has decreased from almost 100 % to less than 40 %, largely due to improvements in ICU management [1]. The mortality rate is higher with ARDS than ALI [5].

The risk factors for perioperative ALI most consistently reported are more extensive resections (such as pneumonectomy) and fluid overload [5, 9]. Other pre- and intraoperative factors have also been implicated, including ASA class [12, 13], alcohol abuse [9, 13], previous radiotherapy [14], low predicted postoperative lung function [15], non-protective ventilation strategies [16], and right pneumonectomy [7, 17].

5.2.1 Fluid Administration as a Risk Factor

In the landmark study by Zeldin et al. [4], patients who received a large fluid load (4913 ± 1169 mL, $n = 10$) in the first 24 h following pneumonectomy had a higher incidence of PPPE than those receiving less fluid (3483 ± 984, $n = 15$ controls). These findings were corroborated by a canine right pneumonectomy model, which compared three groups: a liberal crystalloid load (100 mL/kg bolus preoperatively, followed by >100 ml/kg postoperative balance), a judicious load (50 mL/kg bolus preoperatively followed by <100 mL/kg balance), and a control group (the same fluid regimen as the liberal pneumonectomy group and sham thoracotomy). Pulmonary edema ensued in all of the liberal pneumonectomy dogs, however, in neither of the other groups. This implies that it is not only the volume of fluid administered that predisposes to ALI but that the local and systemic changes that occur at lung resection contribute significantly to the pathophysiology of the condition.

Subsequently, fluid administration, both intra- and postoperatively, has repeatedly been found to be a risk factor for the development of ALI after lung resection [9, 12, 14–17] (see Table 1). Fluid in excess of 2 L total volume administered during pneumonectomy is linked with negative effects on postoperative respiratory outcomes [3, 12, 14, 16], and similar results have been demonstrated with high perioperative fluid loads and lesser pulmonary resections [3, 9, 15]. In patients with pulmonary fibrosis, higher perioperative fluid volumes and balance are linked to an increased risk of postoperative respiratory compromise after lung resection surgery, a devastating complication [18]. Similar findings have also been demonstrated in esophagectomy; however, in these patients, larger volumes of fluid (in the order of 5 L) are implicated [6, 19].

The incremental volume of fluid required to increase the risk of ALI is not large. It is evident from the study by Licker et al. [9] that there may be a small margin between a more "liberal" strategy (the volume of fluid administered that is associated with ALI) and a "conservative" approach (the volume of administered fluid not associated with ALI) [20]: while there was a significant difference in outcomes between patients receiving larger volumes of intraoperative fluid (9.1 v 7.2 ml/kg/h), higher positive fluid balance in the 24 h following surgery (2.0 v 1.52 L), and

Table 5.1 Fluid administration in lung resection and esophagectomy patients with and without postoperative acute lung injury

Authors (publication year)	Procedure	Number of patients	Study design	Timing	Acute lung injury fluid volume	No acute lung injury fluid volume	*P* value
Zeldin et al. (1984) [4]	Pneumonectomy	25	Retrospective	24 h postoperative infusion	37 mL/kg	27 mL/kg	<0.05
Parquin et al. (1996) [14]	Pneumonectomy	146	Prospective (observational)	Intraoperative	≥2.0 L	<2.0 L	<0.01
Licker et al. (2003) [9]	Pulmonary resection	879	Retrospective	Intraoperative	9.1 mL/kg/h	7.2 mL/kg/h	0.023
				Cumulated intra- and 24 h postoperative	2.6 mL/kg/h	2.0 mL/kg/h	0.003
				Fluid balance 24 h postoperation	2.0 L	1.52 L	0.026
Fernández-Pérez et al. (2006) [16]	Pneumonectomy	170	Retrospective	Intraoperative	2.2 L	1.3 L	0.001
Alam et al. (2007) [15]	Pulmonary resection	1428	Retrospective	Intraoperative and 12 h postoperative	2.775 L	2.5 L	<0.05
Marret et al. (2010) [12]	Pneumonectomy	1200	Retrospective	Intraoperative	3.8 L	2.5 L	<0.0001
Mizuno et al. (2012) [18]	Pulmonary resection (pulmonary fibrosis patients)	52	Retrospective	Intraoperative total volume	7.71 mL/kg/h	10.3 mL/kg/h	0.049
				Intraoperative fluid balance	4.99 mL/kg/h	8.00 mL/kg/h	0.035
Casado et al. (2010) [6]	Esophagectomy	45	Retrospective	Intraoperative fluid balance	5.415 L	4.174 L	0.01
				Fluid balance 5 day postoperatively	7.873 L	5.928 L	0.03
Tandon et al. (2001) [19]	Esophagectomy	168	Retrospective	Intraoperative	5.0 L	4.4 L	<0.027

higher accumulated intra- and postoperative fluid volume (2.6 v 2.0 L), the differences are not great. Furthermore, a "dose-dependent" relationship between perioperative fluid administration and ALI was demonstrated by Alam et al. [15], who found that for every 500 mL of perioperative fluid administration, there was a significant increase in the rate of primary lung injury (OR 1.2 (1–1.4), $p=0.02$).

5.3 Pathophysiology

A "multiple-hit hypothesis" for lung injury is well described for ARDS [21]. It describes a number of pathophysiological insults, which, in isolation, may not result in lung injury, however, when accumulated result in the clinical syndrome of ALI or ARDS. The "multiple-hit hypothesis" is likely to also be relevant in perioperative ALI. The "first hit" is an activation of the systemic inflammatory response by surgical trauma, manipulation, or atelectasis [22], which subclinically injures the lung, rendering it more susceptible to subsequent insults. The successive hits then damage the already vulnerable alveolar-capillary membrane, leading to overt ALI or ARDS. The putative second hit may be a variety of known risk factors for postoperative ALI such as FFP administration [13], mediastinal lymphatic damage [23], non-protective ventilation strategies [16], and oxygen toxicity [24].

This multiple-hit model for perioperative ALI is supported by a rodent model, which used intratracheal lipopolysaccharide to mimic sepsis-induced lung injury. A small lung injury was observed with either OLV and pneumonectomy or lipopolysaccharide alone, but an exaggerated injury was triggered when OLV, pneumonectomy, and lipopolysaccharide were combined in one animal [25]. This suggests that the lung is "primed" by the initial insult, and then a subsequent insult will potentially result in a more severe, clinically evident manifestation.

5.3.1 Revised Starling Equation and the Endothelial Glycocalyx

For generations, the axiom guiding transcapillary fluid behavior was Starling's model, first proposed in 1896 [26]. The model expresses fluid flux as a balance between opposing hydrostatic and oncotic pressures. Along the length of the capillary filtration is favored at the arteriolar end and reabsorption at the venular end.

However, in vitro and in vivo deviations from the classic Starling principle have been noted [27], such as absence of the venous reabsorption [28] and lymphatic flow [29] required to prevent interstitial edema, and lack of importance of the interstitial colloid osmotic pressure in determining transendothelial fluid balance [30]. This led to further investigation into non-Starling mechanisms of barrier regulation involving the endothelial glycocalyx layer (EGL) [31].

Danielli first proposed the existence of the EGL in 1942 [32]. It is a dynamic, fragile, and complex layer of membrane-bound macromolecules at the luminal surface of the vascular endothelium [31]. The composition and thickness of the glycocalyx change constantly, as it is continually sheared by plasma flow and replaced

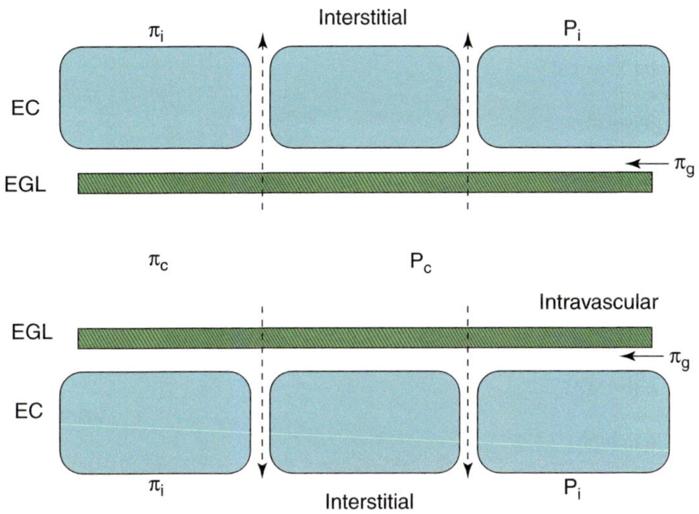

Fig. 5.1 The glycocalyx model for fluid exchange between the intravascular (*c*) and interstitial (*i*) spaces. The various components of the endothelial glycocalyx layer (*EGL*) and revised Starling's forces are shown. In steady state, net filtration into the interstitium occurs and is subsequently removed by the lymphatic system. *EC* endothelial capillary cells, *π* oncotic pressure, *P* hydrostatic pressure, *g* subglycocalyx space (Reproduced with permission from: Ashes and Slinger [3])

[33]. Its components have a net negative charge and therefore repel negatively charged molecules and blood cells [34].

A primary function of EGL is to regulate and influence vascular permeability [35]. Together with circulating substances, it forms a barrier that prevents circulating cells and macromolecules from entering the interstitium. In contrast to the original Starling model, which explained regulation of fluid balance occurring across the entire endothelial cell, a revised model has been proposed whereby the hydrostatic and osmotic forces act only across the EGL surface layer on the luminal aspect of the endothelium [30]. These forces reach equilibrium very quickly, resulting in a much lower fluid flux than predicted by the traditional Starling equation (see Fig. 5.1).

The EGL has other functions. It regulates blood cell-endothelial interaction by its negative charge and via specific adhesion molecules for leukocytes and platelets. These are normally hidden deep within the glycocalyx structure, but become exposed following damage to the EGL [35]. It also protects the vascular endothelium from shear stress and oxidative damage, via nitric oxide-induced vasodilation [36] and scavenging of oxygen free radicals [34].

The EGL may be injured by inflammatory cytokines [37], surgical trauma, and ischemia-reperfusion [38]. Hypervolemia damages the EGL, both by dilution of plasma proteins and via release of atrial natriuretic peptide, which strips the EGL [38]. Loss of the intact EGL causes increased vascular permeability and fluid extravasation. Loss of plasma proteins further compounds this. Leukocyte adhesion molecules are exposed, promoting cellular adhesion, migration, and further inflammation [39]. This vicious cycle of increased permeability, extravasation, and inflammation leads to pulmonary edema, as is observed in ALI.

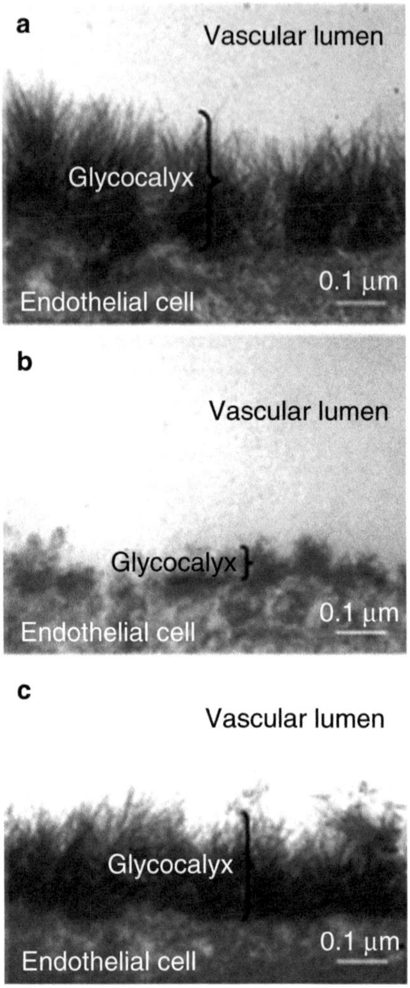

Fig. 5.2 Electron microscopic views of hearts stained to reveal the glycocalyx. (**a**) An intact glycocalyx after 25 min. Of nonischemic perfusion. (**b**) A residual endothelial glycocalyx after 20 min of warm ischemia and 10 min consecutive reperfusion. (**c**) The glycocalyx after pretreatment with 1MAC of sevoflurane followed by 20 min of warm no-flow ischemia and 10 min reperfusion (Reproduced with permission from: Chappell et al. [46])

Several empiric strategies, based on animal experiments, have been proposed to protect the EGL, including avoiding hypervolemia, albumin infusion [40], corticosteroids [41], antithrombin III [42], and direct inhibitors of inflammatory cytokines [43]. Volatile anesthetic agents, when compared with propofol, have been associated with less local release of inflammatory mediators [44, 45] and less glycocalyx destruction [46] (see Fig. 5.2).

5.3.2 Pulmonary Endothelial Damage

The alveolar endothelium also plays a role in the regulation of pulmonary interstitial fluid balance. Fluid transport across the endothelium may occur via tight junctions, breaks in tight junctions and vesicular transport [47]. Leaky junctions are associated with cell death and allow passage of larger molecules. Epithelial sodium channels (ENaCs) are able to enhance the clearance of alveolar fluid [47], and they may be stimulated by beta-adrenergic agonists [48].

Endothelial damage has therefore been implicated in the pathogenesis ALI after lung resection surgery. Endothelial injury maybe induced by activation of systemic and local inflammatory mediators, related to positive pressure ventilation; "volutrauma;" oxygen toxicity; ischemia-reperfusion injury; surgical trauma; and preexisting lung disease [1, 3]. Endothelial cell injury results in disruption of intercellular endothelial cell junctions, cytoskeleton contraction, and cell death, leading to increased permeability of the alveolar-capillary barrier and decreased lung compliance [1].

5.3.3 Lymphatics and RV Dysfunction

Although fluid overload is well recognized as a risk factor for ALI after thoracic surgery, there also appear to be other factors at play. ALI may still occur when very strict fluid-restrictive strategies are implemented [49].

Lung lymphatics play a key role in fluid clearance from the lung [47]. Capillary filtrate that enters the interstitium is drained by lymphatics, and when their capacity to drain fluid is exceeded, pulmonary edema will occur [3]. Although lymph flow can increase sevenfold in response to elevated interstitial pressure [50], in the perioperative setting, this capacity may be reduced. Surgical trauma related to lung resection surgery is thought to be an important factor influencing this [3]. Pulmonary lymphatic drainage is not symmetrical: the drainage of the right lung is essentially ipsilateral (>90 %), whereas the left lung has a significant contralateral contribution (>55 %) [51]. Therefore, right pneumonectomy confers a significantly higher risk of pulmonary edema in the left lung, as over half its lymphatic drainage will be lost, which has been demonstrated clinically [7, 17].

Lymphatic drainage may be further impaired by postoperative right ventricular (RV) dysfunction: the resultant elevation in central venous pressure will reduce the drainage capacity of the lymphatic system [52]. RV dysfunction is very common after lung resection surgery, particularly pneumonectomy [53], and is thought to relate to increased RV afterload and tachycardia [54, 55].

5.4 Risks of Restrictive Approach: Tissue Hypoperfusion and AKI

A restrictive approach to fluid management has been widely adopted to prevent ALI after thoracic surgery [47]. However, a restrictive fluid regimen may incur the risks associated with hypovolemia, which include impaired end-organ perfusion, in particular, acute kidney injury (AKI) [3, 47].

Recent data suggest the incidence of AKI after lung resection surgery is 5.9–6.8 % [56, 57]. It is associated with increased hospital length of stay [56] and cardiopulmonary complications [57]. A link to increased mortality has been inconsistent [56], although a recent study demonstrated a mortality of 19.8 % in those with AKI [57].

Many risk factors for AKI have been identified. Studies by Licker et al. [1] and Ishikawa et al. [56] each identified multiple factors associated with AKI after lung resection surgery. Preoperative patient characteristics include ASA class 3 or 4, FEV1, hypertension, peripheral vascular disease, preoperative renal dysfunction, and preoperative use of angiotensin II receptor antagonists. Intraoperatively, use of vasopressor, duration of anesthesia, use of colloids, and open procedures were implicated. The amount of fluid given intra- and postoperatively was not found to be associated with an increased incidence of AKI: Licker et al. [57] found that patients with and without AKI received similar volumes of fluid both intraoperatively (4.8 v 4.9 mL/kg/h) and on postoperative day 1 (1.1 v 1.1 mL/kg/h), respectively. Similarly, Ishikawa et al. [56] found similar volumes of fluid administered intraoperatively in patients with and without AKI (1450 v 1276 mL).

Maintenance of adequate perfusion pressure is an important factor in preventing AKI [3], especially in those at increased preoperative risk related to chronic kidney disease, hypertension, or peripheral vascular disease. Hypotension related to excessive anesthesia should be avoided, and depth of anesthesia monitoring may allow more accurate dose titration. Adequate perfusion pressure should be maintained through judicious use of vasopressors, and invasive hemodynamic monitors may provide valuable information to help guide therapy [3].

5.5 Esophagectomy

In esophagectomy, the traditional approach involved aggressive fluid resuscitation, due to postulated "third space" losses [3]. The third space, first described in 1961 in major abdominal surgery [58], is classically thought to be a fluid compartment anatomically and functionally separate to the intravascular space, not involved in the exchange of fluid between the vascular space and the interstitium [59]. However, the exact location of this hypothetical compartment, thought to be the gastrointestinal tract or traumatized tissues, has never been fully elucidated. Its existence has recently been challenged due to weak initial evidence, flawed methodology, and the emergence of new data measuring extracellular fluid volume in surgery and hemorrhage [60].

There is an association between fluid balance and postoperative complications after esophagectomy. A link between higher perioperative positive fluid balance and cardiorespiratory complications and death has been demonstrated [61]. Fluid restriction seems protective against respiratory complications following esophagectomy, both as a sole factor [62], and as part of a standardized multimodal regimen including thoracic epidural analgesia, early extubation, and modest fluid restriction [63]. Due to the systemic inflammatory state that occurs following major surgery, and the increased capillary permeability that ensues, irrational replacement of putative "third space" losses during esophagectomy will lead to fluid accumulation in the interstitial space and therefore pulmonary edema [3].

Fluid administration may adversely affect surgical outcomes. There is a growing pool of data suggesting that surgical outcomes [64, 65] including anastomotic complications [66, 67], following gastrointestinal surgery, may be improved with a restrictive fluid strategy or multimodal perioperative management protocol that includes fluid restriction. There is no specific evidence of anastomotic protection by a restrictive fluid regimen in esophageal resection; however, extrapolation of these findings suggests that there may be some additional benefit incurred by fluid restriction in esophagectomy, both improving surgical outcomes and reducing the risk of ALI.

There has been concern regarding use of vasopressors in esophagectomy, due to fear of anastomotic ischemia, a major cause of postoperative mortality. In a porcine model, norepinephrine, when used to treat hypotension caused by hemorrhage, has been associated with severe graft hypoperfusion [68]. However, a small human study found that epinephrine, used to treat hypotension caused by thoracic epidural bupivacaine, restored the resultant decrease in anastomotic blood flow [69]. Similarly, in another small human study, phenylephrine infusion was found to correct epidural bolus-induced reduction of blood flow at the anastomotic end of the newly formed gastric tube [70]. Therefore, it is likely that vasoactive agents, when used to counteract hypotension induced by general or neuraxial anesthesia, can be used without jeopardizing the viability of the surgical anastomosis.

5.6 Goal-Directed Approaches

Goal-directed therapy has been used with variable success in cardiac, vascular, orthopedic, and major abdominal surgery. Interest was generated by Shoemaker et al. [71], who demonstrated morbidity and mortality benefits when a goal-directed approach was applied to the perioperative care of high-risk surgical patients. Some subsequent studies have shown reduced risk of infective complications [72], AKI [73], cardiovascular complications [74], pneumonia, and hospital length of stay [73]. However, others have found no benefit, in abdominal aortic surgery [75] or colorectal surgery [76]. In fact, a goal-directed approach was associated with negative effects on hospital length of stay and readiness for discharge in a subset of aerobically fit colorectal surgical patients [76].

It has been suggested that using clinical assessment of cardiac preload to guide fluid therapy may reduce the risk of ALI after thoracic surgery [3, 47, 77]: by optimizing the volume of fluid infused, the risks of both fluid overload and ALI and hypovolemia and AKI may be reduced. However, it should be noted that studies of goal-directed therapy in non-thoracic surgery frequently feature more "aggressive" fluid resuscitation in the treatment arm, with patients undergoing goal-directed therapy receiving significantly more fluid than those in the control arms [78–80]. This is at odds to the traditional approach of fluid restriction in thoracic surgical patients already discussed.

Preload estimation is notoriously challenging. Commonly used pressure measurements, such as central venous pressure (CVP) and pulmonary artery occlusion pressure (PAOP), are indirect surrogates for LVEDV and as such are influenced by many other factors, including intrathoracic pressure variation (such as in positive pressure ventilation and OLV), open chest surgery, RV function, and cardiovascular compliance [77]. Most goal-directed strategies utilize monitoring of hemodynamic parameters that predict fluid responsiveness, defined as a significant increase in cardiac output with fluid loading, which theoretically allows maximization of cardiac performance and avoids unnecessary volume administration.

5.6.1 Cardiac Index Estimation

Many goal-directed protocols target cardiac index, which may be measured using a variety of modalities, including the pulmonary artery catheter, transpulmonary thermodilution (e.g., PiCCO monitor), pulse contour analysis (e.g., FloTrac-Vigileo system), and transesophageal Doppler measurement. Although use of esophageal Doppler is impractical in esophageal surgery, it has been used with good effect in lung resection surgery. Esophageal Doppler was able to detect a reduction in stroke volume index in lung resection surgery, despite unchanged heart rate and mean arterial pressure, and was used to guide hemodynamic support and fluid therapy [81].

5.6.2 Dynamic Variables: Stroke Volume Variation (SVV) and Pulse Pressure Variation (PVV)

SVV and PPV both use the heart-lung interaction, integrating the effects of preload, respiratory variation, and blood pressure to assess fluid responsiveness [3, 47]. There are some theoretical limitations to the use of these indices during thoracic surgery. Firstly, there has been concern regarding their validity during open chest conditions [82]. Secondly, due to the dependence of these measurements on respiratory variation, their accuracy also is dependent on tidal volume. At relatively large tidal volumes of 8–10 mL/kg during two lung ventilation (TLV), SVV $\geq$ 12 ml/kg and PPV $\geq$ 10 mL/kg correlate highly with fluid responsiveness [83]; however, ventilation with a lung protective strategy may not have the same correlation. Thirdly, the volume of shunted blood through the non-ventilated lung should not contribute to the generation of SVV and PVV, necessitating a lower threshold value during OLV than that used during TLV [3, 84]. In one study examining SVV during OLV, it was shown only to be acceptably predictive of volume responsiveness with tidal volumes >8 mL/kg, with a threshold for fluid responsiveness of 10.5 % [85]. At the upper limits of fluid responsiveness, small increases in cardiac output are associated with large increases in extravascular lung water. This is particularly a problem in conditions of increased endothelial capillary permeability (see Fig. 5.3) [84].

SVV has been used successfully to guide fluid therapy in thoracic surgery. A randomized study in thoracoscopic lobectomy found that the goal-directed therapy group, who received fluid boluses guided by SVV using the FloTrac-Vigileo system, had higher PaO_2/FiO_2 ratios at the end of OLV, earlier extubation time, and received less overall fluid (1385 $\pm$ 350 mL vs. 985 $\pm$ 135 mL) [86]. During esophagectomy, SVV accurately predicted hypovolemia, was useful as a guide to appropriately time perioperative fluid therapy, and correlated better with cardiac output than CVP [87].

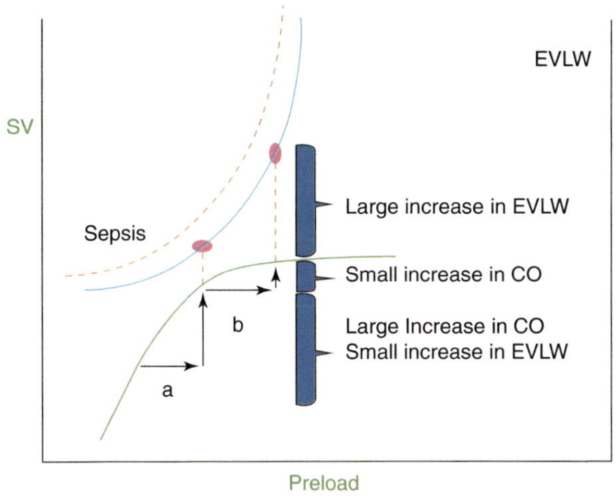

Fig. 5.3 Superimposition of the Frank-Starling (*green*) and Marik-Phillips (*blue*) curves demonstrating the effects of increasing preload on stroke volume (*SV*) and extravascular lung water (*EVLW*) in a patient who has a large increase in preload responsiveness (*a*) vs. a small increase in preload responsiveness (*b*). With conditions of increased capillary permeability such as sepsis, the EVLW curve is shifted to the left, and small increase in preload can result in large increases in EVLW. *CO* cardiac output (Reproduced with permission from: Marik and Lemson [84])

5.6.3 Early Detection of Pulmonary Edema

Transpulmonary thermodilution technology has the added advantage of enabling calculation of extravascular lung water (EVLW) and therefore quantification of pulmonary edema [88]. EVLW has been shown to be an independent predictor of prognosis and survival in critically ill patients [89] and in esophagectomy has been found to correlate with PaO_2/FiO_2 ratio, pulmonary compliance, lung injury score [90], and pulmonary complications [91]. EVLW is derived by subtracting the pulmonary blood volume (PBV) from the pulmonary thermal volume (PTV); there has therefore been concern regarding the use of EVLWI after lung resection, as both PBV and PTV may change [92]. However, EVLWI measured by PiCCO has been shown to correlate well with a double-dye technique for up to 12 h after following major lung resection [93]. A study assessing a goal-directed approach to fluid management for thoracic surgery requiring lateral thoracotomy and OLV found that their strategy, fluid management guided by SVV, did not result in pulmonary fluid overload as assessed by PiCCO EVLWI [94].

Lung ultrasound has been used to diagnose pulmonary edema by the presence of ultrasound B-lines (previously "ultrasound lung comets") with a high degree of sensitivity and specificity (97 % and 95 % respectively) [95]. B-lines may also be quantified, with good inter-rater reliability [96], and there is a correlation between the number of B-lines and EVLW in patients following cardiac surgery [97]. In ARDS, a significant correlation between ultrasound B-lines score and EVLW was shown, with a B-lines score ≥ 6 indicating a pathologic

EVLW >10 mL/kg (sensitivity 82 %, specificity 77 %) [98]. There is very little data evaluating this technique for quantitative assessment of ALI [99], and no study to date addresses its application in the perioperative setting. However, lung ultrasound represents a promising noninvasive bedside modality to rapidly assess EVLW of patients at risk of perioperative lung injury, including those undergoing thoracic surgery, and as such warrants further investigation in the perioperative setting.

5.7 Fluid Choice

Fluid choice in thoracic surgery remains controversial, with concerns regarding unwanted extravascular distribution of crystalloids to the interstitial space balanced against known adverse effects of the various colloid solutions, including AKI, coagulopathy, and anaphylaxis.

Hyperoncotic colloids have been advocated for use in ALI, due to their potential to promote shift of extravascular lung water into the intravascular space [47]. Some beneficial effects on pulmonary parameters have been demonstrated, including pulmonary permeability [100, 101], histological findings [102], reductions in VILI and pulmonary edema [103], and more rapid hemodynamic stabilization [101]. However, in a large systematic review of burns, trauma, and surgical patients, no outcome benefit of colloids could be demonstrated, and hydroxyethyl starch (HES) was found to possibly increase mortality [104].

There is particular concern regarding HES and the risk of AKI: in a multicenter RCT of patients with severe sepsis, HES was shown to increase risk of mortality and use of renal replacement therapy [105]. These findings were seemingly confirmed when a recent systematic review and meta-analysis of HES in critically ill patients found that HES use was associated with a significantly increased risk of AKI, use of renal replacement therapy, and death [106].

Due to concerns regarding synthetic colloid therapy, interest in human albumin has been renewed, as there is no evidence of adverse effects on renal function, and it is generally felt not to affect coagulation [107]. The SAFE trial [108] failed to demonstrate any difference between 4 % albumin and saline therapy in a variety of outcomes in a mixed population of critically ill patients. A recent systematic review and meta-analysis comparing albumin to saline therapy in patients with ARDS found no significant mortality difference, but improved PaO_2/FiO_2 in the first 48 h and after 7 days in patients receiving albumin [109]. However, an overall paucity of evidence was noted, and there is clearly a need for more randomized controlled trials to address this question.

Conclusion

Postoperative ALI is a devastating complication of thoracic surgery. New insights into its pathophysiology include the multifactorial risk profile and the role of the EGL. Excessive fluid administration is harmful, and the risk of ALI may be reduced by fluid restriction, without jeopardizing end-organ perfusion. Several new concepts will continue to be explored, including goal-directed therapy, bedside assessment of EVLW, and fluid selection.

References

1. Licker M, Fauconnet P, Villiger Y, Tschopp J-M (2009) Acute lung injury and outcomes after thoracic surgery. Curr Opin Anaesthesiol 22(1):61–67
2. Slinger PD (1995) Perioperative fluid management for thoracic surgery: the puzzle of postpneumonectomy pulmonary edema. J Cardiothorac Vasc Anesth 9(4):442–451
3. Ashes C, Slinger P (2014) Volume management and resuscitation in thoracic surgery. Curr Anesthesiol Rep 4:386–396
4. Zeldin RA, Normandin D, Landtwing D, Peters RM (1984) Postpneumonectomy pulmonary edema. J Thorac Cardiovasc Surg 87:359–365
5. Gothard J (2006) Lung injury after thoracic surgery and one-lung ventilation. Curr Opin Anaesthesiol 19(1):5–10
6. Casado D, López F, Martí R (2010) Perioperative fluid management and major respiratory complications in patients undergoing esophagectomy. Dis Esophagus 23(7):523–528
7. Turnage WS, Lunn JJ (1993) Postpneumonectomy pulmonary edema. A retrospective analysis of associated variables. Chest 103(6):1646–1650
8. Bernard GR, Artigas A, Brigham KL, Carlet J, Falke K, Hudson L et al (1994) The American-European consensus conference on ARDS. Definitions, mechanisms, relevant outcomes, and clinical trial coordination. Am J Respir Crit Care Med 149:818–824
9. Licker M, de Perrot M, Spiliopoulos A, Robert J, Diaper J, Chevalley C et al (2003) Risk factors for acute lung injury after thoracic surgery for lung cancer. Anesth Analg 97(6):1558–1565
10. Ruffini E, Parola A, Papalia E, Filosso PL, Mancuso M, Oliaro A et al (2001) Frequency and mortality of acute lung injury and acute respiratory distress syndrome after pulmonary resection for bronchogenic carcinoma. Eur J Cardiothorac Surg 20(1):30–36, –discussion36–7
11. Kutlu CA, Williams EA, Evans TW, Pastorino U, Goldstraw P (2000) Acute lung injury and acute respiratory distress syndrome after pulmonary resection. Ann Thorac Surg 69(2):376–380
12. Marret E, Miled F, Bazelly B, El Metaoua S, de Montblanc J, Quesnel C et al (2010) Risk and protective factors for major complications after pneumonectomy for lung cancer. Interact Cardiovasc Thorac Surg 10(6):936–939
13. Sen S, Sen S, Sentürk E, Kuman NK (2010) Postresectional lung injury in thoracic surgery pre and intraoperative risk factors: a retrospective clinical study of a hundred forty-three cases. J Cardiothorac Surg 5(1):62
14. Parquin F, Marchal M, Mehiri S, Hervé P, Lescot B (1996) Post-pneumonectomy pulmonary edema: analysis and risk factors. Eur J Cardiothorac Surg 10(11):929–932
15. Alam N, Park BJ, Wilton A, Seshan VE, Bains MS, Downey RJ et al (2007) Incidence and risk factors for lung injury after lung cancer resection. Ann Thorac Surg 84(4):1085–1091
16. Fernández-Pérez ER, Keegan MT, Brown DR, Hubmayr RD, Gajic O (2006) Intraoperative tidal volume as a risk factor for respiratory failure after pneumonectomy. Anesthesiology 105(1):14–18
17. Verheijen-Breemhaar L, Bogaard JM, van den Berg B, Hilvering C (1988) Postpneumonectomy pulmonary oedema. Thorax 43(4):323–326
18. Mizuno Y, Iwata H, Shirahashi K, Takamochi K, Oh S, Suzuki K et al (2012) The importance of intraoperative fluid balance for the prevention of postoperative acute exacerbation of idio-

pathic pulmonary fibrosis after pulmonary resection for primary lung cancer. Eur J Cardiothorac Surg 41(6):e161–e165
19. Tandon S, Batchelor A, Bullock R, Gascoigne A, Griffin M, Hayes N et al (2001) Perioperative risk factors for acute lung injury after elective oesophagectomy. Br J Anaesth 86(5):633–638
20. Evans RG, Naidu B (2012) Does a conservative fluid management strategy in the perioperative management of lung resection patients reduce the risk of acute lung injury? Interact Cardiovasc Thorac Surg 15(3):498–504
21. Litell JM, Gong MN, Talmor D, Gajic O (2011) Acute lung injury: prevention may be the best medicine. Respir Care 56(10):1546–1554
22. Guarracino F (2012) Perioperative acute lung injury: reviewing the role of anesthetic management. J Anesth Clin Res 4:312
23. Slinger P (1999) Post-pneumonectomy pulmonary edema: is anesthesia to blame? Curr Opin Anaesthesiol 12(1):49–54
24. Lases EC, Duurkens VA, Gerritsen WB, Haas FJ (2000) Oxidative stress after lung resection therapy: a pilot study. Chest 117(4):999–1003
25. Evans RG, Ndunge OBA, Naidu B (2013) A novel two-hit rodent model of postoperative acute lung injury: priming the immune system leads to an exaggerated injury after pneumonectomy. Interact Cardiovasc Thorac Surg 16(6):844–848
26. Starling EH (1896) On the absorption of fluids from the connective tissue spaces. J Physiol (Lond) 19(4):312–326
27. Levick JR, Michel CC (2010) Microvascular fluid exchange and the revised starling principle. Cardiovasc Res 87(2):198–210
28. Bates DO, Levick JR, Mortimer PS (1994) Starling pressures in the human arm and their alteration in postmastectomy oedema. J Physiol 477:355–363
29. Aukland K, Reed RK (1993) Interstitial-lymphatic mechanisms in the control of extracellular fluid volume. Physiol Rev 73:1–78
30. Chau EHL, Slinger P (2014) Perioperative fluid management for pulmonary resection surgery and esophagectomy. Semin Cardiothorac Vasc Anesth 18(1):36–44
31. Collins SR, Blank RS, Deatherage LS, Dull RO (2013) The endothelial glycocalyx. Anesth Analg 117(3):664–674
32. Danielli JF (1940) Capillary permeability and oedema in the perfused frog. J Physiol 98(1):109–129
33. Lipowsky HH (2005) Microvascular rheology and hemodynamics. Microcirculation 12(1):5–15
34. Reitsma S, Slaaf DW, Vink H, van Zandvoort MAMJ, Oude egbrink MGA (2007) The endothelial glycocalyx: composition, functions, and visualization. Eur J Physiol 454(3):345–359
35. Alphonsus CS, Rodseth RN (2014) The endothelial glycocalyx: a review of the vascular barrier. Anaesthesia 69(7):777–784
36. Jacob M, Rehm M, Loetsch M, Paul JO, Bruegger D, Welsch U et al (2007) The endothelial glycocalyx prefers albumin for evoking shear stress-induced, nitric oxide-mediated coronary dilatation. J Vasc Res 44(6):435–443
37. Chappell D, Hofmann-Kiefer K, Jacob M, Rehm M, Briegel J, Welsch U et al (2009) TNF-alpha induced shedding of the endothelial glycocalyx is prevented by hydrocortisone and antithrombin. Basic Res Cardiol 104(1):78–89
38. Bruegger D, Jacob M, Rehm M, Loetsch M, Welsch U, Conzen P et al (2005) Atrial natriuretic peptide induces shedding of endothelial glycocalyx in coronary vascular bed of guinea pig hearts. Am J Physiol Heart Circ Physiol 289(5):H1993–H1999
39. Ait-Oufella H, Maury E, Lehoux S, Guidet B, Offenstadt G (2010) The endothelium: physiological functions and role in microcirculatory failure during severe sepsis. Intensive Care Med 36(8):1286–1298
40. Jacob M, Paul O, Mehringer L, Chappell D, Rehm M, Welsch U et al (2009) Albumin augmentation improves condition of guinea pig hearts after 4 hr of cold ischemia. Transplantation 87(7):956–965

41. Chappell D, Jacob M, Hofmann-Kiefer K, Bruegger D, Rehm M, Conzen P et al (2007) Hydrocortisone preserves the vascular barrier by protecting the endothelial glycocalyx. Anesthesiology 107(5):776–784
42. Chappell D, Jacob M, Hofmann-Kiefer K, Rehm M, Welsch U, Conzen P et al (2009) Antithrombin reduces shedding of the endothelial glycocalyx following ischaemia/reperfusion. Cardiovasc Res 83(2):388–396
43. Nieuwdorp M, Meuwese MC, Mooij HL, van Lieshout MHP, Hayden A, Levi M et al (2009) Tumor necrosis factor-alpha inhibition protects against endotoxin-induced endothelial glycocalyx perturbation. Atherosclerosis 202(1):296–303
44. De Conno E, Steurer MP, Wittlinger M, Zalunardo MP, Weder W, Schneiter D et al (2009) Anesthetic-induced improvement of the inflammatory response to one-lung ventilation. Anesthesiology 110(6):1316–1326
45. Schilling T, Kozian A, Senturk M, Huth C, Reinhold A, Hedenstierna G et al (2011) Effects of volatile and intravenous anesthesia on the alveolar and systemic inflammatory response in thoracic surgical patients. Anesthesiology 115(1):65–74
46. Chappell D, Heindl B, Jacob M, Annecke T, Congong C, Rehm M et al (2011) Sevoflurane reduces leukocyte and platelet adhesion after ischemia-reperfusion by protecting the endothelial glycocalyx. Anesthesiology 115:483–491
47. Assaad S, Popescu W, Perrino A (2013) Fluid management in thoracic surgery. Curr Opin Anaesthesiol 26(1):31–39
48. Downs CA, Kriener LH, Yu L, Eaton DC, Jain L, Helms MN (2012) β-Adrenergic agonists differentially regulate highly selective and nonselective epithelial sodium channels to promote alveolar fluid clearance in vivo. Am J Physiol Lung Cell Mol Physiol 302(11):L1167–L1178
49. Slinger P (2002) Fluid management during pulmonary resection surgery. Ann Card Anaesth 5(2):220–224
50. Zarins CK, Rice CL, Peters RM, Virgilio RW (1978) Lymph and pulmonary response to isobaric reduction in plasma oncotic pressure in baboons. Circ Res 43(6):925–930
51. Nohl-Oser HC (1972) An investigation of the anatomy of the lymphatic drainage of the lungs as shown by the lymphatic spread of bronchial carcinoma. Ann R Coll Surg Engl 51(3):157–176
52. Laine GA, Allen SJ, Katz J, Gabel JC, Drake RE (1986) Effect of systemic venous pressure elevation on lymph flow and lung edema formation. J Appl Physiol 61(5):1634–1638
53. Pedoto A, Amar D (2009) Right heart function in thoracic surgery: role of echocardiography. Curr Opin Anaesthesiol 22(1):44–49
54. Reed CE, Dorman BH, Spinale FG (1996) Mechanisms of right ventricular dysfunction after pulmonary resection. Ann Thorac Surg 62(1):225–231
55. Okada M, Ota T, Matsuda H, Okada K, Ishii N (1994) Right ventricular dysfunction after major pulmonary resection. J Thorac Cardiovasc Surg 108(3):503–511
56. Ishikawa S, Griesdale DEG, Lohser J (2012) Acute kidney injury after lung resection surgery: incidence and perioperative risk factors. Anesth Analg 114(6):1256–1262
57. Licker M, Cartier V, Robert J, Diaper J, Villiger Y, Tschopp J-M et al (2011) Risk factors of acute kidney injury according to RIFLE criteria after lung cancer surgery. Ann Thorac Surg 91(3):844–850
58. Shires T, Williams J, Brown F (1961) Acute change in extracellular fluids associated with major surgical procedures. Ann Surg 154:803–810
59. Chappell D, Jacob M, Hofmann-Kiefer K, Conzen P, Rehm M (2008) A rational approach to perioperative fluid management. Anesthesiology 109(4):723–740
60. Brandstrup B, Svensen C, Engquist A (2006) Hemorrhage and operation cause a contraction of the extracellular space needing replacement—evidence and implications? A systematic review. Surgery 139(3):419–432
61. Wei S, Tian J, Song X, Chen Y (2008) Association of perioperative fluid balance and adverse surgical outcomes in esophageal cancer and esophagogastric junction cancer. Ann Thorac Surg 86(1):266–272

62. Kita T, Mammoto T, Kishi Y (2002) Fluid management and postoperative respiratory disturbances in patients with transthoracic esophagectomy for carcinoma. J Clin Anesth 14(4):252–256
63. Neal JM, Wilcox RT, Allen HW, Low DE (2003) Near-total esophagectomy: the influence of standardized multimodal management and intraoperative fluid restriction. Reg Anesth Pain Med 28(4):328–334
64. Lobo DN, Bostock KA, Neal KR, Perkins AC, Rowlands BJ, Allison SP (2002) Effect of salt and water balance on recovery of gastrointestinal function after elective colonic resection: a randomised controlled trial. Lancet 359:1812–1818
65. Brandstrup B, Tønnesen H, Beier-Holgersen R, Hjortsø E, Ørding H, Lindorff-Larsen K et al (2003) Effects of intravenous fluid restriction on postoperative complications: comparison of two perioperative fluid regimens: a randomized assessor-blinded multicenter trial. Ann Surg 238(5):641–648
66. Marjanovic G, Villain C, Juettner E, Hausen Zur A, Hoeppner J, Hopt UT et al (2009) Impact of different crystalloid volume regimes on intestinal anastomotic stability. Ann Surg 249(2):181–185
67. Schnüriger B, Inaba K, Wu T, Eberle BM, Belzberg H, Demetriades D (2011) Crystalloids after primary colon resection and anastomosis at initial trauma laparotomy: excessive volumes are associated with anastomotic leakage. J Trauma 70(3):603–610
68. Theodorou D, Drimousis PG, Larentzakis A, Papalois A, Toutouzas KG, Katsaragakis S (2008) The effects of vasopressors on perfusion of gastric graft after esophagectomy. An experimental study. J Gastrointest Surg 12(9):1497–1501
69. Al-Rawi OY, Pennefather SH, Page RD, Dave I, Russell GN (2008) The effect of thoracic epidural bupivacaine and an intravenous adrenaline infusion on gastric tube blood flow during esophagectomy. Anesth Analg 106(3):884–887
70. Pathak D, Pennefather SH, Russell GN, Rawi Al O, Dave IC, Gilby S et al (2013) Phenylephrine infusion improves blood flow to the stomach during oesophagectomy in the presence of a thoracic epidural analgesia. Eur J Cardiothorac Surg 44(1):130–133
71. Shoemaker WC, Appel PL, Kram HB, Waxman K, Lee TS (1988) Prospective trial of supranormal values of survivors as therapeutic goals in high-risk surgical patients. Chest 94(6):1176–1186
72. Dalfino L, Giglio MT, Puntillo F, Marucci M, Brienza N (2011) Haemodynamic goal-directed therapy and postoperative infections: earlier is better. A systematic review and meta-analysis. Crit Care 15(3):R154
73. Corcoran T, Rhodes JEJ, Clarke S, Myles PS, Ho KM (2012) Perioperative fluid management strategies in major surgery: a stratified meta-analysis. Anesth Analg 114(3):640–651
74. Arulkumaran N, Corredor C, Hamilton MA, Ball J, Grounds RM, Rhodes A et al (2014) Cardiac complications associated with goal-directed therapy in high-risk surgical patients: a meta-analysis. Br J Anaesth 112(4):648–659
75. Bisgaard J, Gilsaa T, Rønholm E, Toft P (2013) Optimising stroke volume and oxygen delivery in abdominal aortic surgery: a randomised controlled trial. Acta Anaesthesiol Scand 57(2):178–188
76. Challand C, Struthers R, Sneyd JR, Erasmus PD, Mellor N, Hosie KB et al (2012) Randomized controlled trial of intraoperative goal-directed fluid therapy in aerobically fit and unfit patients having major colorectal surgery. Br J Anaesth 108(1):53–62
77. Rocca Della G, Costa MG (2003) Preload indexes in thoracic anesthesia. Curr Opin Anaesthesiol 16:69–73
78. Goepfert MSG, Reuter DA, Akyol D, Lamm P, Kilger E, Goetz AE (2007) Goal-directed fluid management reduces vasopressor and catecholamine use in cardiac surgery patients. Intensive Care Med 33(1):96–103
79. Benes J, Chytra I, Altmann P, Hluchy M, Kasal E (2010) Intraoperative fluid optimization using stroke volume variation in high risk surgical patients: results of prospective randomized study. Crit Care 14:R118
80. Lopes MR, Oliveira MA, Pereira VOS, Lemos IPB, Auler JOC, Michard F (2007) Goal-directed fluid management based on pulse pressure variation monitoring during high-risk surgery: a pilot randomized controlled trial. Crit Care 11(5):R100

81. Diaper J, Ellenberger C, Villiger Y, Robert J, Tschopp J-M, Licker M (2008) Transoesophageal Doppler monitoring for fluid and hemodynamic treatment during lung surgery. J Clin Monit Comput 22(5):367–374
82. Wyffels PAH, Sergeant P, Wouters PF (2010) The value of pulse pressure and stroke volume variation as predictors of fluid responsiveness during open chest surgery. Anaesthesia 65(7):704–709
83. Marik PE, Cavallazzi R, Vasu T, Hirani A (2009) Dynamic changes in arterial waveform derived variables and fluid responsiveness in mechanically ventilated patients: a systematic review of the literature. Crit Care Med 37(9):2642–2647
84. Marik PE, Lemson J (2014) Fluid responsiveness: an evolution of our understanding. Br J Anaesth 112:617–620
85. Suehiro K, Okutani R (2011) Influence of tidal volume for stroke volume variation to predict fluid responsiveness in patients undergoing one-lung ventilation. J Anesth 25(5):777–780
86. Zhang J, Chen CQ, Lei XZ, Feng ZY, Zhu SM (2013) Goal-directed fluid optimization based on stroke volume variation and cardiac index during one-lung ventilation in patients undergoing thoracoscopy lobectomy operations: a pilot study. Clinics (Sao Paulo) 68(7):1065–1070
87. Kobayashi M, Koh M, Irinoda T, Meguro E, Hayakawa Y, Takagane A (2009) Stroke volume variation as a predictor of intravascular volume depression and possible hypotension during the early postoperative period after esophagectomy. Ann Surg Oncol 16(5):1371–1377
88. Katzenelson R, Perel A, Berkenstadt H, Preisman S, Kogan S, Sternik L et al (2004) Accuracy of transpulmonary thermodilution versus gravimetric measurement of extravascular lung water. Crit Care Med 32(7):1550–1554
89. Sakka SG, Klein M, Reinhart K, Meier-Hellmann A (2002) Prognostic value of extravascular lung water in critically ill patients. Chest 122(6):2080–2086
90. Oshima K, Kunimoto F, Hinohara H, Hayashi Y, Kanemaru Y, Takeyoshi I et al (2008) Evaluation of respiratory status in patients after thoracic esophagectomy using PiCCO system. Ann Thorac Cardiovasc Surg 14(5):283–288
91. Sato Y, Motoyama S, Maruyama K, Okuyama M, Hayashi K, Nakae H et al (2007) Extravascular lung water measured using single transpulmonary thermodilution reflects perioperative pulmonary edema induced by esophagectomy. Eur Surg Res 39(1):7–13
92. Michard F (2007) Bedside assessment of extravascular lung water by dilution methods: temptations and pitfalls. Crit Care Med 35(4):1186–1192
93. Naidu BV, Dronavalli VB, Rajesh PB (2009) Measuring lung water following major lung resection. Interact Cardiovasc Thorac Surg 8(5):503–506
94. Haas S, Eichhorn V, Hasbach T, Trepte C, Kutup A, Goetz AE et al (2012) Goal-directed fluid therapy using stroke volume variation does not result in pulmonary fluid overload in thoracic surgery requiring one-lung ventilation. Crit Care Res Pract 2012:1–8
95. Lichtenstein DA, Meziere GA (2008) Relevance of lung ultrasound in the diagnosis of acute respiratory failure: the BLUE protocol. Chest 134:118–125
96. Anderson KL, Fields JM, Panebianco NL, Jenq KY, Marin J, Dean AJ (2013) Inter-rater reliability of quantifying pleural B-lines using multiple counting methods. J Ultrasound Med 32(1):115–120
97. Agricola E, Bove T, Oppizzi M, Marino G, Zangrillo A, Margonato A et al (2005) "Ultrasound comet-tail images": a marker of pulmonary edema: a comparative study with wedge pressure and extravascular lung water. Chest 127(5):1690–1695
98. Bataille B, Rao G, Cocquet P, Mora M, Masson B, Ginot J et al (2015) Accuracy of ultrasound B-lines score and E/Ea ratio to estimate extravascular lung water and its variations in patients with acute respiratory distress syndrome. J Clin Monit Comput 29:169–176
99. Corradi F, Brusasco C, Pelosi P (2014) Chest ultrasound in acute respiratory distress syndrome. Curr Opin Crit Care 20(1):98–103
100. Verheij J (2005) Effect of fluid loading with saline or colloids on pulmonary permeability, oedema and lung injury score after cardiac and major vascular surgery. Br J Anaesth 96(1):21–30

101. Huang C-C, Kao K-C, Hsu K-H, Ko H-W, Li L-F, Hsieh M-J et al (2009) Effects of hydroxyethyl starch resuscitation on extravascular lung water and pulmonary permeability in sepsis-related acute respiratory distress syndrome. Crit Care Med 37(6):1948–1955
102. Margarido CB, Margarido NF, Otsuki DA, Fantoni DT, Marumo CK, Kitahara FR et al (2007) Pulmonary function is better preserved in pigs when acute normovolemic hemodilution is achieved with hydroxyethyl starch versus lactated Ringer's solution. Shock 27(4):390–396
103. Li L-F, Huang C-C, Liu Y-Y, Lin H-C, Kao K-C, Yang C-T et al (2011) Hydroxyethyl starch reduces high stretch ventilation-augmented lung injury via vascular endothelial growth factor. Transl Res 157(5):293–305
104. Perel P, Roberts I (2013) Colloids versus crystalloids for fluid resuscitation in critically ill patients. Cochrane Database Syst Rev 28:CD000567
105. Perner A, Haase N, Guttormsen AB (2012) Hydroxyethyl starch 130/0.42 versus Ringer's acetate in severe sepsis. N Engl J Med 367:124–134
106. Zarychanski R, Abou-Setta AM, Turgeon AF (2013) Association of hydroxyethyl starch administration with mortality and acute kidney injury in critically ill patients requiring volume resuscitation: a systematic review and meta-analysis. JAMA 309:678–688
107. Lange M, Ertmer C, Van Aken H (2011) Intravascular volume therapy with colloids in cardiac surgery. J Cardiothorac Vasc Anesth 25:847–855
108. Finfer S, Bellomo R, Boyce N, French J, Myburgh J (2004) A comparison of albumin and saline for fluid resuscitation in the intensive care unit. N Engl J Med 350:2247–2256
109. Uhlig C, Silva PL, Deckert S, Schmitt J, de Abreu MG (2014) Albumin versus crystalloid solutions in patients with the acute respiratory distress syndrome: a systematic review and meta-analysis. Crit Care 18(2):R10

6 How to Organise the PACU? What to Treat in the PACU?

Mohamed R. El Tahan

6.1 How to Organise the PACU?

The implementation of the PACUs has gained the attention of healthcare providers since 1942 to improve patient safety and reduce the incidence of postoperative anaesthesia-related complications, mortality and length of hospital stay [1]. The economic structure of the PACU is likely to decrease the hospital costs [2]. The PACU's advantages are extended to patients undergoing thoracic procedures, because the PACU has highly specialised facilities and essentially functions as an ICU. Thus, increased availability of the PACU beds resulted in reduced utilisation of ICU resources without compromising patient care after major thoracic surgery [3].

6.1.1 PACU Location

Importantly, the PACU should be located in immediate proximity to the OR, assuming that both are on the same floor, to provide instant access to essential supplies and equipment and allow the surgical and anaesthesia personnel who recently cared for the patient, in timely identification and treatment of any significant complications during the PACU stay. Unfortunately, this may not always be possible due to pre-existing architecture or construction limitations.

The straight path versus multiple turns as well as the short distance should be considered during the construction of the PACU to facilitate the transfer from the OR to the PACU. Whereas the elevator trips during the transfer from the OR to the PACU should be avoided as much as possible to minimise the potential delay and harm for the patients. Before finalising the construction plans, the responsible

M.R. El Tahan
Anaesthesiology Department, College of Medicine, University of Dammam, Dammam, Saudi Arabia
e-mail: moham-edrefaateltahan@hotmail.com

© Springer International Publishing Switzerland 2017

M. Şentürk, M.O. Sungur (eds.), *Postoperative Care in Thoracic Surgery*,
DOI 10.1007/978-3-319-19908-5_6

anaesthesiologists should determine the time needed to transfer from the most distant OR to the PACU door while pushing a stretcher and several IV poles with infusion pumps [4].

6.1.2 Number of PACU Bed Slots

The appropriate number of PACU bed slots varies with the type and length of surgical cases (e.g. the first cases are likely be discharged from the PACU before second cases are finished), and the usual turnover time of both the OR and PACU beds. Thus, it is recommended that 1.5–2 PACU slots should be available for each room in the OR suite [4].

6.1.3 PACU Floor Plan

A traditional design is a square open-ward design with one wall accommodating the nurses' desk and support areas (e.g. medication carts or cabinets, seating area for order writing or dictation, equipment and supply storage, linen carts, etc.) and the other three walls having patient bed slots (Fig. 6.1). Supplies are usually stored on shelves or in baskets on the head wall (Fig. 6.2). This design offers direct, simultaneous sight lines to the patients and the shortest distance between the PACU beds to avoid untoward clinical events or demand to increase nursing staff.

The available designs for the patient's bed slots include:

- Lined up along a wall where the utilities come from the wall by the patient's head (Fig. 6.1).
- "Pods" of four beds at 90° angles located in the middle of a large space. The utilities drop from the ceiling or come up into a tower-like utility tree at the centre of the four patients' heads allowing one or two nurses to have immediate access to deliver care with little time or effort lost walking from bed to bed [4].

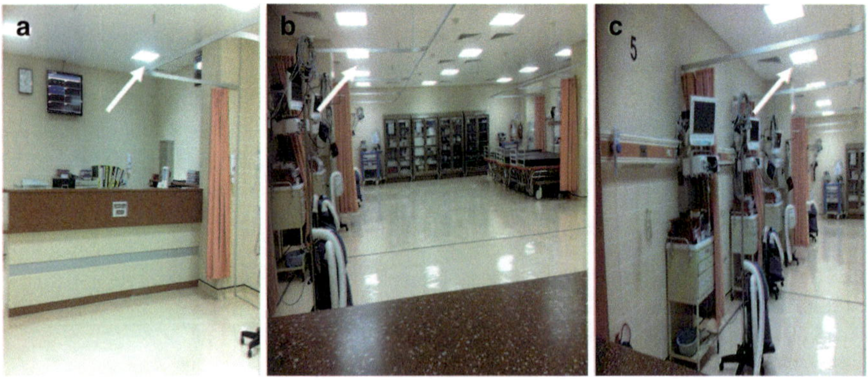

Fig. 6.1 (**a**, **b**) A traditional PACU square open-ward design, (**c**) the PACU bed-spaces and [*white arrows*] the standard bright fluorescent ceiling lights

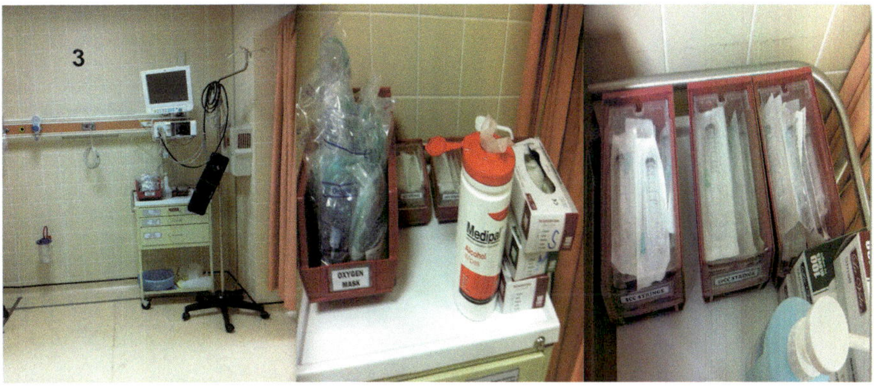

Fig. 6.2 The stored PACU supplies in baskets on the head wall

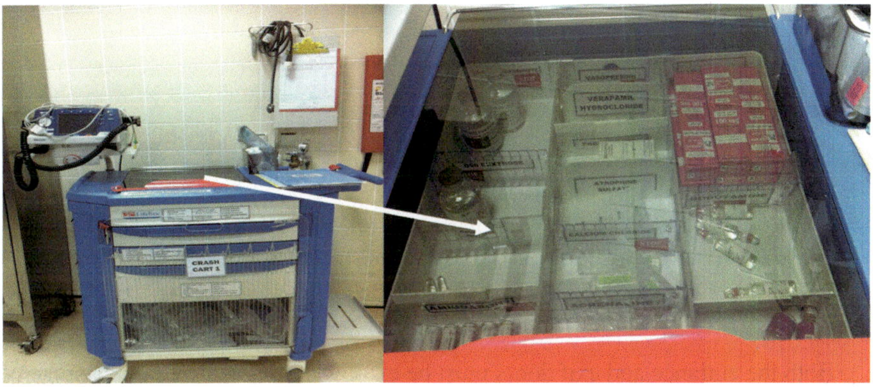

Fig. 6.3 The emergency PACU cart

Additionally, the design of the PACU must accommodate permanent and prominent places for emergency carts (resuscitation, airway and surgical equipment particularly for thoracic patients) (Fig. 6.3) and a significant storage space (Fig. 6.4a–c).

Ideally, there should be at least one isolation room that has a connecting door with the main PACU area and another door opening out to a hospital corridor, allowing separation patients with resistant infections or severely immunocompromised patients from the general PACU population. It can be equipped with an air-handling system that can be changed literally [4].

6.1.4 PACU Traffic

The orientation of the PACU should facilitate the flow of patients allowing direct entrance to the PACU from an OR corridor and a preferably separate exit to a main hospital corridor. Whereas, the use of the same PACU door for both entrance and exit may inevitably lead to traffic jams and potentially dangerous situations [4].

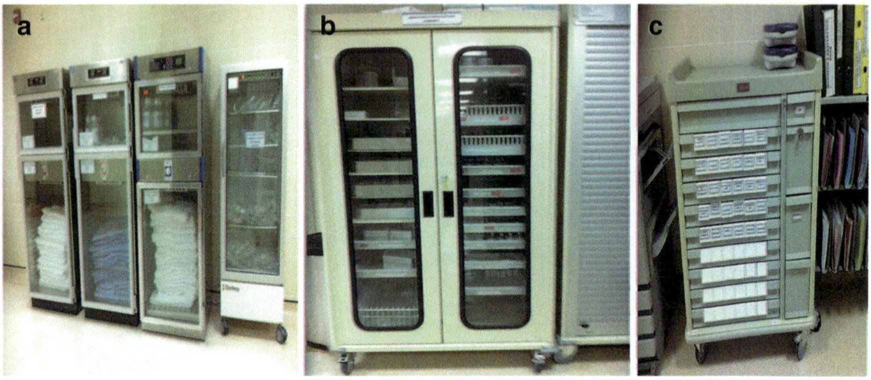

Fig. 6.4 The storage space in the PACU. (**a**) Cabinets including blankets, linens and fluids; (**b**) drawers including commonly used medications in the PACU; and (**c**) a cabinet and a cart including medications

Table 6.1 PACU bed-space

A floor space to the actual bed slot itself	≥100–120 sq. ft.
A working space to the nurses around all four sides of a bed	≥3 sq. ft.
A shelf space to supplies and equipment	≥12 sq. ft.
A writing surface nearby such as a rolling tray table	
A floor space to IV poles or more convenient ceiling-track-mounted IV poles	

Haret et al. [4]

Both the entrance and exit doors must be extra wide to guarantee the passage of a full-sized hospital bed with an ECMO/intra-aortic balloon pump console and people pushing IV poles on both sides. The doors could be automatically opened by a push button on the wall or by motion sensors [4].

It would be desirable to include a separate "pedestrian entrance" distinct from the doors used for patient entrance and exit. This could facilitate movement of staff and visitors and minimise distracting traffic jams, "whooshing" of the doors and the introduction of contaminated air from other parts of the facility [4].

6.1.5 PACU Bed-Spaces

It is a standard to budget a total of about 150–200 sq. ft. for each patient bed slot separated with ceiling-to-floor privacy curtains between the bed-spaces to ensure the patient privacy in the PACU as shown in Table 6.1 and Fig. 6.1c. Each bed slot needs to be equipped with a pull-chain emergency call buzzer, allowing patient to call the PACU nurse when step away from the side of the bed or allowing the PACU nurse to call attention in emergency without yelling and alarming other patients in the room [4].

6.1.6 General Considerations of the PACU

6.1.6.1 Layout

- Two fire exits at opposite ends of the room are recommended in addition to compliance with the institutional fire codes.
- A nonslip tile floor in one neutral colour allowing finding dropped objects (e.g. needle), and light, neutral, "warm" colours for the walls are usually suggested (Fig. 6.5a).
- Multiple synchronised clocks to the same time should be readily visible from all locations in the PACU.
- A handwashing sink for each six bed slots is strongly recommended (Fig. 6.5b).
- A medication room or area including a cabinet or carts is required (Fig. 6.4c).
- Two separate utility rooms with storage areas should be incorporated into the plan:
  - The clean utility area includes a large blanket warmer (Fig. 6.4a).
  - The dirty utility area should have three separate sinks for regular use, instrument washing and flushing and a separate door to an outside corridor, allowing removal of trash and contaminated waste and dirty linen without carrying it past patients in the PACU.
- Staff support space including:
  - Adequate number of staff lavatories to the size of the staff, which should be separate from any patient facilities.
  - A staff break area is necessary and it could be equipped with a sleeve patient's monitor and alarms heard allowing continuous patient's observation while staff members are on break.
  - An adequate desk space for physicians and staff to write notes or dictate, including adequate number of terminals, if a computerised information system is in use (Fig. 6.6a).
  - Office space for the head nurse is a highly desirable addition (Fig. 6.6a).

6.1.6.2 Equipment and Drugs

- The equipment and drug supplies should be stored and available in the PACU, including suction equipment and oxygen supply sources at each bed (Figs. 6.2, 6.4c and 6.6b, c).
- A respiratory oxygen delivery system should be available for use in the transport from the OR to the ward, to high-dependency area or the ICU.

6.1.6.3 PACU Lighting

- It is desirable to have some daylight visible to patients in the PACU that has the potential to reduce the postoperative cognitive dysfunction (POCD) [5]. Otherwise, the standard bright fluorescent lights are used in ceiling fixtures (Fig. 6.1c).
- Each bed-space needs enough levels of controllable lighting within the bed-space.
- A low-level night light is required for observation of a sleeping patient when the unit is otherwise quiet to minimise the incidence of POCD [5].
- In addition, the PACU should have at least one portable light that can be moved to any bed slot to facilitate any needed procedures.

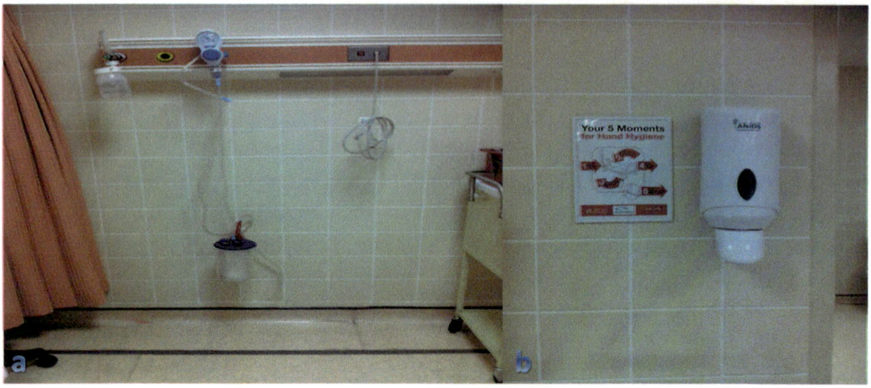

Fig. 6.5 (**a**) A nonslip tile floor of the PACU and (**b**) a handwashing tool in the PACU

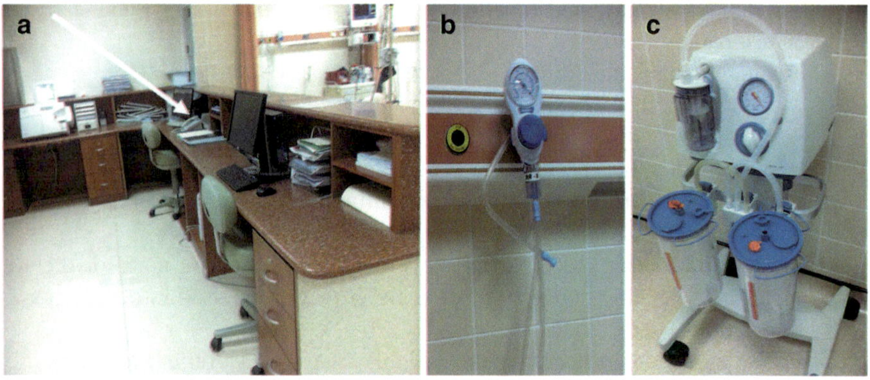

Fig. 6.6 (**a**) A PACU desk space for physicians and nursing staff to write notes, a telephone line [*A white arrow*], a computer terminal and a central patients monitor and (**b**) a bedside and (**c**) portable suction equipment

6.1.6.4 PACU Environment

- (The average temperature in a PACU should be about 75 °F (24 °C) to avoid aggravating OR- induced hypothermia, despite cooler temperatures, may be favoured by the staff.)
- The relative humidity should be maintained at 40–60 %.
- The heating, ventilation and air conditioning system of the PACU should be set to include a slight positive air pressure in the PACU, discouraging entering bacteria from outside the PACU. There should be a minimum of six air changes per hour, two of which are fresh outside air.

6.1.6.5 Electrical Power

- At least six to eight regular outlets should be available on the head wall or on the utility centre for each bed-space. At least two of them should be clearly marked with red face plates and connected to an emergency power system that has a kick-in time of <10 s following a power failure.

- A supply of flashlights and battery-powered lanterns should be available to avoid total darkness in the case of the power failure in which the emergency power also fails.
- Ventilators and infusion pumps for vasoactive drugs should always be plugged into emergency outlets.
- Additionally, several 240-volt plugs allowing the use of portable X-ray machines should be available.

6.1.6.6 Medical Gases

- The standard regulations for all medical gas installations must be considered.
- There should be at least two to three oxygen outlets (one having a flow meter installed at all times) on the head wall or utility tree for each bed slot.
- Three to five suction outlets should be available at the head of each bed slot for tracheal suction, gastrointestinal suction, chest tubes, drains and airway or surgical emergencies (Fig. 6.6b, c).
- There should be one compressed air outlet at each bed-space to be used as a blender for a ventilator.

6.1.6.7 Central Equipment in the PACU

- One or more full resuscitation or "code" cart, including external and internal defibrillating paddles, is needed for the thoracic patients depending on the size of the unit (Fig. 6.3).
- Both external and transvenous pacing electrodes and generators should be available.
- The difficult airway cart that should be kept in every PACU containing a complete array of airway equipment, including a videolaryngoscope, a fibre-optic bronchoscope and a light source.
- A mechanical ventilator could be permanently kept in the PACU or to be ready for rapid deployment when needed.
- A number of surgical trays and supplies should be available at the PACU at all times, including thoracostomy and tracheostomy trays and chest reopening set because there is usually not enough time to have them brought in from the OR in crisis cases.

6.1.6.8 Essential Equipment for Each Bed-Space

- All stretchers used for patients in the PACU should be capable of a head-down and semi-setting positions. Usually, having one stretcher per bed-space is not enough, because it is unlikely the left stretcher with the discharged patient to be returned in time to be ready for the next patient to be transferred from the OR to that PACU bed-space.
- A self-inflating resuscitator bag, a stethoscope and a warming device rather than the traditional heated blankets should be available near the head of each bed-space at all times.

- Spirometers and negative inspiratory force meters must be enough so that they are readily available when needed.
- Other items that should be immediately at hand include a pressure bag for rapid IV infusion, blood tubes, blood gas kits, basic nursing equipment (e.g. emesis basin, gauze, gloves, eye protectors, pads, tape, IV equipment, etc.) and tools (e.g. scissors, a clamp set, possibly a suture set, etc.).

6.1.6.9 Patient Monitoring

- The recommended ASA standard monitors for all admitted PACU patients include an electrocardiogram monitor, heart rate, a non-invasive blood pressure module, a pulse oximeter, respiratory rate and a rapid-acting electronic thermometer [6].
- All of the PACU monitors should have invasive pressure channels for patients undergoing thoracic procedures. Vital signs are recorded as often as necessary but at least every 15 min while the patient is in the PACU.
- At least one capnograph immediately should be available to monitor ventilation in a seriously ill patient or verify correct tracheal intubation.
- A dedicated cardiac output computer must be available if pulmonary artery catheters are used.
- There should be at least one peripheral nerve stimulator with TOF and double-burst capability in the PACU to identify patients with PORC, defined as a TOF ratio <0.9, which may occur in 22–60 % of patients in the PACU.
- Computerised patient data management systems have been widely used, into which data can be entered by either direct capture of monitor signals or entry by the PACU nurses or physicians.

6.1.6.10 PACU Communications

- An inadequate number of telephones is a common problem in the PACUs. Cordless telephones can be quite useful, since they allow the nurse to talk on the telephone without leaving the bedside.
- Of note, the main telephone at the PACU desk needs to be as free as possible for incoming calls.
- It is advisable to have a different telephone number from the main number to be used only by the OR circulating nurses to inform the PACU about impending patient transfers to the PACU.
- A dedicated intercom system exclusive to the surgical suite area is a potential alternative, which may or may not tie into the OR overhead paging system.
- Another option is to use two-way voice communication devices utilising the hospital wireless network, voice recognition and wearable equipment allowing the PACU nurse to continue taking care of the patient at the bedside without a cordless phone.
- More recently, a dedicated alarm system that would summon help in a crisis (e.g. code situation) involving a large (often red) button under a clear plastic cover at the desk or on the wall in a central location in the PACU is considered to activate

light and bell alarm in the OR and in the place most likely to be populated by anaesthesia personnel who can respond immediately.

6.1.7 Staff

Ideal staff should consist of:

- An anaesthesiologist should be assigned to be responsible for final medical decisions in the PACU (i.e. respiration, circulation, fluid, metabolic balance and analgesia).
- An expert charge nurse in the advanced cardiac life support directs the PACU, acts as a backup care nurse when the PACU gets busy and supervises the minute-to-minute operation [7].
- Skilled PACU nurses trained in airway management, basic life support and dealing with the unique patients emerging from anaesthesia after thoracic procedures (e.g. caring for acute surgical wounds and a variety of chest drains) should be capable to provide the direct early postoperative patient care. Usually, it is necessary to have one PACU nurse caring exclusively for each patient undergoing thoracic procedure, at least for the initial 15 min in the PACU. After that, patients who are conscious and stable can usually be monitored by a nurse who is simultaneously watching one similar patient. Patients who are stable, awake, alert and uncomplicated who have been in the PACU for more than 30 min can be watched even less closely. On contrary, patients who are unstable or who have complications (e.g. hypoventilation) require constant close monitoring regardless how long they have been in the PACU [8]. Classically, the PACU nurses take at least 60 min to admit a patient, manage the patient's recovery, get the patient ready for discharge from the PACU and complete all the paperwork.
- The operating surgeon is responsible for decisions about the results of the performed thoracic procedure.

6.1.8 PACU Discharge Criteria

Discharge of patients after thoracic procedures from the PACU to the ward or high-dependency unit is usually the responsibility of the physician or PACU nurse according to the institutional policy and discharge criteria (Table 6.2) [4]. Brown et al. reported shortening the PACU stay by 24 % with using these predetermined discharge criteria [11].

6.2 What to Treat in PACU?

There is an emphasis on the adverse events occurring in the PACU after thoracic procedures such as airway obstruction, aspiration of vomitus and inadequate ventilation from residual curarisation. Interdisciplinary rounds in the PACU can

Table 6.2 Discharge criteria from the PACU to the ward

1. He/she is alert
2. Oriented to the time and place
3. Conversant and cooperative
4. If vital signs have been stable for at least 30 min
5. The patient could sit up without dizziness or nausea
6. The pain is considered tolerable, and the modified Aldrete score is ≥ 9 [10]
7. Outpatients should be discharged to a responsible adult who will accompany them home
8. Outpatients should be provided with written instructions regarding postoperative diet, medications, activities and a phone number to call in case of emergency

Haret et al. [4, 9]

potentially reduce these complications through improved quality of care and effective communications between physicians, house and nursing staff [12].

6.2.1 Early Postoperative Complications

6.2.1.1 Postoperative Nausea and Vomiting (PONV)

The PONV has an overall 20–30 % incidence of patients undergoing general anaesthesia. PONV has a significant negative effect on patient satisfaction with anaesthesia, and even it may cause severe complications such as Boerhaave syndrome, airway compromise and emphysema [13]. Independent predictors for PONV include female gender, young age, non-smoking status, history of motion sickness or past PONV, intraoperative using volatile anaesthetics or nitrous oxide, prolonged duration of anaesthesia and postoperative use of opioids [13, 14]. Considering a multimodal approach can be effective for preventing PONV.

Many varieties of antiemetics could be used for treatment of the PONV as shown in Table 6.3 and Fig. 6.7.

6.2.1.2 Postoperative Residual Curarisation (PORC)

PORC is commonly observed in the PACU when neuromuscular blocking drugs are used intraoperatively. TOF ratios <0.70–0.90 are associated with upper airway obstruction, inadequate recovery of pulmonary function, reduced pharyngeal muscle coordination, an increased risk for aspiration and an impaired hypoxic ventilatory response [15]. Conventional neuromuscular monitoring and standard clinical tests (e.g. 5-s head lift) are unreliable in detecting PORC; thus, incomplete neuromuscular recovery can be minimised with acceleromyographic monitoring in the PACU [16].

6.2.1.3 Emergence Delirium and Postoperative Dysfunction

Emergence from anaesthesia could be accompanied by signs of delirium, including fluctuating mental status and inattention, with reported prevalence rates of approximately 5–19 %[17]. Emergence delirium, primarily manifesting with a hypoactive subtype, may be associated with prolonged PACU stays and worse outcomes [18–20]. Preventable determinants for emergence delirium include high postoperative pain scores, long fasting times, premedication with benzodiazepines [17] and receiving opioids [18].

6.2.1.4 Anxiety in the PACU

Risk factors for postoperative anxiety in adults include the ASA physical status, preoperative anxiety, minor psychiatric disorders, moderate to intense postoperative pain and negative future perception. In contrast, the neural-block anaesthesia, systemic multimodal analgesia and neuraxial opioids are protective factors against postoperative anxiety [21]. Benzodiazepines in controlled concentrations can be used to reduce postoperative anxiety even in elderly patients. Of note, alternative therapies may include administering dexmedetomidine or clonidine or considering acupressure, relaxation techniques or massage therapy [22].

6.2.1.5 Glycaemic Control

Diabetes mellitus is the strongest risk factor for mortality following lung transplant [hazard ratio 3.96 (2.85–5.51)] [23]. Hyperglycaemia as a result of neuroendocrine and the stress response to surgical procedures is most notable in the postoperative period in both diabetic and non-diabetic patients. Glycaemic control in the postoperative period has been shown to reduce wound infections and hyperglycaemia-associated poor outcomes [24]. Thus avoidance of severe hyperglycaemia (>10 mmol/l (>180 mg/dl)) is important in adults after thoracic surgery through continuous IV infusion of insulin in conjunction with glycaemic monitoring every 30–60 min. Additionally, the preoperative ingestion of clear fluids containing 50–100 g of carbohydrate until two hours before surgery, unless contraindicated, and avoiding hypothermia and bleeding could minimise postoperative insulin resistance [25]. Additionally, cautious should be exerted to avoid hypoglycaemia during the postoperative period that may go unrecognised and resulting in irreversible brain injury and mortality.

6.2.1.6 Pain in the PACU

Inadequate control of acute pain after thoracic surgery can potentially result in postoperative pulmonary complications because of impaired sputum clearance and reduced ventilatory capacity [26] or experiencing post-thoracic surgery chronic pain [27].

A multimodal analgesia approach using different modalities with different mechanism of actions such as regional (e.g. thoracic epidural analgesia (TEA), paravertebral blockade (PVB), intercostal nerve block, intrapleural block, cryoanalgesia, transcutaneous electrical nerve stimulation (TENS)) and systemic analgesic techniques (e.g. opioids, ketamine, dexmedetomidine, clonidine, non-steroidal antiinflammatory drugs (NSAIDs), paracetamol and local anaesthetic) is commonly used for pain control in the PACU [28]. Of note, post-thoracic surgery shoulder pain is usually refractory to TEA and requires NASIDs, pregabalin and sometimes opioids [29, 30].

Table 6.3 Classes of commonly used antiemetics

Group	Drug	Adverse effects
1. 5-HT3 receptor antagonists	Ondansetron Dolasetron Palonosetron Tropisetron Granisetron Palonosetron	Headache Elevated transaminases QT prolongation Palonosetron shows fewer side effects
2. Glucocorticoids	Dexamethasone	Hypotension
		Increases blood sugar
3. Antihistamines	Dimenhydrinate Cyclizine	Drowsiness
		Dry mouth
		Tachycardia
		QT prolongation
		Visual disturbances
		Dysuria
4. Cholinergic antagonists	Scopolamine	Visual disturbances
		Dry mouth
		Confusion
		Hallucinations
5. Neurokinin-1 receptor antagonists (*Off-label use*)	Aprepitant Fosaprepitant	Headache
		Elevated transaminases
		Dry mouth
		Drowsiness
6. Butyrophenone	Droperidol Haloperidol	QT prolongation
		Hypotension
		Reflexive tachycardia
		Drowsiness
		Dystonia
		Anxiety
		Agitation
		Insomnia
		Akathisia
		Dyskinesia
		Headache
		Hypotension
		Dry mouth
		Visual disturbances
		QT prolongation
7. Benzamide	Metoclopramide	Hypotension
		Reflexive tachycardia
		Dyskinesia

Modified from Haret et al. [4], Jokinen et al. [13]

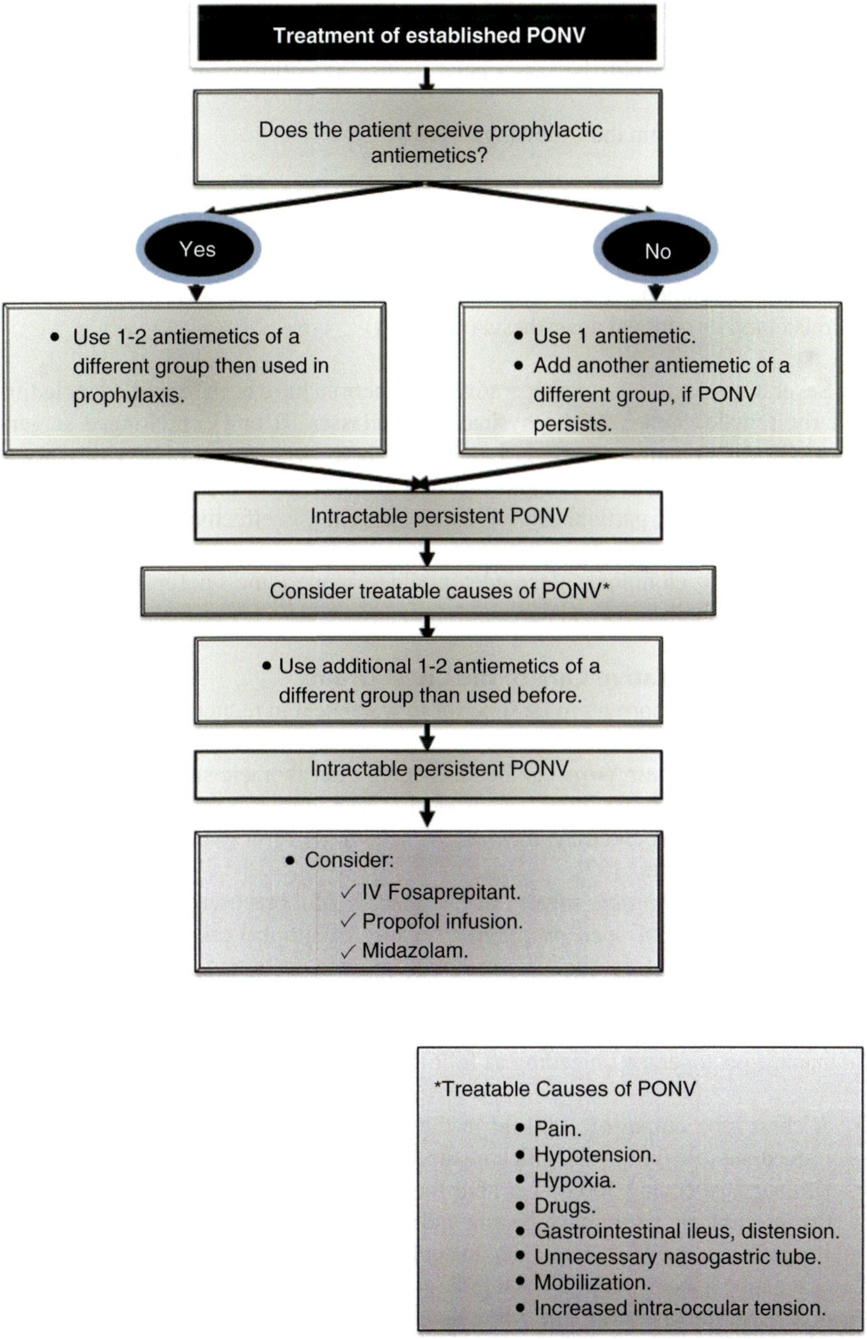

Fig. 6.7 Approach for treatment of established PONV (Modified from Jokinen et al. [13], Haret et al. [4])

6.2.1.7 Hypothermia in the PACU

Inadvertent postoperative hypothermia is common among 60– 90 % of patients in the PACU that could be associated with 300–400 % increase in oxygen consumption.

It could result from the following:

- Excessive heat loss due to exposure of the body surface to a low-temperature environment, particularly during open thoracotomy and clam-shell incisions
- Affecting of normal thermoregulatory mechanisms secondary to the action of general anaesthetic agents (e.g. intravenous and volatile anaesthetics, muscle relaxants) or regional anaesthesia (e.g. TEA)

Several risk factors for postoperative hypothermia have been identified including elderly, female gender, ASA physical status classes III or IV, prolonged surgery >2 h, OR temperature <26 °C (78.8 °F), low body weight and history of chronic endocrine diseases and intravenous infusion of cold fluids [31].

Active warming, particularly forced air warming, is effective in treating hypothermia [32]. Numerous drugs have been described to minimise postoperative shivering such as clonidine, dexmedetomidine, meperidine, nefopam, tramadol, ondansetron, granisetron and parecoxib [33, 34].

6.2.1.8 Postoperative Care of the Chest Drains

Chest tube suction appears to be superior to water seal in reducing the incidence of pneumothorax [35].

Postoperative chest X-ray can be considered after thoracic surgery only if complete expansion of the lung (pleurodesis, pneumothorax) is warranted [36]. Postoperative ultrasound may alleviate the need to perform routine chest X-rays to rule out pneumothorax [37].

Bleeding after thoracic surgery occurs in <2 % of thoracoscopic procedures and around 1 % to 3 % of open procedures because of surgical complications, coagulopathy, receiving of antiplatelets or anticoagulants or certain comorbidities (e.g. diabetes, renal or hepatic insufficiency) [38, 39].

Hourly observation of chest tube output with vital sign monitoring are important to manage postoperative bleeding as follows [40]:

- A chest tube output of 1000 ml in the first postoperative hour necessitates an immediate re-exploration with concurrent correction of coagulopathy.
- Drainage exceeding 200 ml per hour for 2 to 4 h after correction of a coagulopathy also indicates surgical bleeding and dictates re-exploration.
- If a patient is haemodynamically unstable but the chest tube output does not suggest active haemorrhage, a chest radiograph is usually required to rule out radio-opacity of the operative side with clotted chest tubes.
- If a patient is haemodynamically stable but the chest output is high, checking the haematocrit on the chest tube drainage can be helpful in distinguishing active bleeding from a lymphatic leak.

The significant *postoperative air leak after pulmonary resections* can be expiratory, forced expiratory, inspiratory (on positive pressure ventilation) or continuous.

Management in the PACU [35]:

- If there is no pleural space, then they are managed by underwater seal.
- If there is a pleural space, negative suction is applied to the underwater seal.

6.2.1.9 Early Postoperative Hypoxemia and Oxygen Therapy

Early tracheal extubation following thoracic procedures favours shorter stays in the PACU and lower hospital costs [41]. The causes of postoperative hypoxaemia (SpO_2 <90 %, PaO_2 <60 mmHg) are presented in Table 6.4 [42, 43].

Intraoperative use of lung recruitment strategy, short-acting opioids and neuromuscular blocking drugs, TEA or PVB and allowing patients to lay down in the semi-setting position in conjunction with using supplemental oxygen in the PACU can potentially prevent postoperative hypoxaemia [44–46]. NIV has been established to treat postoperative pulmonary dysfunction to avoid re-intubation in conscious patients with stable haemodynamics [47].

6.2.1.10 Cardiovascular Complications

They occur in 10–15 % of patients after major lung resection [48]. Most important cardiovascular complications can be listed as arrhythmia, right-to-left shunt, heart failure, cardiac herniation, cardiac tamponade and myocardial ischaemia.

Postoperative SVT including AF is a common complication after pulmonary resection, in 24–67 % of patients undergoing pneumonectomy and 12.3 % after lobectomy. If patients have AF with compromised haemodynamic parameters, then electrical cardioversion should be carried out immediately. If patients have symptomatic AF, amiodarone could be used without increased incidence of respiratory complications [49].

Heart failure occurs in 8.2 % after thoracic procedures [50]. In the PACU, transthoracic echocardiography and functional class and N-terminal B-type natriuretic peptide levels are parts of a multimodality approach to diagnose the postoperative RV dysfunction [51, 52]. Pharmacological, ventilatory and mechanical supports for the RV are used in order to optimise RV function by controlling preload, decreasing afterload and providing inotropic support for both ventricles.

Cardiac herniation is most commonly seen after pneumonectomy associated with pericardiotomy or pericardiectomy [53].

Pericardial tamponade, though rare after open lobectomy, should be considered along with other complications when a patient repeatedly develops hypotension alongside an equalisation of CVP with pulmonary artery diastolic pressure. Echocardiography is the diagnostic study of choice to visualise impaired filling of the RV because of increased pericardial pressure.

Patients with significant coronary artery disease within 1 year of coronary stenting pose high risks for postoperative myocardial ischaemia/infarction after thoracic surgery [54, 55].

Table 6.4 Causes of postoperative hypoxaemia

1. Inadequate pain relief
2. Hypothermia
3. Shivering
4. Hypoventilation
5. PORC
6. Use of opioids
7. Atelectasis
8. Pneumothorax
9. Post-pnuemonectomy or post-expansion pulmonary oedema
10. Activation of the inflammatory cascade
11. Excessive air leak
12. Aspiration of gastric contents
13. Excessive fluid therapy
14. Tachyarrhythmia (particularly AF)
15. RV dysfunction
16. Right-to-left shunt
17. Injury to the phrenic nerve

6.2.1.11 Fluid Therapy and Acute Kidney Injury

One of the independent risk factors for ALI after surgery for lung cancer is excessive fluid infusion (odds ratio, 2.9; 95 % confidence interval, 1.9–7.4) [56].

IV fluids should be infused judiciously in the PACU at a recommended rate of 1–2 ml/kg/h [57]. A fluid restriction after thoracic procedures could be guided with using minimally invasive haemodynamic monitoring of pulse pressure/stroke volume variation, extravascular lung water and intra-thoracic blood volume index variables, but it is not clear whether the use of these methods protects against development of postoperative AKI [58]. Decreased urine output less than <0.5 mL/kg/h is a common occurrence in the PACU, whereas AKI is uncommon in the PACU. Early postoperative AKI is associated with more need for tracheal re-intubation, postoperative mechanical ventilation and prolonged hospital stay.

Acknowledgements The authors want to express his appreciation for Ms. Angelin Jeba Suja, PACU staff nurse, King Fahd Hospital of the University of Dammam, for preparing the included photographs in this chapter.

References

1. Simpson JC, Moonesinghe SR (2013) Introduction to the postanaesthetic care unit. Perioper Med (Lond) 2:5
2. Macario A, Glenn D, Dexter F (1999) What can the postanesthesia care unit manager do to decrease costs in the postanesthesia care unit? J Perianesth Nurs 14:284–293
3. Schweizer A, Khatchatourian G, Ho¨hn L, Spiliopoulos A, Romand J, Licker M (2002) Opening of a new postanesthesia care unit: impact on critical care utilization and complications following major vascular and thoracic surgery. J Clin Anesth 14:486–493

4. Haret D, Kneeland M, Ho E (2012) Postanesthesia care units. In: Operating room design manual 2012. American Society of Anesthesiologists, Park Ridge. 14. pp 57–72. Permission to use was obtained
5. Krenk L, Rasmussen LS, Kehlet H (2010) New insights into the pathophysiology of postoperative cognitive dysfunction. Acta Anaesthesiol Scand 54:951–956
6. Practice guidelines for postanesthetic care: a report by the American Society of Anesthesiologists Task Force on Postanesthetic Care (2002). Anesthesiology 96:742–745
7. Frederico A (2007) Innovations in care: the nurse practitioner in the PACU. J Perianesth Nurs 22:235–242
8. Nicholau D (2009) The postanesthesia care unit. In: Miller RD (ed) Miller's anesthesia, 6th edn. Elsevier Chruchill Livingstone, Philadelphia
9. El Tahan MR (2011) Effects of aminophylline on cognitive recovery after sevoflurane. J Anesth 25:648–656
10. Aldrete JA (1995) The post-anaesthesia recovery score revisited. J Clin Anesth 7:89–91
11. Brown I, Jellish WS, Kleinman B, Fluder E, Sawicki K, Katsaros J et al (2008) Use of postanesthesia discharge criteria to reduce discharge delays for inpatients in the postanesthesia care unit. J Clin Anesth 20:175–179
12. Hoke N, Falk S (2012) Interdisciplinary rounds in the post-anesthesia care unit: a new perioperative paradigm. Anesthesiol Clin 30:427–431
13. Jokinen J, Smith AF, Roewer N, Eberhart LHJ, Kranke P (2012) Management of postoperative nausea and vomiting. How to deal with refractory PONV? Anesthesiol Clin 30:481–493
14. Leslie K, Myles PS, Chan MT, Paech MJ, Peyton P, Forbes A et al (2008) Risk factors for severe postoperative nausea and vomiting in a randomized trial of nitrous oxide-based vs nitrous oxide-free anaesthesia. Br J Anaesth 101:498–505
15. Murphy GS, Szokol JW, Marymont JH, Greenberg SB, Avram MJ, Vender JS (2008) Residual neuromuscular blockade and critical respiratory events in the post-anesthesia care unit. Anesth Analg 107:130–137
16. Murphy GS, Szokol JW, Marymont JH, Greenberg SB, Avram MJ, Vender JS et al (2008) Intraoperative acceleromyographic monitoring reduces the risk of residualneuromuscular blockade and adverse respiratory events in the post-anesthesia care unit. Anesthesiology 109:389–398
17. Radtke FM, Franck M, Hagemann L, Seeling M, Wernecke KD, Spies CD (2010) Risk factors for inadequate emergence after anesthesia: emergence delirium and hypoactive emergence. Minerva Anestesiol 76:394–403
18. Card E, Pandharipande P, Tomes C, Lee C, Wood J, Nelson D et al (2014) Emergence from general anaesthesia and evolution of delirium signs in the post-anaesthesia care unit. Br J Anaesth. pii: aeu442
19. Neufeld KJ, Leoutsakos JM, Sieber FE, Wanamaker BL, Gibson Chambers JJ, Rao V et al (2013) Outcomes of early delirium diagnosis after general anesthesia in the elderly. Anesth Analg 117:471–478
20. Xará D, Silva A, Mendonça J, Abelha F (2013) Inadequate emergence after anesthesia: emergence delirium and hypoactive emergence in the post-anesthesia care unit. J Clin Anesth 25:439–446
21. Caumo W, Schmidt AP, Schneider CN, Bergmann J, Iwamoto CW, Bandeira D et al (2001) Risk factors for preoperative anxiety in adults. Acta Anaesthesiol Scand 45:298–307
22. Jellish WS, O'Rourke M (2012) Anxiolytic use in the postoperative care unit. Anesthesiol Clin 30:467–480
23. Hackman KL, Bailey MJ, Snell GI, Bach LA (2014) Diabetes is a major risk factor for mortality after lung transplantation. Am J Transplant 14:438–445
24. Russo N (2012) Perioperative glycemic control. Anesthesiol Clin 30:445–466
25. Lena D, Kalfon P, Preiser JC, Ichai C (2011) Glycemic control in the intensive care unit and during the postoperative period. Anesthesiology 114:438–444
26. Wenk M, Schug SA (2011) Perioperative pain management after thoracotomy. Curr Opin Anaesthesiol 24:8–12. doi:10.1097/ACO.0b013e3283414175
27. Khelemsky Y, Noto CJ (2012) Preventing post-thoracotomy pain syndrome. Mt Sinai J Med 79:133–139

28. Buvanendran A, Kroin JS (2009) Multimodal analgesia for controlling acute postoperative pain. Curr Opin Anaesthesiol 22:588–593
29. Bunchungmongkol N, Pipanmekaporn T, Paiboonworachat S, Saeteng S, Tantraworasin A (2014) Incidence and risk factors associated with ipsilateral shoulder pain after thoracic surgery. J Cardiothorac Vasc Anesth 28:991–994
30. Imai Y, Imai K, Kimura T, Horiguchi T, Goyagi T, Saito H et al (2015) Evaluation of postoperative pregabalin for attenuation of postoperative shoulder painafter thoracotomy in patients with lung cancer, a preliminary result. Gen Thorac Cardiovasc Surg 63:99–104
31. Kiekkas P, Poulopoulou M, Papahatzi A, Souleles P (2005) Effects of hypothermia and shivering on standard PACU monitoring of patients. AANA J 73:47–53
32. Warttig S, Alderson P, Campbell G, Smith AF (2014) Interventions for treating inadvertent postoperative hypothermia. Cochrane Database Syst Rev 11, CD009892
33. Alfonsi P (2003) Postanaesthetic shivering. Epidemiology, pathophysiology and approaches to prevention and management. Minerva Anestesiol 69:438–442
34. Li X, Zhou M, Xia Q, Li W, Zhang Y (2014) Effect of parecoxib sodium on postoperative shivering: a randomised, double-blind clinical trial. Eur J Anaesthesiol 31:225–230
35. Coughlin SM, Emmerton-Coughlin HM, Malthaner R (2012) Management of chest tubes after pulmonary resection: a systematic review and meta-analysis. Can J Surg 55:264–270
36. Leschber G, May CJ, Simbrey-Chryselius N (2014) Do thoracic surgery patients always need a postoperative chest X-ray? Zentralbl Chir 139(Suppl 1):S43–S49
37. Goudie E, Bah I, Khereba M, Ferraro P, Duranceau A, Martin J et al (2012) Prospective trial evaluating sonography after thoracic surgery in postoperative careand decision making. Eur J Cardiothorac Surg 41:1025–1030
38. Imperatori A, Rotolo N, Gatti M, Nardecchia E, De Monte L, Conti V et al (2008) Perioperative complications of video-assisted thoracoscopic surgery (VATS). Int J Surg 6(Suppl 1):S78–S81
39. Sirbu H, Busch T, Aleksic I, Lotfi S, Ruschewski W, Dalichau H (1999) Chest re-exploration for complications after lung surgery. Thorac Cardiovasc Surg 47:73–76
40. Litle VR, Swanson SJ (2006) Postoperative bleeding: coagulopathy, bleeding, hemothorax. Thorac Surg Clin 16:203–207, v
41. Browne SM, Halligan PW, Wade DT, Taggart DP (2003) Postoperative hypoxia is a contributory factor to cognitive impairment after cardiac surgery. J Thorac Cardiovasc Surg 126:1061–1064
42. Bosînceanu M, Sandu C, Ionescu LR, Roată C, Miron L (2014) Clinical-epidemiological study on the incidence of postoperative complications after pulmonary resection for lung cancer. Rev Med Chir Soc Med Nat Iasi 118:1040–1046
43. Siddiqui N, Arzola C, Teresi J, Fox G, Guerina L, Friedman Z (2013) Predictors of desaturation in the postoperative anesthesia care unit: an observational study. J Clin Anesth 25:612–617
44. Martin DS, Grocott MPW (2013) Oxygen therapy in anaesthesia: the yin and yang of O2. Br J Anaesth 111:867–871
45. Aust H, Eberhart LH, Kranke P, Arndt C, Bleimüller C, Zoremba M et al (2012) Hypoxemia after general anesthesia. Anaesthesist 61:299–309
46. Pai VB, Vallurupalli S, Kasula SR, Hakeem A, Bhatti S (2014) A change of heart: reopening of a foramen ovale. Can J Cardiol 30:1250. e17-8
47. Jaber S, De Jong A, Castagnoli A, Futier E, Chanques G (2014) Non-invasive ventilation after surgery. Ann Fr Anesth Reanim 33:487–491
48. Ferguson MK, Saha-Chaudhuri P, Mitchell JD, Varela G, Brunelli A (2014) Prediction of major cardiovascular events after lung resection using a modified scoring system. Ann Thorac Surg 97:1135–1140
49. Berry MF, D'Amico TA, Onaitis M (2014) Use of amiodarone after major lung resection. Ann Thorac Surg 98:1199–1206
50. Hernandez AF, Whellan DJ, Stroud S, Sun JL, O'Connor CM, Jollis JG (2004) Outcomes in heart failure patients after major noncardiac surgery. J Am Coll Cardiol 44:1446–1453

51. Pedoto A, Amar D (2009) Right heart function in thoracic surgery: role of echocardiography. Curr Opin Anaesthesiol 22:44–49
52. Ho SY, Nihoyannopoulos P (2006) Anatomy, echocardiography, and normal right ventricular dimension. Heart 92:i2–i13
53. Mehanna MJ, Israel GM, Katigbak M, Rubinowitz AN (2007) Cardiac herniation after right pneumonectomy: case report and review of the literature. J Thorac Imaging 22:280–282
54. Wang Z, Zhang J, Cheng Z, Li X, Wang Z, Liu C et al (2014) Factors affecting major morbidity after video-assisted thoracic surgery for lung cancer. J Surg Res 192:628–634
55. Fernandez FG, Crabtree TD, Liu J, Meyers BF (2013) Incremental risk of prior coronary arterial stents for pulmonary resection. Ann Thorac Surg 95:1212–1218, discussion 1219–20
56. Licker M, de Perrot M, Spiliopoulos A, Robert J, Diaper J, Chevalley C et al (2003) Risk factors for acute lung injury after thoracic surgery for lung cancer. Anesth Analg 97:1558–1565
57. Evans RG, Naidu B (2012) Does a conservative fluid management strategy in the perioperative management of lung resection patients reduce the risk of acute lung injury? Interact Cardiovasc Thorac Surg 15:498–504
58. Haase O, Raue W, Neuss H, Koplin G, Mielitz U, Schwenk W (2013) Influence of postoperative fluid management on pulmonary function after esophagectomy. Acta Chir Belg 113:415–422

7 Should I Blame the Surgeon: Surgical Complications and Surgical Treatment of the Complications

Jelena Grusina-Ujumaza and Alper Toker

7.1 Introduction

In this chapter, authors try to clarify the postoperative major complications seen after thoracic surgery, mainly after lung resections, mediastinal mass resections, and lung transplantations. However this chapter did not deal with postoperative arrhythmias and pulmonary edema, since they were discussed in other chapters in this book.

7.2 Postoperative Hemorrhage and Residual Hemothorax

Chest tubes placed at the end of the operation help to prevent pneumothorax and monitor air leaks and bleeding in early postoperative period. The incidence of postoperative hemorrhage after thoracic surgery is variable and depends on the type of operation: it can occur in 4 % of the cases after pulmonary resections and just 0.33 % after mediastinoscopy [1, 2]. Most of the surgical bleedings (no disorders of coagulation factors – normal INR (international normalized ratio), prothrombin time, and thrombocyte count) are small in amount and generally resolve spontaneously. Just a very few percent of bleeding (up to 2.6 %) needs emergency surgery [3]. Criteria for

J. Grusina-Ujumaza
Department of Thoracic Surgery, Pauls Stradins Clinical University Hospital, Riga, Latvia
Department of Thoracic Surgery, Group Florence Nightingale Hospitals, Istanbul, Turkey

A. Toker (✉)
Department of Thoracic Surgery, Group Florence Nightingale Hospitals, Istanbul, Turkey
Department of Thoracic Surgery, Istanbul University, Istanbul Faculty of Medicine, Istanbul, Turkey
e-mail: ae-toker@superonline.com

© Springer International Publishing Switzerland 2017

M. Şentürk, M.O. Sungur (eds.), *Postoperative Care in Thoracic Surgery*,
DOI 10.1007/978-3-319-19908-5_7

postoperative bleeding control are the amount of drainage and the hemodynamic effects of the drainage. A continuing thoracic hemorrhagic drainage of more than 1000 ml or 200 ml/h for 4–6 h or a sudden drainage of 400 ml may be a sign for a need of an emergency intervention [4, 5]. A blood count should be obtained to detect any changes in the hemoglobin and hematocrit levels, and a chest X-ray should be taken to exclude hemothorax. Hematocrit of the blood obtained from chest tube may indicate the severity of the drainage. If the hematocrit level of the chest drain blood is more than 50 % of the blood hematocrit level, this may be a sign of continuing hemorrhage. During early postoperative course, the thoracic drainage system should be checked – it should be left open (except drainage after pneumonectomy) and should work normal (we have to see oscillation in the drainage tube). Following pneumonectomy, chest tube is recommended to keep clamped and declamped for a few minutes in every hour to control the bleeding. In an intubated patient, with a high positive end-expiratory pressure, the presence of an air leak may be considered as normal. Also, a drain without any oscillation may be normal in such patients.

Recently, due to increase of the patients with coronary artery stents, lung resection candidates are more complicated because of perioperative anticoagulation and antiplatelet therapy (APT). Bertolaccini et al. [6] found that there were no statistically significant differences between the outcomes for the 38 patients receiving APT compared with the controls, in terms of the operative time, the hospital stay, the estimated blood loss, or the morbidity when stratified by the procedure [6]. On the other hand, in Foroulis's study [7], it was shown that APT use was a predisposing factor for postoperative bleeding.

In our experience, with increasing use of video-assisted surgery (VATS) and vascular staplers, massive bleeding due to slipping of ligature is extremely uncommon.

Residual hemothorax, which is not associated with an active bleeding, may occur after thoracic surgery. Up to 15 % of the lung transplant recipients may have this complication. Although thrombolytics may be recommended for a successful treatment, authors prefer VATS for the evacuation of the retained hemothorax [8]. In some patients, changing the location of the chest tube may help in resolving of the residual hemothorax (Fig. 7.1).

7.3 Cardiac Herniation and Tamponade

Cardiac herniation and tamponade are rare complications which may occur after extended pulmonary resections – pneumonectomy or lobectomy – for malignant diseases or pleuropneumonectomy for malignant mesothelioma or thymoma surgery or when pericardiotomy or pericardiectomy is performed in addition to any type of thoracic surgery. It may also occur after lung transplantation [9–11]. Cardiac herniation has a high mortality rate. Thirty to 50 % of cases may be fatal because of a delay either in the diagnosis or the treatment. It is 100 % fatal, if undetected [12].

The incidence of cardiac herniation after pulmonary resections for lung cancer is about 1.7 % [13]. Cardiac herniation after right-sided pneumonectomy is more frequent. It generally occurs in the first 3 postoperative days [14, 15]. It presents with

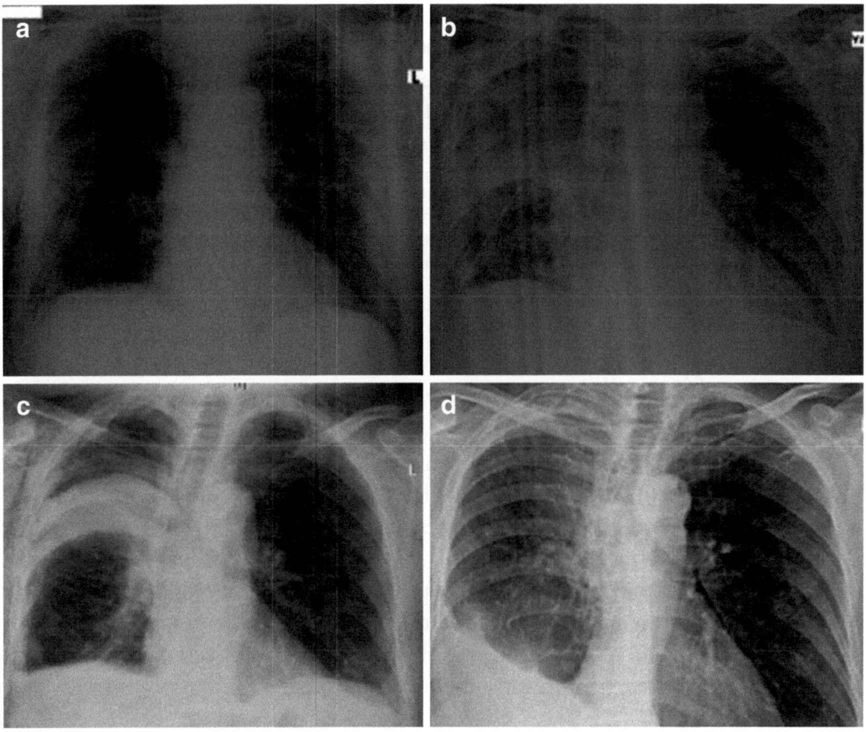

Fig. 7.1 VATS for the evacuation of the retained hemothorax or revising the location of chest tube may help in resolving of the residual hemothorax. (**a**) Early postoperative period. (**b**) Right sided hemothorax, several hours later. (**c**) Residual hemothorax prior to indicated VATS evacuation. (**d**) One week after the VATS with the upper displacement of the residual lung tissue

acute symptoms; there is a critical moment for cardiac herniation and/or tamponade after pneumonectomy. It may occur even in the operation room when patient is turned from the lateral decubitus to the supine position. Acutely significant hypotension may present. The cause of this could be cardiac strangulation (the size of the pericardial graft may be small), cardiac herniation (after pericardiectomy without the closure of the pericardium or patch dehiscence), or tamponade. Transesophageal echocardiography can assist in decision-making before leaving the operating room without reopening the thoracotomy [9]. During the early postoperative period, risk factors for a cardiac herniation could be increased due to the increased intrathoracic pressure with cough and sputum expectoration, the positive-pressure ventilation, the negative suction from drain, and the changes in patient's position (e.g., lying on the side of surgery) [5]. Symptoms start suddenly with the presentation of superior vena cava syndrome, low cardiac output, dysrhythmias, hypotension, cardiac arrest, and shock. For diagnosis, chest X-ray (shadows of the heart and apex), electrocardiography (ECG), and echocardiogram have to be performed for the diagnosis. The clues of the herniation include axis change on ECG, cardiac malrotation on echocardiogram, and hemodynamic collapse [16]. Thorax computed tomography

(CT) (if hemodynamics of patient allows) is also recommended. Treatment should be started immediately – the patient should lie opposite to the surgical side and emergency reoperation has to be performed.

Cardiac tamponade as a complication after extrapleural pneumonectomy may occur in 3.6% of the patients [9]. Postoperative bleeding into the pericardial sac may occur even after lobectomy without pericardiectomy. The patient may have acute clinical presentation and needs an urgent surgery [17]. It was proposed that an intrapericardial retraction of the suture line of the divided pulmonary vein could cause a bleeding from the malfunctioning staple line, and this could lead to a cardiac tamponade [18–20]. It can be treated just with a transcutaneous pericardial drainage and/or immediate surgery.

Cardiac tamponade is characterized by a low cardiac output and a classical Beck's triad (hypotension, muffled heart sounds, and distended neck veins). The chest X-ray, ECG, and echocardiogram should be performed. Surgical treatment is recommended in most of the cases.

These complications might be the cause of cardiac arrest and could have fatal results. Sugarbaker [9] wrote that a cardiac arrest within 10 days postoperatively needs emergency thoracotomy (sometimes in the intensive care unit), open cardiac massage, and pericardial patch removal. Closed cardiac massage is not effective enough after pneumonectomy, since the heart has shifted out of the midline, and it cannot be properly compressed by the sternum and vertebral column. All the members of the postoperative care team must be educated on this point to avoid losing valuable time performing futile closed-chest compressions [9].

7.4 Lobar torsion and gangrene

Lobar, segmental or common basal pyramid torsion is a rare complication which may occur after different type of pulmonary resections and lung transplantation with an incidence rate less than 0.1% [21–23]. Usually torsion occurs in the middle lobe or in the left lower lobe following upper lobe resections. Lobar torsion may develop in the first postoperative 2 weeks [21, 23, 24]. The rotation of the bronchovascular pedicle results with bronchial obstruction and vascular compromise is the cause of gangrene and potential mortality if left untreated [25]. Recognition of pulmonary torsion may be difficult. Clinical presentations vary from slight hypoxemia to septic shock. The clinical findings depend on the degree of rotation in the lobar hilum, generally the rotation is 180 degrees although 90 and 360 degree torsions have been reported [26]. Symptoms of pulmonary torsion can start suddenly with an unexplained dyspnea, productive cough, hemoptysis, tachycardia, and fever, diminished breathing sounds on the effected side or presence of air leak. Chest radiographs may show opacification of the lobe. Findings do not change after nasotracheal aspiration. Chest X ray may demonstrate pneumothorax or collapsed lobe in an unusual position. High resolution chest computed tomography with pulmonary angiogram may confirm the diagnosis - opacification, complete obstruction – "cut-off"- of the bronchus, stenosis or obstruction of kinking vessels are the radiological findings [23]. Flexible bronchoscopy should be performed and diagnosis may be confirmed if "fish mouth" like appearance is noticed. The trans-esophageal echocardiography may reveal a presence of potential lethal thrombus in pulmonary vein. Urgent reoperation is indicated, reposition and fixation with following anticoagulant therapy to or complete resection could be performed, if pulmonary infarction or gangrene is suspected. Good analgesia, aggressive antibiotics treatment and mini-tracheostomy to aid suctioning of the secretions may help to reduce the infectious complications after torsion [25].

7.5 Air Leak and Subcutaneous Emphysema

An air leak after pulmonary resection is the most commonly seen finding. In the early postoperative period, it may be seen at a rate of 28–60 % of the patients; however, in the immediate postoperative period, an air leak should not be considered as a pathological condition. A pathological "air leak" may refer to any leakage of the air from the lung identified by noting bubbles in a chest drainage system, by progressive subcutaneous emphysema, or by expanding pneumothorax [27, 28]. On the morning of the postoperative day (POD) 1, an air leak is present in 26–48 % of the patients, with a decreasing incidence toward the POD 4 to as low as 8 % [29–31]. But, in some specific procedures such as bilateral lung volume reduction surgery, an air leak may occur in 90 % of the patients [32]. If an air leak is longer than 7 days (some consider more than 4 days and more than 10 days), it may be considered as prolonged air leak (PAL) [27]. The incidence of PAL is between 9.6 and 15 %, and also it was suggested that PAL may increase the rate of other pulmonary complications, including atelectasis, pneumonia, and empyema, but it is not associated with an increased incidence of cardiopulmonary morbidity [31, 34]. As a result of PAL, the postoperative length of stay is increased [28, 35]. An empyema can develop in 11 % of the patients with PAL [31]. Among the most important risk factors of PAL are an underlying COPD, an inhaled steroid treatment, an active pulmonary infection, insulin-dependent diabetes, a low body mass index (<25.5 kg/m^2), a reduced forced expiratory volume in the first second (FEV1) or reduced predicted postoperative FEV1, an upper lung field resection, lung volume reduction surgery, and intraoperative pleural adhesions [32, 36]. As previously mentioned, chest tube drainage systems may help to monitor the air leak after pulmonary surgery. Different chest tube modalities can be used in postoperative period – water seal or negative pressure drainage system −20 cm H_2O or −10 cm H_2O suction. Chest tubes placed on water seal after pulmonary lobectomy are generally well tolerated and safe; however, they do not reduce the duration of the air leak or the incidence of prolonged air leak when compared with negative suction tubes [33]. Air leak volume can be seen easily, if digital drainage system is used. If a high volume of air leak persists, a pneumothorax and/or subcutaneous emphysema may develop, and negative pressure drainage system should be used in this situation. Chest tube can be removed, if there is no air leak and drainage is less than 200 ml in the last 24 h, but generally drainage volume depends on the underlying disease and the surgery performed. For instance, in our practice we remove chest tube, when there is no drainage and air leak after radical pleurectomy and decortication surgery for mesothelioma. We may remove chest tubes when the daily drainage is around 400 ml or the drainage is less than 50 ml in the past 12 h in conventional lung resections like a lobectomy.

If there is a small air leak and the lungs are totally expanded, the chest tube may be clamped (which is named as "provocative clamping"), and a chest X-ray should be taken to determine whether the lung remains expanded or not. The tube can be removed if the lung remains expanded, but if the lung collapses and subcutaneous emphysema develops, then the clamp should be opened and the patient can be discharged with a Heimlich valve connected to chest tube. Operation for PAL is rarely necessary. Sometimes talc pleurodesis or an autologous blood patch via chest tube can be tried, or an endobronchial valve may effectively solve this problem especially in high-risk patients [29, 37, 38].

Subcutaneous emphysema (SE) as a complication of air leak may occur when air enters into the subcutaneous space of the chest wall and the soft tissues of the face, neck, upper chest, and shoulder and may change voice. SE could expand to the abdomen subcutaneous space or even into the peritoneum. Cerfolio [30] reported that SE occurs in 6.3 % of the patients after pulmonary resections. Although nonlethal, it may be difficult to convince the family members and other colleagues from the intensive care unit. A CT scan to identify an air pocket and to guide additional percutaneous drainage catheters may be helpful. Bronchoscopy may be required to exclude a bronchopleural fistula or a possible tracheal laceration during the intubation. Depending on the severity of SE, there are different methods of management, including observation, reoperation, and usage of pop-off valves. If reoperation is necessary, VATS or thoracotomy can be performed [30].

7.6 Chylothorax

A chylothorax is a leak of lymphatic fluid with chylomicrons and fats into the thoracic cavity. Chylothorax could be observed as milky or creamy pleural effusion coming from the chest tube in the early postoperative period or several days after surgery. It may occur as a result of a laceration of lateral branches of the lymphatic duct or direct iatrogenic duct injury and/or incomplete ligation of the lymphatic duct during some procedures, among which are extended mediastinal lymph node dissection, mediastinal tumor resection, esophageal resection, or extrapleural pneumonectomy [39]. The incidence after pulmonary resection is between 0.2 and 2.1 % and after esophagectomy 3.8 %, and the incidence rate also depends on the preference of mediastinal lymph node dissection techniques [39–43]. The diagnosis of a chylothorax is established if pleural effusion has a high level of triglyceride (>110 mg/dL), but if the level is between 50 and 100 mg/dL, lipoprotein analysis should be performed [41]. If triglyceride concentration is lower than 50, it is probably not a chylothorax. A persistent leakage may lead to albumin and antibody loss, malnutrition, and lymphocytopenia and increase the risk of bacterial and viral infections which is associated with significant postoperative morbidity and mortality [43]. In addition, an average daily chest tube output exceeding 400 mL in the early postoperative period should prompt fluid analysis for chylothorax to facilitate early diagnosis and consideration of thoracic duct ligation [43]. The first choice in the treatment is to stop oral diet intake and immediately to start parenteral feeding. Daily drainage volume has been controlled, and decision whether to continue conservative treatment or to perform surgery has been made. Most of the postoperative chylothorax may be resolved by conservative therapy including octreotide/somatostatin infusion [42, 44, 45]. If the amount of the leak is low, it could stop at seal on its own, but before removing the chest tube, the patient should be given a fatty meal diet for two days, and if output is still nonchylous and the volume is low, then the chest tube is removed [40]. But if chylous leakage is greater than 2000 ml for the first 2 days, or as suggested by some authors greater than 1000 ml/per day for 5 days, reoperation should be performed without waiting any further [46, 47]. Lymphangiography and lymphoscintigraphy are useful to localize the leak [44, 45]. The alternative method of the management of the chylothorax is percutaneous catheterization of the thoracic duct and embolization [48].

7.7 Nerve Injury

Extended thoracic surgery may cause intrathoracic nerve injury (phrenic or recurrent laryngeal nerves). Most of the phrenic nerve injuries in literature are described after cardiac surgery, but it may also develop after thoracic surgery such as extended pulmonary resection, esophageal or mediastinal surgery, and cervical rib resection for thoracic outlet syndrome [49]. It may present with unilateral or bilateral diaphragm palsy and results in atelectasis, pneumonia, decreased pulmonary function, sleep-disordered breathing, and pulmonary effusion. It usually can be suspected when patient has decreased exercise tolerance or dyspnea. An intubated patient may have difficulties in weaning. X-ray demonstrates elevation of the affected hemidiaphragm, and ultrasound examination confirms the diagnosis [50]. The best treatment of choice is surgery, either diaphragmatic plication or phrenic nerve reconstruction for unilateral injury or diaphragmatic pacemakers in cases of bilateral injury [50–54]. In Fig. 7.2, you may see a patient with phrenic nerve paralysis and chest X-ray after VATS plication.

The recurrent laryngeal nerve has a high risk of injury during the dissection of the subaortic region, especially during pneumonectomy and esophagectomy, or in cases where patients received preoperative radiotherapy [55]. Recurrent laryngeal nerve palsy after mediastinal lymph node dissection may occur in up to 1.5 % and after esophagectomy up to 8 % but after left-sided pneumonectomy up to 30 % of cases [56–58]. The result of the injury is vocal cord paralysis, which is suspected if the patient has a weak or whispery voice or a weak cough or if the patient aspirates after water intake in early postoperative period; the last symptom should be differentiated from vocal cord edema in the very early postextubation period. When vocal cord paralysis is suspected, laryngoscopy or flexible fiber-optic laryngoscopy should be performed and followed by laryngostroboscopy and laryngeal electromyography. The management involves pulmonary physiotherapy to decrease risk of aspiration, medialization laryngoplasty with or without implant material, or

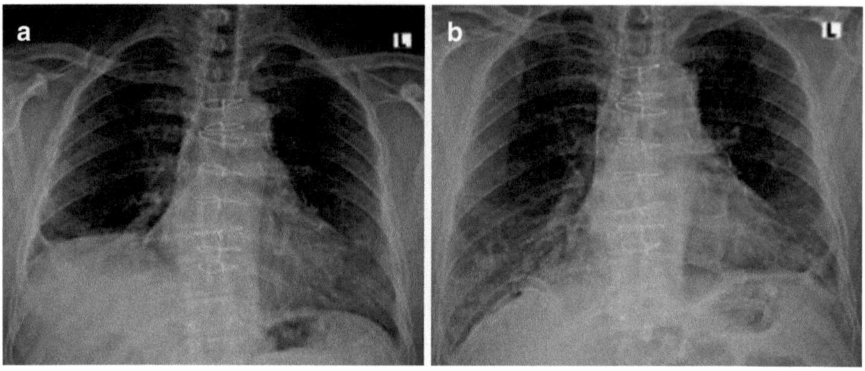

Fig. 7.2 (**a**) Chest X-ray view of a patient with phrenic nerve paralysis. (**b**) Chest X-ray view of a patient after VATS diaphragmatic plication

injection medialization [59–61]. Bilateral vocal cord paralysis is a catastrophe, which may occur after tracheal stenosis resection at the subglottic level. Experienced tracheal surgeons know the pitfalls and generally never have this complication.

7.8 Right-to-Left Shunt

Right-to-left shunt or platypnea-orthodeoxia syndrome is rarely observed after right-sided pneumonectomy operation or after an elevated right hemidiaphragm. The presence of a persistent foramen ovale (PFO) or open atrial septal defect can cause this syndrome. It is diagnosed by echocardiography or MRI. PFO is found in about 20 % of the normal population. Patients with PFO after pneumonectomy may not suffer from dyspnea and desaturation in supine position, but they may occur in sitting or upright position. Though PFO is normally asymptomatic, it is a potential source for a right-to-left shunt when the pulmonary artery and right heart pressure are increased [62–66].

Perkins [63] recommended including cardiac shunt in the differential diagnosis of hypoxemia, even in the presence of normal cardiac pressures, once other more common causes have been excluded. Transesophageal echocardiography may confirm the diagnosis. If the shunt persists, it needs percutaneous or surgical closure.

7.9 Atelectasis

Atelectasis is the collapse or incomplete expansion of the lung or part of the lung. It is one of the commonest abnormalities in chest X-ray after thoracic surgery, and it may be life threatening if not treated correctly. Atelectasis can occur in 15 % of the patients, and it is seen more frequently following right upper pulmonary resections [1, 67]. The cessation of smoking before surgery and preoperative bronchodilators can help to prevent atelectasis. Predisposing factors for atelectasis after surgery are secretion retention, hypoventilation, pulmonary edema due to volume overload, decreased ciliary activity after sleeve resection, and COPD. Symptoms of the atelectasis are dyspnea, tachypnea, decreased respiratory sounds, tachycardia, and fever. Defined opacity, volume loss, fissure displacement, heightened hemidiaphragm, and mediastinal shift can be seen on a chest radiograph. Early pulmonary physiotherapy and nasotracheal aspiration are usually helpful in the postoperative period. Endobronchial aspiration and lavage with bronchoscopy may be performed (Fig. 7.3). The Thoracic Surgery Database had informed that about 3.7 % of atelectasis cases require bronchoscopy after lobectomy. Another helpful technique may be noninvasive positive-pressure ventilation and also effective pain management [5, 68, 69].

7.10 Postsurgical Empyema

Postsurgical empyema is the development of infection in the pleural space after esophageal, pulmonary, or mediastinal surgery. The incidence is higher in pneumonectomy (2–12 %) and may occur in 3 % of patients after lobectomy; the majority of these patients also present with a bronchopleural fistula (BPF) [5]. The incidence of the postsurgical empyema increases according to the indication of resection – inflammatory or neoplastic disease and the presence of a neoadjuvant therapy [70]. Risk factors include older age, cardiopulmonary impairment, malnutrition, induction therapy (especially chemoradiotherapy), diabetes, steroids, right-sided pneumonectomy, extended resections, postoperative pneumonia, and prolonged mechanical ventilation giving rise to barotrauma. Empyema can occur secondary to a spontaneous pneumothorax with persistent bronchopleural fistula [71]. PAL increases the risk of empyema up to 11 % [11]. Most of the cases develop in the early postoperative period (generally in first 3 months) but may occur also later (Fig. 7.4). The contamination of the pleural space develops from a BPF or esophagopleural fistula or from blood-borne sources. Clinical symptoms are mostly age specific and related to the general condition of the patient. The patient may be asymptomatic but may also have fever, fatigue, chest pain, dyspnea, and purulent or serosanguinous expectoration. The first sign of empyema is a change in the drainage pattern from serous to purulent, if the chest tube is still in place. And if it continues with air leak, the diagnosis of the BPF can be suspected. A pleural opacity with or without fluid level is usually detected on postoperative chest X-ray after lobectomy or segmentectomy. But after pneumonectomy, a decrease in the fluid level is visible. The most common bacterial pathogens are *Staphylococcus*, *Pseudomonas*, and anaerobic microorganisms. The treatment of the pleural empyema depends on the time of the diagnosis and the presence of the BPF and patients' general condition. The management includes antibiotic therapy and adequate chest tube thoracostomy with sensitive antibiotic solution irrigation to clean the remaining cavity [71]. After patient is stabilized (usually in 1–2 weeks), surgery may be performed. For empyema treatment,

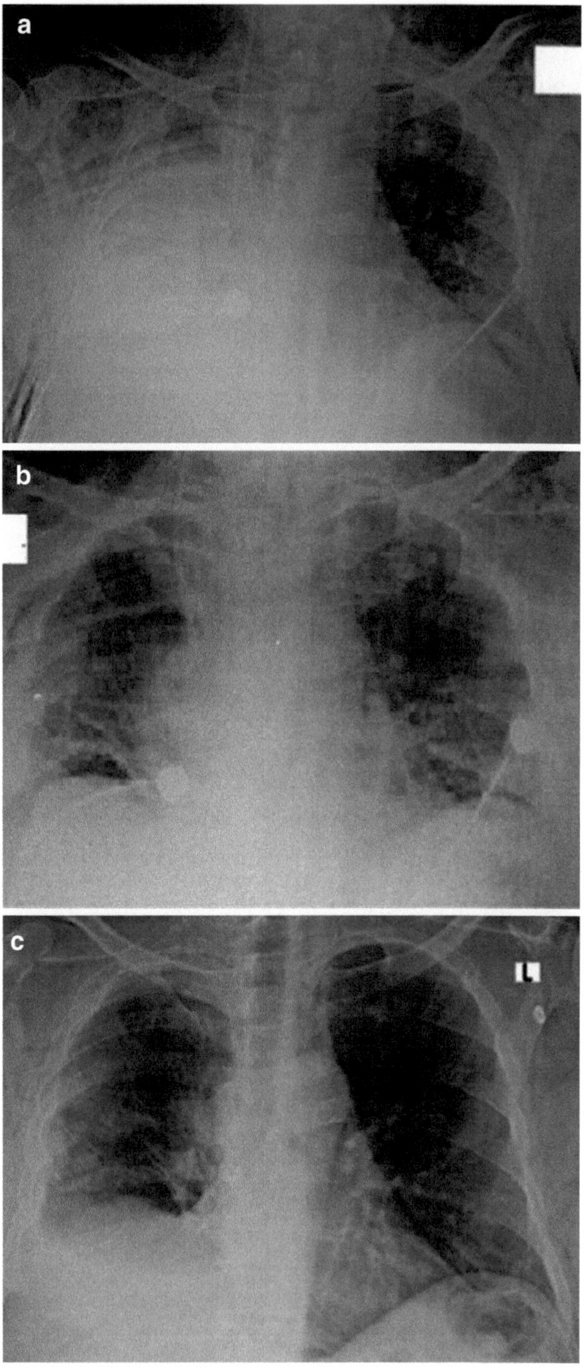

Fig. 7.3 Early pulmonary physiotherapy and nasotracheal aspiration are usually helpful in the prevention of postoperative atelectasis. Endobronchial aspiration and lavage with bronchoscopy help in the treatment of atelectasis. (**a**) Right lung atelectasis. (**b**) Immediately after the nasotracheal suction. (**c**) The next day with aggressive physiotherapy

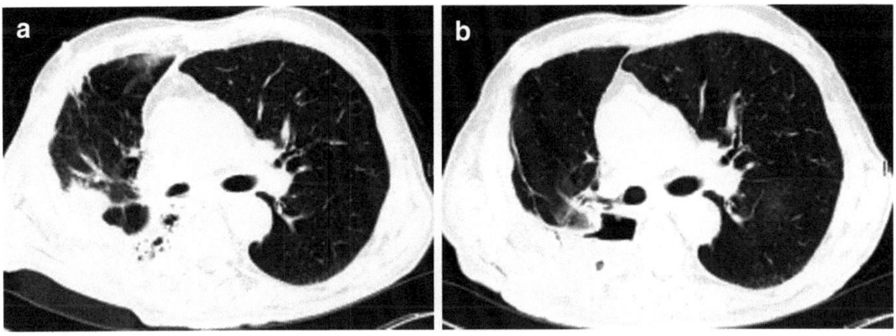

Fig. 7.4 CT scan view of a patient with empyema after lung resection (a–b)

surgeon may perform Eloesser procedure, myoplasty with muscle flap closure, thoracoplasty, or modified Clagett or Eloesser procedure [72].

7.11 Bronchopleural Fistula

BPF is a connection between the bronchus and pleural space. BPF ranges from small to large, the latter being a nightmare for thoracic surgeons often leading to life-threatening events. This complication leads to an increased morbidity and mortality after pulmonary resection. The overall incidence is 4.4 %, and it depends on the resection type [73]. Mortality rate is between 40 and 70 % of the patients with BPF after pulmonary resection [74, 75]. Risk factors of BPF include right-sided or completion pneumonectomy, surgery for infectious or inflammatory diseases, high-dose induction radiotherapy, prolonged mechanical ventilation, empyema, infected postresectional space, and residual tumor at the bronchial stump (Fig. 7.5). Most deaths are due to sepsis facilitated by aspiration pneumonia, ARDS, and malnutrition. Massive hemoptysis may be seen very rarely as a result of pulmonary artery erosion due to an infective inflammation. Most frequently a BPF is seen in 1 week after surgery [71, 72].

Small fistulas may be asymptomatic and close without any special treatment, but some BPF can lead to tension pneumothorax, aspiration pneumonia, and asphyxia. It can start with sudden dyspnea, excessive coughing, fever, fatigue, bloody sputum, and subcutaneous emphysema. In the case of tension pneumothorax, emergency chest tube drainage should be performed. If there is a suspicion of a BPF after pneumonectomy, the patient should be laid down on the operation side for protection of the opposite lung from contamination, and adequate chest drainage and antibacterial treatment should be performed [72]. Bronchoscopy is useful to confirm the diagnosis by demonstrating the presence of the BPF (Fig. 7.5). If there is no visible fistula and the suspicion continues, methylene blue injection to the bronchial stump may be performed; the drainage of the methylene blue via the chest tube is then diagnostic. During bronchoscopy, a balloon catheter may be inserted to see whether it stops the air leak. There is a typical decrease in the fluid level on the operated side after

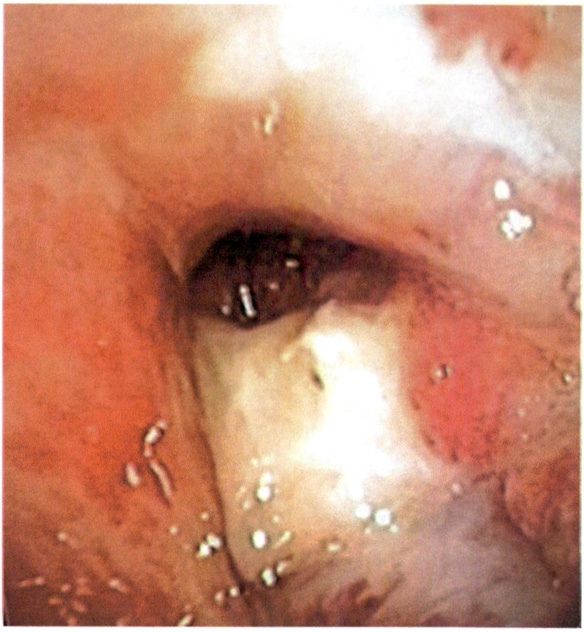

Fig. 7.5 Risk factors of bronchopleural fistula include right-sided or completion pneumonectomy, surgery for infectious or inflammatory diseases, high-dose induction radiotherapy, prolonged mechanical ventilation, empyema, infected postresectional space, and residual tumor at the bronchial stump. Bronchoscopic demonstration is the key to a definitive diagnosis

pneumonectomy. Also ventilation scintigraphy with inhalation of a radionuclide can be helpful for diagnosis. The definitive treatment should be chosen according to a diameter of the fistula and general conditions of the patient. The repair of the bronchial stump may be considered in pneumonectomy patients with early BPF (i.e., within 2 weeks). Open-window thoracoscopy can be performed for BPF with empyema treatment [71, 72].

7.12 Complications After Lung Transplantation

7.12.1 Vascular Anastomotic Complications

Complications of the arterial and venous anastomoses include stenosis, arterial kinking, and thrombus formation. Pulmonary artery stenosis has been reported in the early and late period after lung transplantation. There may be dyspnea, signs of pulmonary hypertension, and right heart failure (e.g., systemic hypotension, peripheral edema). Echocardiography may demonstrate an increased right ventricular pressure or right ventricular dysfunction. Quantitative ventilation/perfusion scan shows unequally distributed blood flow between the lungs after bilateral transplantation or disproportionate flow to the native lung after single-lung transplantation. Pulmonary angiography is usually necessary to confirm the diagnosis and helps in balloon dilatation or stent placement. Surgical reconstruction is the final option for stenosis not amenable to other interventions [73–77].

Kinking of the pulmonary artery is associated with decreased flow in the pulmonary vein, as assessed by transesophageal echocardiography [78]. Percutaneous placement of a metallic stent is recommended.

Pulmonary vein thrombosis occurs in the early postoperative period. Thrombus formation at the pulmonary venous/left atrial anastomotic suture line carries the risk of systemic embolization and cerebrovascular accident, and also it may obstruct pulmonary venous outflow and cause severe pulmonary edema refractory to medical management [79–81].

Clinical features include hypoxemia, decreased lung compliance, and diffuse radiographic opacities in the allograft. The diagnosis is made by transesophageal echocardiography.

There is no standardized management of the pulmonary vein thrombosis after lung transplantation. Fibrinolytic therapy can be useful, if the bleeding risk is not high [82]. Refractory hypoxemia and/or hemodynamic instability may require emergent surgical thrombectomy, but outcomes are usually poor. On the other hand, small venous anastomotic thrombi can resolve spontaneously [5, 83, 84].

7.12.2 Airway Complications

With the improvements in the surgical techniques and perioperative management of lung transplantation, the incidence of airway complications (AC) decreased to 10–20 % with a related mortality rate at 2–3 % [85–87]. Several risk factors for AC were identified: surgical technique, infections, and several immunosuppressive medications. The current recommendations are to avoid sirolimus at least 90 days after transplantation because of its antiproliferative properties. Donor and recipient risk factors could cause AC such as duration of donor's mechanical ventilation (50–70 h before organ retrieval) or difference between donor and recipient's bronchial diameters. Other risk factors may be primary graft dysfunction, acute cellular rejection, positive-pressure mechanical ventilation and need for a high positive end-expiratory pressure (PEEP), organ preservation technique, acute kidney injury, etc. Primary graft dysfunction, which is a type of reperfusion injury, may compromise pulmonary flow and increase the length of mechanical ventilation, and the high level of PEEP may be required. Positive-pressure mechanical ventilation and PEEP have a potential to increase the bronchial wall, and anastomosis stress and graft perfusion might be impaired when high inflation pressures are needed [88–92].

Bronchial stenosis is one of the common complications with a reported incidence between 6 and 23 % [93, 94]. It may be asymptomatic and diagnosed by routine bronchoscopy or may have a slight clinical symptom or manifestation of bronchial stenosis more frequently with increasing dyspnea, cough, post-obstructive pneumonia, or radiographic abnormalities. Bronchoscopy is a standard method for diagnosis. Management of bronchial stenosis includes balloon dilatation, ablation with cryotherapy, electrocautery or laser argon plasma coagulation, and stent placement [92, 95, 96].

7.12.3 Necrosis and Dehiscence

Isolated necrotic changes of the anastomosis may develop in patients undergoing transplantation, between first and fifth weeks. Necrosis can resolve quickly or can progress to the dehiscence. Early diagnosis is important. And if there is clinical presentation of prolonged air leak, pneumothorax, or pneumomediastinum, there exists the possibility of anastomosis dehiscence being a suspect too. Flexible bronchoscopy is a gold standard for diagnosis, and view of significant necrosis and loose sutures may be seen. Management of anastomotic dehiscence is surgical repair or even retransplantation [97].

Airway fistulas after lung transplantation are uncommon. Fistulas have been described between the airway and the pleura, mediastinum, aorta, pulmonary arteries, and left atrium. BPF is rare and may present with dyspnea, hypotension, sepsis, pneumothorax, subcutaneous emphysema, or persistent air leak. Endoscopic techniques for closing of fistula or surgical options can be used. Bronchomediastinal fistula has a high mortality, and the clinical presentation can be bacteremia, sepsis, mediastinitis, mediastinal abscess, or cavitation. Surgical treatment is recommended. Bronchovascular fistulas can present with minimal hemoptysis to fatal bleeding. These complications are rare but associated with high mortality. It should be suspected at the case of *Aspergillus* infection [97].

References

1. Stephan F, Bouchesel S, Hollande J et al (2000) Pulmonary complications following lung resection: a comprehensive analysis of incidence and possible risk factors. Chest 118(5):1263–1270
2. Lemaire A, Nikolic I, Petersen T et al (2006) Nine-year single center experience with cervical mediastinoscopy: complications and false negative rate. Ann Thorac Surg 82(4):1185–1189; discussion 1189–90
3. Peterffy A, Henze A (1983) Hemorrhagic complications during pulmonary resection: a retrospective review of 1428 resections with 113 hemorrhagic episodes. Scand J Thorac Cardiovasc Surg 17(3):283–287
4. Haithcock BE, Feins RH (2009) Complications of pulmonary resection. In: Shields TW (ed) General thoracic surgery, 7th edn. Lippincott Williams & Wilkins, Philadelphia, pp 557–559
5. Gebitekin C, Varela G, Aranda JL et al (2014) Early postoperative complications. In: Kuzdzal J, Asamura H, Detterberck F, Goldstaw P, Lerut A, Thomas P, Treasure T (eds) ESTS textbook, 1st ed. Medycyna Praktyczna, Cracow, p 85–93
6. Bertolaccini L, Terzia A, Rizzardia G et al (2012) Risk is not our business: safety of thoracic surgery in patients using antiplatelet therapy. Interact Cardiovasc Thorac Surg 14:162–166
7. Foroulis CN, Kleontas A, Karatzopoulos A et al (2014) Early reoperation performed for the management of complications in patients undergoing general thoracic surgical procedures. J Thorac Dis 6(S1):S21–S31
8. Ferrer J, Roldan J, Roman A et al (2003) Acute and chronic pleural complications in lung transplantation. J Heart Lung Transplant 22:1217–1225
9. Sugarbaker DJ, Jaklitsch MT, Bueno R et al (2004) Prevention, early detection, and management of complications after 328 consecutive extrapleural pneumonectomies. J Thorac Cardiovasc Surg 128(1):138–146
10. Karalapillai D, Larobina M, Stevenson K et al (2008) A change of heart: acute cardiac dextroversion with cardiogenic shock after partial lung resection. Crit Care Resusc 10(2): 140–143

11. Mohite PN, Sabashnikov A, Rao P et al (2013) Single lung retransplantation for graft infarction due to herniation of heart. Thorac Cardiovasc Surg Rep 2(1):40–42
12. Veronesi G, Spaggiari L, Solli PG et al (2001) Cardiac dislocation after extended pneumonectomy with pericardioplasty. Eur J Cardiothorac Surg 19(1):89–91
13. Deslauriers J, Ginsberg RJ, Piantadosi S et al (1994) Prospective assessment of 30-Day operative morbidity for surgical resections in lung cancer. Chest 106(6 Suppl): 329S–330S
14. Terauchi Y, Kitaoka H, Tanioka K et al (2012) Inferior acute myocardial infarction due to acute cardiac herniation after right pneumonectomy. Cardiovasc Interv Ther 27(2):110–113
15. Baisi A, Cioffi U, Nosotti M et al (2002) Intrapericardial left pneumonectomy after induction chemotherapy: the risk of cardiac herniation. J Thorac Cardiovasc Surg 123:1206–1207
16. Fenstad ER, Anavekar NS, Williamson E et al (2014) Acute right ventricular failure secondary to cardiac herniation and pulmonary artery compression. Circulation 129:e409–e412
17. Pillai JB, Barnard S (2003) Cardiac tamponade: a rare complication after pulmonary lobectomy. Interact Cardiovasc Thorac Surg 2(4):657–659
18. Ozawa Y, Ichimura H, Sato T et al (2013) Cardiac tamponade due to coronary artery rupture after pulmonary resection. Ann Thorac Surg 96(4):e97–e99
19. Chen J, Chen Z, Pang L et al (2012) A malformed staple causing cardiac tamponade after lobectomy. Ann Thorac Surg 94(6):2107–2108
20. McLean RH, Paradian BB, Nam MH (1999) Pericardial tamponade: an unusual complication of lobectomy for lung cancer. Ann Thorac Surg 67:545–546
21. Cable DG, Deschamps C, Ailen MS et al (2001) Lobar torsion after pulmonary resection: presentation and outcome. J Thorac Cardiovasc Surg 122(6):1091–1093
22. Stephens G, Bhagwat K, Pick A et al (2015) Lobar torsion following bilateral lung transplantation. J Card Surg 30:209–214
23. Apostolakis E, Koletsis EN, Panagopoulos N et al (2006) Fatal stroke after completion pneumonectomy for torsion of left upper lobe following left lower lobectomy. J Cardiothorac Surg 1:25
24. Crijns K, Jansen FH, van Straten AHM et al (2012) A pulmonary shadow after lobectomy: an unexpected diagnosis. Neth J Med 70(5):232–235
25. Alassar A, Marchbank A (2014) Left lower lobe torsion following upper lobectomy-prompt recognition and treatment improve survival. J Surg Case Rep 8, jju078
26. Hennink S, Wouters MWJM, Klomp HM et al (2008) Necrotizing pneumonitis caused by postoperative pulmonary torsion. Interact Cardiovasc Thorac Surg 7(1):144–145
27. Singhal S, Ferraris VA, Bridges CR et al (2010) Management of alveolar air leaks after pulmonary resection. Ann Thorac Surg 89:1327–1335
28. Brunelli A, Xiume F, Al Refai M et al (2006) Air leaks after lobectomy increase the risk of empyema but not of cardiopulmonary complications: a case-matched analysis. Chest 130(4):1150–1156
29. Cerfolio RJ, Tummala RP, Holmann WL et al (1998) A prospective algorithm for the management of air leaks after pulmonary resections. Ann Thorac Surg 66:1726–1731
30. Cerfolio RJ, Bryant AS, Maniscalco LM (2008) Management of subcutaneous emphysema after pulmonary resections. Ann Thorac Surg 85:1759–1765
31. Brunelli A, Monteverde M, Borri A et al (2004) Predictors of prolonged air leak after pulmonary lobectomy. Ann Thorac Surg 77(4):1205–1210; discussion 1210
32. DeCamp MM, Blackstone EH, Naunheim KS et al (2006) Patient and surgical factors influencing air leak after lung volume reduction surgery: lessons learned from the National Emphysema Treatment Trial. Ann Thorac Surg 82(1):197–206; discussion 206–7
33. Brunelli A, Monteverde M, Borri A et al (2004) Comparison of water seal and suction after pulmonary lobectomy: a prospective, randomized trial. Ann Thorac Surg 77(6):1932–1937; discussion 1937
34. Isowa N, Hasegawa S, Bando T et al (2002) Preoperative risk factors for prolonged air leak following lobectomy or segmentectomy for primary lung cancer. Eur J Cardiothorac Surg 21:951–954

35. Varela G, Jimenez MF, Novoa N et al (2005) Estimating hospital costs attributable to prolonged air leak in pulmonary lobectomy. Eur J Cardiothorac Surg 27(2):329–333
36. Brunelli A, Varela G, Refai M et al (2010) A scoring system to predict the risk of prolonged air leak after lobectomy. Ann Thorac Surg 90:204–209
37. Lang-Lazdunski L, Coonar AS (2004) A prospective study of autologous 'blood patch' pleurodesis for persistent air leak after pulmonary resection. Eur J Cardiothorac Surg 26(5):897–900
38. Gkegkes ID, Mourtarakos S, Gakidis I (2015) Endobronchial valves in treatment of persistent air leaks: a systematic review of clinical evidence. Med Sci Monit 21:432–438
39. Wang W, Yin W, Shao W et al (2014) Comparative study of systematic thoracoscopic lymphadenectomy and conventional thoracotomy in resectable non-small cell lung cancer. J Thorac Dis 6(1):45–51
40. Bryant AS, Minnich DJ, Wei B et al (2014) The incidence and management of postoperative chylothorax after pulmonary resection and thoracic mediastinal lymph node dissection. Ann Thorac Surg 98(1):232–235; discussion 235–7
41. Cho HJ, Kim DK, Lee GD et al (2014) Chylothorax complicating pulmonary resection for lung cancer: effective management and pleurodesis. Ann Thorac Surg 97(2):408–413
42. Fujita T, Daiko H (2014) Efficacy and predictor of octreotide treatment for postoperative chylothorax after thoracic esophagectomy. World J Surg 38(8):2039–2045
43. Shah RD, Luketich JD, Schuchert MJ et al (2012) Postesophagectomy chylothorax: incidence, risk factors, and outcomes. Ann Thorac Surg 93(3):897–903; discussion 903–4
44. Bender B, Murthy V, Chamberlain RS (2015) The changing management of chylothorax in the modern era. Eur J Cardiothorac Surg 49(1):18–24
45. Uchida S, Suzuki K, Hattori A et al (2016) Surgical intervention strategy for postoperative chylothorax after lung resection. Surg Today 46(2):197–202
46. Cerfolio RJ, Allen MS, Deschamps C et al (1996) Postoperative chylothorax. J Thorac Cardiovasc Surg 112(5):1361–1365
47. Lagarde SM, Omloo JM, de Jong K et al (2005) Incidence and management of chyle leakage after esophagectomy. Ann Thorac Surg 80(2):449–454
48. Marcon F, Irani K, Aquino T et al (2011) Percutaneous treatment of thoracic duct injuries. Surg Endosc 25(9):2844–2848
49. Kitagawa N, Shinkai M, Take H et al (2015) Mediastinoscopic extended thymectomy for pediatric patients with myasthenia gravis. J Pediatr Surg 50(4):528–530
50. Simansky DA, Paley M, Refaely Y et al (2002) Diaphragm plication following phrenic nerve injury: a comparison of paediatric and adult patients. Thorax 57:613–616
51. Kaufman MR, Elkwood AI, Rose MI et al (2011) Reinnervation of the paralyzed diaphragm: application of nerve surgery techniques following unilateral phrenic nerve injury. Chest 140(1):191–197
52. Brouillette RT, Hahn YS, Noah ZL et al (1986) Successful reinnervation of the diaphragm after phrenic nerve transection. J Pediatr Surg 21(1):63–65
53. Onders RP, Dimarco AF, Ignagni AR et al (2004) Mapping the phrenic nerve motor point: the key to a successful laparoscopic diaphragm pacing system in the first human series. Surgery 136(4):819–826
54. Kawashima S, Kohno T, Fujimori S et al (2015) Phrenic nerve reconstruction in complete video-assisted thoracic surgery. Interact Cardiovasc Thorac Surg 20:54–59
55. Bakhos C, Oyasiji T, Elmadhun N et al (2014) Feasibility of minimally invasive esophagectomy after neoadjuvant chemoradiation. J Laparoendosc Adv Surg Tech A 24(10):688–692
56. Watanabe A, Nakazawa J, Miyajima M et al (2012) Thoracoscopic mediastinal lymph node dissection for lung cancer. Semin Thorac Cardiovasc Surg 24(1):68–73
57. Luketich JD, Pennathur A, Awais O et al (2012) Outcomes after minimally invasive esophagectomy: review of over 1000 patients. Ann Surg 256(1):95–103
58. Welter S, Cheufou D, Darwiche K et al (2015) Tracheal injuries, fistulae from bronchial stump and bronchial anastomoses and recurrent laryngeal nerve paralysis: management of complications in thoracic surgery. Chirurg 86(5):410–418

59. Schneider B, Bigenzahn W, End A et al (2003) External vocal fold medialization in patients with recurrent nerve paralysis following cardiothoracic surgery. Eur J Cardiothorac Surg 23(4):477–483
60. Bhattacharyya N, Batirel H, Swanson SJ (2003) Improved outcomes with early vocal fold medialization for vocal fold paralysis after thoracic surgery. Auris Nasus Larynx 30(1):71–75
61. Krasna MJ, Forti G (2006) Nerve injury: injury to the recurrent laryngeal, phrenic, vagus, long thoracic, and sympathetic nerves during thoracic surgery. Thorac Surg Clin 16(3):267–275
62. Smeenk FW, Postmus PE (1993) Interatrial right-to-left shunting developing after pulmonary resection in the absence of elevated right-sided heart pressures. Review of the literature. Chest 103(2):528–531
63. Perkins LA, Costa SM, Boethel CD et al (2008) Hypoxemia secondary to right-to-left interatrial shunt through a patent foramen ovale in a patient with an elevated right hemidiaphragm. Respir Care 53(4):462–465
64. Bellato V, Brusa S, Balazova J et al (2008) Platypnea-orthodeoxia syndrome in interatrial right to left shunt postpneumonectomy. Minerva Anestesiol 74:271–275
65. Godart F, Rey C, Prat A et al (2000) Atrial right-to-left shunting causing severe hypoxaemia despite normal right-sided pressures. Report of 11 consecutive cases corrected by percutaneous closure. Eur Heart J 21:483–489
66. Bhattacharya K, Birla R, Northridge D et al (2009) Platypnea-orthodeoxia syndrome: a rare complication after right pneumonectomy. Ann Thorac Surg 88(6):2018–2019
67. Sanchez PG, Vendrame GS, Madke GR et al (2006) Lobectomy for treating bronchial carcinoma: analysis of comorbidities and their impact on postoperative morbidity and mortality. J Bras Pneumol 32(6):495–504
68. Korst RJ, Humphrey CB (1997) Complete lobar collapse following pulmonary lobectomy. Its incidence, predisposing factors, and clinical ramifications. Chest 111(5):1285–1289
69. Stolz AJ, Schutzner J, Lischke R et al (2008) Predictors of atelectasis after pulmonary lobectomy. Surg Today 38(11):987–992
70. Crabtree TD, Denlinger CE (2010) Complications of surgery for lung cancer. In: Pass HI, Carbone DP, Johnson DH et al (eds) Principles and practice of lung cancer. Lippincott Williams & Wilkins, Philadelphia, pp 531–546
71. Van Schil PE, Jeroen M, Hendriks JM et al (2014) Focus on treatment complications and optimal management surgery. Transl Lung Cancer Res 3(3):181–186
72. Miller Jr JI (2009) General Thoracic Surgery 7th ed. Lippincott Williams & Wilkins, Philadelphia, p 784–787
73. Waurick PE, Kleber FX, Ewert R et al (1999) Pulmonary artery stenosis 5 years after single lung transplantation in primary pulmonary hypertension. J Heart Lung Transplant 18:1243
74. Banerjee SK, Santhanakrishnan K, Shapiro L et al (2011) Successful stenting of anastomotic stenosis of the left pulmonary artery after single lung transplantation. Eur Respir Rev 20:59
75. Lumsden AB, Anaya-Ayala JE, Birnbaum I et al (2010) Robot-assisted stenting of a high-grade anastomotic pulmonary artery stenosis following single lung transplantation. J Endovasc Ther 17:612
76. Soriano CM, Gaine SP, Conte JV et al (1999) Anastomotic pulmonary hypertension after lung transplantation for primary pulmonary hypertension: report of surgical correction. Chest 116:564
77. Ahya VN, Kawut SM (2005) Noninfectious complications following lung transplantation. Clin Chest Med 26(4):613–622
78. Miyaji K, Nakamura K, Maruo T et al (2004) Effect of a kink in unilateral pulmonary artery anastomosis on velocities of blood flow through bilateral pulmonary vein anastomoses in living-donor lobar lung transplantation. J Am Soc Echocardiogr 17:998
79. Uhlmann EJ, Dunitz JM, Fiol ME (2009) Pulmonary vein thrombosis after lung transplantation presenting as stroke. J Heart Lung Transplant 28:209
80. Schulman LL, Anandarangam T, Leibowitz DW et al (2001) Four-year prospective study of pulmonary venous thrombosis after lung transplantation. J Am Soc Echocardiogr 14:806

81. Leibowitz DW, Smith CR, Michler RE et al (1994) Incidence of pulmonary vein complications after lung transplantation: a prospective transesophageal echocardiographic study. J Am Coll Cardiol 24:671
82. González-Fernández C, González-Castro A, Rodríguez-Borregán JC et al (2009) Pulmonary venous obstruction after lung transplantation diagnostic advantages of transesophageal echocardiography. Clin Transplant 23:975
83. Shah AS, Michler RE, Downey RJ et al (1995) Management strategies for pulmonary vein thrombosis following single lung transplantation. J Card Surg 10:169
84. Nagahiro I, Horton M, Wilson M et al (2003) Pulmonary vein thrombosis treated successfully by thrombectomy after bilateral sequential lung transplantation: report of a case. Surg Today 33:282
85. Meyers BF, Lynch J, Trulock EP et al (1999) Lung transplantation: a decade of experience. Ann Surg 230(3):362–371
86. Murthy SC, Blackstone EH, Gildea TR et al (2007) Impact of anastomotic airway complications after lung transplantation. Ann Thorac Surg 84:401–409
87. Fernández-Bussy S, Majid A, Caviedes I et al (2011) Treatment of airway complications following lung transplantation. Arch Bronconeumol 47(3):128–133
88. Mulligan MS (2001) Endoscopic management of airway complications after lung transplantation. Chest Surg Clin N Am 11(4):907–915
89. King-Biggs MB, Dunitz JM, Park SJ et al (2003) Airway anastomotic dehiscence associated with use of sirolimus immediately after lung transplantation. Transplantation 75(9):1437–1443
90. Van De Wauwer C, Van Raemdonck D, Verleden GM et al (2007) Risk factors for airway complications within the first year after lung transplantation. Eur J Cardiothorac Surg 31(4):703–710
91. Kshettry VR, Kroshus TJ, Hertz MI et al (1997) Early and late airway complications after lung transplantation: incidence and management. Ann Thorac Surg 63(6):1576–1583
92. Santacruzm JF, Mehta AC (2009) Airway complications and management after lung transplantation: ischemia, dehiscence, and stenosis. Proc Am Thorac Soc 6:79–93
93. Schröder C, Scholl F, Daon E et al (2003) A modified bronchial anastomosis technique for lung transplantation. Ann Thorac Surg 75(6):1697–1704
94. Herrera JM, McNeil KD, Higgins RS et al (2001) Airway complications after lung transplantation: treatment and long-term outcome. Ann Thorac Surg 71(3):989–993
95. De Gracia J, Culebras M, Alvarez A et al (2007) Bronchoscopic balloon dilatation in the management of bronchial stenosis following lung transplantation. Respir Med 101(1):27–33
96. Keller CA, Hinerman R, Singh A et al (2001) The use of endoscopic argon plasma coagulation in airway complications after solid organ transplantation. Chest 119(6):1968–1975
97. Machuzak M, Santacruz JF, Gildea T et al (2015) Airway complications after lung transplantation. Thorac Surg Clin 25(1):55–75

Should Every "Myasthenic Thymectomy" Be Sent to ICU?

8

Zerrin Sungur and Mert Şentürk

8.1 Introduction

In recent years, perioperative approach to patients with myasthenia gravis (MG) has changed substantially as a result of new information obtained about its pathology and improved the therapeutic solutions. Regarding surgical treatment, not only the experience has improved but also new minimally invasive techniques such as "video-assisted thoracoscopic extended thymectomy (VATET)" are associated with a better outcome and decreased incidence of catastrophic complications [1]. Last but not the least, regarding anesthetic approach, new drugs in our armory have challenged the classical encountered problems. Nonetheless, safe and effective treatment of a myasthenic patient in the perioperative period remains multidisciplinary. This review will focus on general information of MG and possible postoperative challenges.

8.2 General Information

Myasthenia gravis (MG) has first been described at the end of the nineteenth century as a progressive decline in the tension of simulated muscles which resolves at rest. Later in the twentieth century, it is called as an autoimmune disease affecting postsynaptic membrane in adulthood. The pediatric or juvenile form of the disease was defined later in the middle of the twentieth century. The term "juvenile MG" (JMG) is currently used for patients between 0 and 19 years old [2]. However this definition excludes neonatal MG which is caused by passive transfer of maternal

Z. Sungur (✉) • M. Şentürk
Department of Anesthesiology and Intensive Care Medicine, Istanbul University, Istanbul Faculty of Medicine, Istanbul, Turkey
e-mail: zerrin_sr@yahoo.com

© Springer International Publishing Switzerland 2017

M. Şentürk, M.O. Sungur (eds.), *Postoperative Care in Thoracic Surgery*,
DOI 10.1007/978-3-319-19908-5_8

AChR antibodies. In neonatal MG, muscle weakness is relieved in 2–4 weeks, and therapy remains mostly symptomatic.

Possibly due to better diagnosis and treatment approaches in the last decades, prevalence and incidence of MG appears to be increased [3]: The pooled incidence rate is reported to be about 5.3 per million person-years and the estimated pooled prevalence rate about 77.7 per million. For JMG, the incidence in Europe is reported to be 0.1–0.5/100.000 per year [4, 5].

MG is caused by pathogenic autoantibodies to components of the postsynaptic muscle end plate. A subgrouping based on the different antibodies has been defined recently [6]. This classification affects also the clinical approach, including surgery. Briefly, there are autoantibodies against the acetylcholine receptor (AChR), muscle-specific kinase (MuSK), and lipoprotein-related protein 4 (LRP4). MG with AChR antibodies is further divided to "early-onset" and "late-onset" MG. Moreover, "thymoma-associated," "antibody-negative generalized," and "ocular" types are also differentiated. Among them, "early-onset MG with AChR antibodies" and "thymoma-associated MG" can profit from surgical treatment. Generally, there is a close relationship between the indication for surgery and cellular abnormalities of thymic gland (hyperplasia or thymoma). JMG is often seropositive with anti-AChR [6].

8.3 Diagnosis

Initially, clinical suspicion of fluctuating muscle weakness leads to further tests of definitional diagnosis, which consists of three tests [7]:

1. Edrophonium test: Edrophonium is a short-acting anticholinesterase (anti-AChE) drug. The test is accepted as positive if patient's muscle weakness is ameliorated 45 s after drug administration and this improvement continues approximately for 5 min.
2. Electromyography: A decremented response of affected muscles for repetitive action potential is a characteristic finding of MG for EMG studies. These findings may also be seen in similar disorders such as Lambert-Eaton syndrome and certain myotonies or motor neuron diseases.
3. Detection of antibodies: The presence of anti-AChR antibodies is pathognomic for MG.

8.4 Clinical Course

Muscle weakness, which is the main feature of disorder, improves at rest and worsens with activity [8]. Therefore, a myasthenic patient who is not undergoing surgery may also require mechanical ventilation support during any exacerbation of the disease.

The common peak for age onset is at third decade and mainly in women; a secondary peak is also reported in older men after fifth decade.

Table 8.1 Myasthenia Gravis Foundation of America Clinical Classification

Stage	Clinical status
I	Only ocular involvement
II	Generalized mild muscle weakness
IIa	Predominantly affects limb and axial muscles
IIb	Predominantly bulbar involvement or respiratory weakness
III	Generalized moderate muscle weakness
IIIa	Predominantly affects limb and axial muscles
IIIb	Predominantly bulbar involvement or respiratory weakness
IV	Generalized severe muscle weakness
IVa	Predominantly affects limb and axial muscles
IVb	Predominantly bulbar involvement or respiratory weakness
V	Tracheal intubation or mechanical ventilation

MGFA Myasthenia Gravis Foundation of America

More than half of subjects have ocular signs like diplopia or ptosis. Extremity muscles are affected in such a way that results in fatigue more prominently at the end of day. In the limbs, proximal muscle groups are more frequently impaired than distal muscle groups. Patients may also present with dysphagia or dysarthria together with bulbar impairment which is an indication of a more severe disease. In such cases, possibility of aspiration or malnutrition should be investigated preoperatively. Table 8.1 summarizes clinical classification originally suggested by Osserman and later modified by the Myasthenia Gravis Foundation of America.

8.4.1 Comorbidities and Drug Interactions

Any patient with MG should be investigated for other autoimmune diseases such as endocrine diseases (thyroid disorders), rheumatoid arthritis, ulcerative colitis, and sarcoidosis, as these disorders are frequently encountered [9]. As previously mentioned, malnutrition due to dysphasia or hypothyroidism as a result of autoimmune disease requires extra attention from the anesthesiologist as they may affect postoperative recovery. If detected, these conditions must be treated prior to surgery.

Several conditions that may exacerbate the course of disease and may even cause the need for mechanical ventilation are reported. Infections, thyroid disorders, radiation, and extreme temperature are frequent pathological risk factors; however, sleep disorders, pain, or menses may also worsen patient's status [6, 9]. Besides drugs which may affect/weaken neuromuscular junction, a large variety may aggravate the course of the disease in a dose-dependent manner with antibiotic [e.g., aminoglycosides], antiarrhythmic [e.g., verapamil], and neuropsychiatric agents (Table 8.2). Although corticosteroid is a part of the therapy, it may paradoxically cause an early exacerbation of MG. If surgery should be performed at initial phase of steroid therapy, anesthetist must be aware of this worsening effect [10].

Besides drugs, electrolyte imbalances may be associated with increased muscle weakness. Hypermagnesemia is the most prominent cause as magnesium acts

Table 8.2 Myasthenia gravis drug medication list (MGFA)

Group	Risk	Drug	Comments
Antibiotics			
Aminoglycosides	2	Gentamicin, amikacin, tobramycin, neomycin, streptomycin	Eye preparation can exacerbate ocular myasthenia
Ketolide	1		
Glycopeptides	2	Telithromycin	
Lincosamide	2	Vancomycin	
Fluoroquinolones	3	Clindamycin Ciprofloxacin, levofloxacin, etc.	Eye preparation generally safe
Penicillins	4	Ampicillin, amoxicillin, penicillin G, etc.	Little evidence of causing problem
Cardiac medications			
Class I antiarrhythmics	2	Procainamide, quinidine, lidocaine, etc.	Avoid use if possible; can be used if arrhythmia is emergent and there's no alternative
Beta-blockers	3		
Calcium canal blockers		Atenolol, labetalol, metoprolol, etc.	Oral, parenteral, and ophthalmic preparations
Statins	3	Verapamil, diltiazem, nifedipine, etc. Atorvastatin, simvastatin	Verapamil is the worst; all should be used with caution
Antiepileptics			
Hydantoin	3	Phenytoin	
Barbiturate	3	Phenobarbital, pentobarbital, etc.	
Other	3	Gabapentin	
Psychiatric medications			
Antimanic	3	Lithium	
Phenothiazine	3	Chlorpromazine, fluphenazine, etc.	
Butyrophenones	3	Haloperidol	
Benzodiazepines	4	Alprazolam, lorazepam, etc.	
Miscellaneous			
Chemotherapeutics	2	Cisplatin, Fludara	
Musculoskeletal agents	2	Botulinum toxin A	Should not be used without discussing with neuromuscular specialist

(1) Contraindicated, avoid in MG even if the disease is controlled; (2) likely to worsen MG, systemic administration only with available ventilation support in a hospital; (3) may worsen MG, usually well tolerated but use with caution; (4) have caused in rare cases, usually not a problem for the majority of MG patients

as an antagonist to calcium during neuromuscular transmission. Hypermagnesemia is mostly iatrogenic like preeclampsia/eclampsia therapy. Serum magnesium levels are not always consistent with clinical course, so weakness should be carefully assessed.

Moreover iatrogenic MG has been defined with penicillamine, interferon therapy, and bone marrow transplantation. Symptoms are usually mild among these subjects, and MG is most often reversible with the discontinuation of the therapy, i.e., penicillamine and interferon. Onset after bone marrow transplantation varies between months to years. These patients require exceptional surgery.

8.4.2 The Myasthenic and the Cholinergic Crises

Crisis is defined as a need for mechanical ventilation due to respiratory muscle weakness. In patients with MG, there is a risk of developing two kinds of crises with different therapeutic approaches: the myasthenic and the cholinergic crises. The myasthenic crisis is rather an exacerbation: It can be caused or provoked by factors like respiratory infections, emotional stress, and surgery. Specific immunotherapies (plasma exchange or intravenous immunoglobulin) are associated with a rapid recovery in few days in most of the cases [6]. A limited group of myasthenic crisis requires weeks to resolve with vigorous immunosuppressive therapy with underlying cause if it exists. Residual effects of long-lasting anesthetic drugs may also impair neuromuscular function in early postoperative course as in myasthenic crisis.

The cholinergic crisis may also appear with muscle weakness with even need for invasive mechanical ventilation. However, the main etiological factor is an overdose with cholinesterase inhibitors, and clinical presentation is with signs or symptoms associated (e.g., excessive salivation, sweating, abdominal cramps, urinary urgency, bradycardia, muscle fasciculation or weakness). Differential diagnosis may be problematic in some cases necessitating a single dose of edrophonium. This agent would improve symptoms in a myasthenic crisis, but they will worsen or not be changed in a cholinergic crisis.

8.4.3 Therapy

The treatment consists of medical and surgical modalities. For an appropriate management of the perioperative period, it is useful to have some information also about the medical treatment of the patient, for it can be crucial in determining the optimal timing for the operation. The most important and common way of treatment is still symptomatic: Improving neuromuscular transmission is the key approach and achieved with an anti-AChE, mainly pyridostigmine [7, 11]. The drug results in increased ACh levels at neuromuscular junction as it decreases ACh degradation. The response to therapy may not be uniform for muscle groups [7].

Patients with anti-MuSK are less likely to respond pyridostigmine therapy [12]. In case of severe muscarinergic side effects, glycopyrronium bromide, atropine sulfate, and loperamide can be used.

Regarding the immunosuppressive therapy, corticosteroid therapy has been shown to be beneficial on slowing the progression [13]. Other alternatives for immunosuppressive therapy include azathioprine, cyclophosphamide, cyclosporine A, tacrolimus, and rituximab [6]. Patients under tacrolimus and cyclosporine therapy should be investigated preoperatively about renal impairment.

Plasma exchange and intravenous immunoglobulin are appropriate for myasthenic crisis or severe myasthenia [14]. However, both modalities can be performed prior to surgery to optimize neuromuscular function. Timing of surgery should be planned close to these aforementioned therapies in order to get the maximum benefit.

Myasthenic crisis is an emergency case and has to be treated under "intensive care" conditions with respiratory support, treatment of infections, and monitoring of vital functions and mobilization. Intravenous immunoglobulin (IVIG) and plasma exchange are options for further treatment; both can be given in sequence if necessary, as patients can respond to one but not to the other [15].

Treatment of cholinergic crisis includes endotracheal intubation, atropine, and cessation of cholinesterase inhibitors until the crisis is over.

8.5 Preoperative Evaluation

Elective surgery for myasthenic patients should be reserved for a stable period of the disease when the medication requirement is minimal for uneventful perioperative course. It is mandatory – although not sufficient – to obtain neurological optimization in order to ensure an early and safe recovery in postoperative period. It should be kept on mind that vigilant preoperative assessment by an experimented anesthetist is the first step to reduce complications and need for ICU. Management with an experienced team would be rational to distinguish high-risk myasthenic patients and to diagnose and to treat acute postoperative complications. If acute cases with a high possibility of myasthenic crisis are presented, more aggressive strategies such as plasmapheresis or intravenous immunoglobulin can be necessary for the operative preparation [15].

Prediction of postoperative myasthenic crisis (POMC) would be very beneficial, both because of possible preventive approaches and also to plan a postoperative ICU admission. A recent article proposes a new predictive score of POMC (Table 8.3) [16]: Regarding this system, patients with a score of <2.5 have the probability of having a POMC of less than 10 %, while a score of >4.0 is associated with a POMC probability of approximately 50 %.

Anti-AChE therapy on the morning of surgery is associated with two different approaches. Suspension of anti-AChE therapy can reduce neuromuscular block requirements, but it may also decrease neuromuscular recovery in early postoperative period [17]. Therefore, maintenance of pyridostigmine is generally accepted as essential for physiologic recovery in adults [18, 19].

Table 8.3 A new postoperative myasthenic crisis score [16]

Variables associated with POMC	Assigned points (0–8.5)
Osserman scale	
Stage I–IIA	0
Stage IIB	1
Stage III–IV	3
Duration of myasthenia gravis (year)	
<1	0
1–2	1
>2	2
Lung resection	
No	0
Yes	2.5
BMI	
<28	
≥28	1

POMC postoperative myasthenic crisis, *BMI* body mass index

Coexisting diseases should be carefully investigated, especially those which would affect patient's recovery such as thyroid disturbances as it affects neuromuscular recovery [7].

Routine premedication with opioids or common sedatives should be avoided or performed very carefully because they can depress the respiration. While sedating these patients, drugs having no effect on respiration (such as dexmedetomidine) can be preferred.

8.6 Perioperative Anesthetic Management

Thymectomy in indicated patients can be performed either via sternotomy ("open") or with minimally invasive methods (video-assisted thoracoscopic extended thymectomy (VATET) or robotic surgery). The advantages of VATET compared to open surgery were defined as reduced stress, lowered pain scores, early mobilization, and diminished length of stay [20–22]. Besides these benefits thoracoscopic surgery presents, a new challenge for the anesthesiologist is the inevitable use of neuromuscular blocking agents (NMBAs) for lung isolation as well as double-lumen tube insertion.

Indeed, in MG, use of NMBAs should be avoided, "if possible." The use of succinylcholine is not recommended at all, as response to depolarizing agent is variable with higher doses than healthy subjects and dual block becomes a potential risk. Regarding the use of nondepolarizing agents, the effects and duration of action can vary depending on the preoperative precautions (such as maintenance or discontinuation of pyridostigmine). Therefore, there are several series and case reports where alternative methods such as high-dose desflurane [23] or thoracic epidural anesthesia [24] have been used to avoid the NMBAs in open thymectomy and in other operations than thymectomy. In a recent cohort study, the success rate of anesthetic management for MG without NMBA was found to be 71.1 %. Interestingly, subjects requiring mechanical ventilation came from NMBA-free groups (5 %) [25]. However in VATET, one-lung ventilation (OLV) is absolutely indicated; as a consequence, NMBAs are necessary for several reasons [19]:

- Successful positioning of double-lumen tubes can be very difficult in patients without NMBAs.
- A totally "silent" lung is obligatory for a successful operation.
- Spontaneous breathing efforts are not desired during OLV as it can confer with surgical comfort.

For lung isolation, successful applications of bronchial blockers have also been reported in complicated cases [26].

The differences in sensitivity between the different types of nondepolarizing NMBAs in MG appear to be very small. Mivacurium, a short-acting NMBA, differs by elimination mechanism (hydrolysis by plasma cholinesterase). Pyridostigmine therapy was suspected to increase elimination of mivacurium. It has been shown that reduced dose of mivacurium is associated with adequate muscle relaxation and safe extubation [19]. Intermediate-acting NMBAs such as rocuronium, cisatracurium, and vecuronium have similar effects on MG patients. Empirically, 50 % of the standard dose is suggested to be adequate, albeit with an increased risk of prolonged recovery. A recent study has shown that baseline train-of-four (TOF) ratio and age of disease onset are determinants of the increased response to rocuronium in MG [27].

Neuromuscular monitoring (i.e., train-of-four or TOF) is crucial both to achieve adequate relaxation and moreover to ensure safe recovery (TOF>90) at the end of surgery. In adult MG, TOF is a part of standard monitoring independent of NMBA administration [18, 27, 28]. When reversal agents are available, TOF would be beneficial to assess objectively timing and dosing. TOF should be an obligatory monitoring in all myasthenic patients (also in other operations than thymectomy). Only a calibration before the administration of NMB can make sense; therefore, the monitoring should start before the induction [29] and continue until a TOF ratio of >0.9 (rather 1.0) has been obtained.

Generally, drugs that can even potentially affect the respiratory effort (e.g., benzodiazepines and opiates) should be avoided. Volatile anesthetics are known to affect neuromuscular transmission in a dose-dependent manner. Inhibition of postsynaptic nicotinic ACh receptors seems to have significant role with other possible mechanisms. This effect is more pronounced among myasthenic patients whose preoperative TOF ratio is less than 90 % [28]. Sevoflurane has been showed to depress T4/T1 ratio at two MAC both in myasthenic and healthy subjects [28]. Similarly desflurane has been shown to achieve comfortable intubation conditions and fast recovery as propofol [17].

Sugammadex (yet not approved by FDA) is a selective NMBA-binding agent designed to reverse the effect of the steroidal NMBA rocuronium and also vecuronium [9]. It decreases the amount of free NMBA molecules by binding the molecules making them ineffective without any intervention with the AChR or the anticholinesterases. The use of sugammadex in MG patients has been described in relative larger series in recent publications [30, 31]. Generally, use of sugammadex after (diminished doses of) rocuronium showed faster reversal and no postoperative complications. However, it must be noted that there are some case reports showing that sugammadex was not effective in the reversal of rocuronium in MG [32, 33]. Obviously, sugammadex is a new drug, and scientific and practical experience is still necessary in different patient populations including MG. For now, it is suggested as a very potential beneficial improvement.

8.6.1 Juvenile MG

Juvenile MG is often anti-AChR type and responds to thymectomy. As in adults, plasmapheresis or intravenous immunoglobulin G is indicated for refractory MG or prior to operation [34].

The benefits of thymectomy in JMG have been reported in recent series [35, 36]; furthermore, another study comparing open and thoracoscopic approaches has reported a significant decrease in hospital stay [38].

The largest series in juvenile MG reported 40 children, about one half (17 of 40) of whom was assessed as severe MG [37]. In this study, TOF monitoring was a part of monitoring of JMG patients, and with the use of reduced dose of rocuronium (1× ED95), TOF recovery greater than 1 h was not observed. Sugammadex was used safely also in this patient group.

An additional challenge for the anesthetic management of JMG is airway management for the pediatric OLV (this is actually also a general problem, even without MG). In one series, thoracoscopic thymectomy was managed without muscle relaxation in 20 children [36], whereby endotracheal intubation was achieved with single-lumen tube which does not necessitate a deep muscle relaxation. On the other hand, the benefits and necessities of lung isolation should also be considered. Double-lumen tubes (left, 28 or 32 Fr) are preferred among relatively older children (i.e., above 30 kg). For smaller children, endobronchial blockers with guidance of pediatric fiber-optic bronchoscope (3.7 mm) constitute a reliable alternative; however, its usage necessitates an experienced thoracic anesthetist familiar with pediatric cases [35].

8.7 Postoperative Follow-Up

Postoperative follow-up for MG begins with total recovery of neuromuscular function. Besides spontaneous breathing efforts, upper airway reflexes should be intact, which can be quite objectively decided by a TOF ratio of >90 %. Monitoring of TOF is also recommended during the immediate postoperative period. Clinical evaluations (such as a head lift>5 s in the conscious patient) are also helpful, but they are inferior to TOF monitoring and tongue-depressor test. Adequate tidal volume, trigger level, or blood gas analysis can also help to assess respiratory muscle function.

Residual curarization should be prevented by TOF monitoring and by reversal drugs if needed. Maintenance of the recent treatment (including anti-AChE therapy) helps physiologic recovery and should be preferred.

Effective analgesia is essential, not only to preserve pulmonary function but also to prevent a postoperative myasthenic crisis. For VATET, paravertebral analgesia with long-acting local anesthetics can be the method of choice. For open thymectomies and other operations, epidural analgesia/anesthesia is associated not only with a decrease in perioperative NMBA use but also an adequate postoperative analgesia. Intercostal blocks can be used solely or – better – as an adjunct to paravertebral or epidural analgesia. Generally, non-opioid analgesics should be preferred; NSAID or acetaminophen or dexmedetomidine can be used, although the interactions of these drugs have also not been examined in studies. If systemic opioids are inevitably required, small doses of short-acting opioids should be desirable.

Respiratory failure is a rare but serious complication. Differential diagnosis consists of residual effects of anesthetics, myasthenic crisis, and cholinergic crisis. Myasthenic crisis can be related to ongoing infection, hormonal factors, and surgical stress. The incidence has been reported between 6 and 34 % [16, 39, 40]. In two large newer series, myasthenic crisis was observed in less than 10 % of the patients [16, 39]. Related factors varied between centers such as history of myasthenic crisis, uncontrolled myasthenia, higher body mass index, combination with lung surgery or severe MG, and also impaired lung function or decremental response of orbicularis oculi muscle [16, 39, 40]. Symptoms present as a consequence of fatigue of the pharyngeal and respiratory muscles. Patients with residual anesthetic effects may benefit from noninvasive ventilation. In case of myasthenic crisis, immunomodulation is preferred with treatment of underlying cause like infection. Plasmapheresis or intravenous immunoglobulin should be administered quickly to limit crisis. In such cases, mechanical ventilation may often be necessary.

Cholinergic crisis is associated with an excess of ACh in both muscarinic and nicotinic receptors. Overstimulation of nicotinic receptors results involuntary twitching, fasciculation, and weakness which can be explained with inability to coordinate contraction and relaxation. Treatment consists on discontinuation of anti-AChE therapy.

Routine admission to the intensive care unit (ICU) with mechanical ventilation should be avoided because of several reasons such as increased infection risk, airway-associated morbidity, and not at least stress-induced myasthenic crisis.

An uneventful course is possible only with a multidisciplinary approach. Patient should be prepared for thymectomy with optimal physiological conditions. This group of patients benefit mostly of minimal invasive alternatives with reduced surgical stress. Preoperative evaluation is the cornerstone of anesthetic management, and the anesthesiologist should be familiar with the clinical course of MG. Weaning from mechanical ventilation begins at preoperative visit when planning perioperative treatment; fast-track strategies are suitable for this group.

Conclusion

The increasing number of thymectomy and especially of VATET in MG necessitates an adequate knowledge of MG. This would help in differential diagnosis of possible postoperative problems. ICU admission is rarely required; however, it may be challenging because of possible interactions of different drugs (i.e., NMBs, anti-AChE, and others), comorbidities, and non-concrete prediction of the treatment facilities. Therefore, ICU admission should be avoided as possible. An appropriate pre- and perioperative approach would help to decrease the postoperative ICU admission and prolonged mechanical ventilation.

References

1. Ozkan B, Toker A (2016) Catastrophes during video-assisted thoracoscopic thymus surgery for myasthenia gravis. pii: ivw144 [Epub ahead of print]
2. Evoli A (2010) Acquired myasthenia gravis in childhood. Curr Opin Neurol 23:536–540
3. Carr AS, Cardwell CR, McCarron PO, McConville J (2010) A systemic review of population based epidemiological studies in myasthenia gravis. BMC Neurol 10:1–9
4. Mc Grogan A, Sneddon S, de Vries CS (2010) The incidence of myasthenia gravis. Neuroepidemiology 34:171–183
5. Della Marina A, Trippe H, Lutsz S, Schara U (2014) Juvenile myasthenia gravis: recommendations for diagnostic and therapeutic approaches. Neuropediatrics 45:75–83
6. Gilhus NE, Verschuuren JJ (2015) Myasthenia gravis: subgroup classification and therapeutic strategies. Lancet Neurol 14:1023–1036
7. Sieb JP (2013) Myasthenia gravis: an update for the clinician. Clin Exp Immunol 175:408–418
8. Abel M, Eisenkraft JB (2002) Anesthetic implication of myasthenia gravis. Mt Sinai J Med 61:31–37
9. Blichfeldt-Lauridsen L, Hansen BD (2012) Anesthesia and myasthenia gravis. Acta Anesthesiol Scand 56:17–22
10. Benzing G, Bove KE (1992) Sedating drugs and neuromuscular blockade during mechanical ventilation. JAMA 267:1775
11. Hirsch NP (2007) Neuromuscular junction in health and disease. Br J Anaesth 99:132–138
12. Ionita CM, Acsadi G (2013) Management of juvenile myasthenia gravis. Pediatr Neurol 48:95–104
13. Monsul NT, Patwa HS, Knorr AM, Lesser RL, Goldstein JM (2004) The effect of prednisone on the progression from ocular to generalized myasthenia gravis. J Neurol Sci 217:131–133
14. Silvestri NJ, Wolfe GE (2014) Treatment-refractory myasthenia gravis. J Clin Neuromuscul Dis 15:167–178
15. Barth D, Nabavi N, Ng E et al (2011) Comparison of IVIg and PLEX in patients with myasthenia gravis. Neurology 76:2017–2023
16. Leuzzi G, Meacci E, Cusumano G et al (2014) Thymectomy in myasthenia gravis: proposal for a predictive score of postoperative myasthenic crisis. Eur J Cardiothorac Surg 45:76–88
17. Gritti P, Sgarzi M, Carrara B et al (2012) A standardized protocol for the perioperative management of myasthenia gravis patients. Experience of 110 patients. Acta Anesthesiol Scand 56:66–75
18. Tripathi M, Kaushik S, Dubey P (2009) The effect of use of pyridostigmine and requirement of vecuronium in patients with myasthenia gravis. J Postgrad Med 49:311–315
19. Sungur Ulke Z, Sentürk M (2009) Mivacurium in patients with myasthenia gravis undergoing video-assisted thoracoscopic thymectomy. Br J Anaesth 103:310–311
20. Toker A, Tanju S, Sungur Z et al (2008) Videothoracoscopic thymectomy for nonthymomatous myasthenia gravis: results of 90 patients. Surg Endosc 22:912–916
21. Diaz A, Black E, Dunning J (2014) Is thymectomy in non-thymomatous myasthenia gravis of any benefit? Interact Cardiovasc Thorac Surg 18:381–389
22. Toker A, Eroglu O, Ziyade S et al (2005) Comparison of early postoperative results of thymectomy: partial sternotomy vs. videothoracoscopy. Thorac Cardiovasc Surg 53:110–113
23. Koda K, Kimura H, Uzawa M et al (2014) Desflurane anesthesia without muscle relaxant for a patient with myasthenia gravis undergoing laparoscopic high anterior resection: a case report. Masui 63:1135–1138

24. Rangasamy V, Kumar K, Rai A, Baidya D (2014) Sevoflurane and thoracic epidural anesthesia for trans-sternal thymectomy in a child with juvenile myasthenia gravis. J Anaesthesiol Clin Pharmacol 30:276–278
25. Fujita Y, Moriyama S, Aoki S et al (2015) Estimation of the success rate of anesthetic management for thymectomy in patients with myasthenia gravis treated without muscle relaxants: a retrospective observational cohort study. J Anesth 29(5):794–797
26. El-Tahan MR, Doyle DJ, Hassieb AG (2014) High-frequency jet ventilation using the Arndt bronchial blocker for refractory hypoxemia during one-lung ventilation in a myasthenic patient with asthma. J Clin Anesth 26:570–573
27. Fujimoto M, Terasaki S, Nishi M, Yamamoto T (2015) Response to rocuronium and its determinants in patients with myasthenia gravis: a case–control study. Eur J Anaesthesiol 32:672–680
28. Nitahara K, Sugi Y, Higa K et al (2007) Neuromuscular effects of sevoflurane in patients with myasthenia gravis patients. Br J Anaesth 98:337–341
29. Unterbuchner C (2016) Is one acceleromyographically measured train-of-four ratio sufficient after sugammadex to identify residual curarization in postoperative, awake patients? Br J Anaesth 116:433–434
30. Sungur Ulke Z, Yavru A, Camci E et al (2013) Use of rocuronium and sugammadex in patients with myasthenia gravis undergoing video-assisted thoracoscopic extended thymectomy. Acta Anesthesiol Scand 57:745–748
31. De Boer H, Shields MO, Booij LHDJ (2014) Reversal of neuromuscular blockade with sugammadex in patients with myasthenia gravis undergoing video-assisted thoracoscopic extended thymectomy. Eur J Anaesth 31:708–721
32. Sugi Y, Nitahara K, Shiroshita T, Higa K (2013) Restoration of train-of-four ratio with neostigmine after insufficient recovery with sugammadex in a patient with myasthenia gravis. A A Case Rep 1:43–45
33. Kiss G, Lacour A, d'Hollander A (2013) Fade of train-of-four ratio despite administration of more than 12 mg kg(−1) sugammadex in a myasthenia gravis patient receiving rocuronium. Br J Anaesth 110:854–855
34. Liew WK, Powell CA, Sloan SR et al (2014) Comparison of plasmapheresis and intravenous immunoglobulin as maintenance therapies for juvenile myasthenia gravis. JAMA Neurol 71(5):575–580
35. Özkan B, Demir A, Kapdağlı M et al (2015) Results of videothoracoscopic thymectomy in children: analysis of 40 patients. Interact Cardiovasc Thorac Surg 1:1–4
36. Kitagawa N, Shinkai M, Take H et al (2015) Mediastinoscopic extended thymectomy for pediatric patients with myasthenia gravis. J Pediatr Surg 50:528–530
37. Goldstein SD, Culbertson NT, Garrett D et al (2015) Thymectomy for myasthenia gravis in children: a comparison of open and thoracoscopic approaches. J Pediatr Surg 50:92–97
38. Christison-Lagay E, Dharia B, Vajsar J, Kim PC (2013) Efficacy and safety of thoracoscopic thymectomy in the treatment of juvenile MG. Pediatr Surg Int 29:583–586
39. Seok Lee H, Sun Lee H, Eun Lee H et al (2015) Predictive factors for myasthenic crisis after videoscopic thymectomy in patients with myasthenia gravis. Muscle Nerve 52(2):216–220
40. Ando T, Omasa M, Kondo T et al (2015) Predictive factors of myasthenic crisis after extended thymectomy for patients with myasthenia gravis. Eur J Cardiothorac Surg 48(5):705–709

9 How About Esophagectomies?

Tamás Végh

9.1 Indications of Esophagectomy

Surgical procedures of the esophagus are very unique and difficult in terms of surgery, anesthesia, and postoperative care. The reason is that esophagus passes through three regions of the body, so surgical procedure may be performed in the cervical, thoracic, and abdominal region or in more than one region in same time.

The most common reason for esophagectomy is cancer; however, it can also be a result of Barrett's esophagus, hiatus hernia, achalasia, stricture, rupture of the esophagus, or congenital conditions.

The two most common types of esophageal cancer are squamous cell carcinoma, originating in the thoracic part of the esophagus, and adenocarcinoma, which arises from the glandular cells lining in the distal part of the esophagus and at the esophagogastric junction.

The preferred treatment for esophageal cancer is surgery. However, for many patients, surgery is combined with chemotherapy, radiation therapy, or hormone therapy. These nonsurgical treatments may be administered before surgery (neoadjuvant therapy) or after surgery (adjuvant therapy) [1–5].

9.2 Types of Esophagectomy

Esophagectomy is a high-risk procedure, and the complication rate is high due to the anatomic challenges of the procedure. Esophagectomy may be done using either of two main types of techniques: open and minimal invasive method. In the

T. Végh
University of Debrecen, Department of Anesthesiology and Intensive Care, Debrecen, Hungary

Outcomes Research Consortium, Cleveland, OH, USA
e-mail: veghdr@gmail.com

© Springer International Publishing Switzerland 2017

M. Şentürk, M.O. Sungur (eds.), *Postoperative Care in Thoracic Surgery*,
DOI 10.1007/978-3-319-19908-5_9

standard, open technique, the surgeon operates through one or more large incisions in the neck, chest, or abdomen.

The choice of surgical approach depends upon the tumor location, submucosal extension, adherence to the surrounding tissues, the conduit to be used to restore gastrointestinal continuity, and the extent of lymphadenectomy [6] (Table 9.1). Although the gastric interposition is most commonly used as a conduit for reconstruction following esophagectomy, the jejunum or the colon can also be used as the conduit. These conduits are resistant to the effects of gastric acid, and they have a shape similar to the native esophagus [21–23].

9.3 Preoperative Preparation for Esophagectomy

Preoperative selection and patient preparation are crucial for esophagectomy because an esophageal resection results in a large physiologic insult to the patient. Although the mortality from esophagectomy has decreased in the last decades, adequate patient selection is an important issue of that reduction in mortality by identifying high-risk patients in whom the procedure would be too hazardous. During the preoperative evaluation, anesthesiologists have to consider many factors, including age, cardiac and pulmonary function, nutritional status, medications, neoadjuvant therapy, and blood transfusion.

Cardiopulmonary function evaluation is the same as for lung resection procedures [24–26].

9.4 Anesthesia for Esophagectomy

Detailed review of anesthesia for esophagectomy has been previously addressed. However, there are factors during the anesthesia which have influence on postoperative period after esophagectomy.

Although the incidence of anastomotic complications decreased in the last decades, anastomotic complications and perfusion of the conduit are important issues after esophagectomy, as it has been accounted for 37 % of all hospital death after esophagectomy. Thoracic anastomoses have lower leak rate than cervical anastomoses but have higher morbidity and mortality. One of the factors that are playing role in the incidence of anastomotic leaks is conduit ischemia. Appropriate tissue oxygenation depends on several variables: vascular anatomy and tone and blood oxygen tension. How can anesthesiologist improve blood supply of the conduit? Thoracic epidural anesthesia and the use of prostaglandins have influence on gastric vasomotor tone; the use of intravenous nitroglycerin and venous bloodletting can reduce venous congestion. Systemic hypotension may impair gastric tube perfusion and must be treated. The use of vasoconstrictors in normovolemic condition has no detrimental effect on gastric blood flow, and the use of short-acting vasopressors as phenylephrine or ephedrine is safe and not associated with postoperative anastomotic leak. Before the use of vasopressors hypovolemia should always be excluded.

Table 9.1 Types of esophagectomy

Resection name	Indication	Surgical resection	Disadvantages
Cervical esophageal resection	Carcinoma of the cervical esophagus	Removal of portions of the pharynx, the larynx, the thyroid gland, and portions of the proximal esophagus. This one-stage, three-phase operation requires cervical, abdominal, and thoracic incisions and a permanent terminal tracheostomy [7, 8]	
Transhiatal esophagectomy	Cervical, thoracic, and esophagogastric junction cancers	Upper midline laparotomy incision and a left neck incision, typically without a thoracotomy. The thoracic esophagus is bluntly dissected through the diaphragmatic hiatus superiorly and via the neck inferiorly. A cervical anastomosis is created most often with a gastric pull-up approach [9, 10]	Inability to perform a full thoracic lymphadenectomy
Ivor-Lewis transthoracic esophagectomy	Cancers in the lower third of the esophagus	Laparotomy with a right thoracotomy and an intrathoracic esophagogastric anastomosis allowing a full thoracic lymphadenectomy	Leak occurring at the intrathoracic anastomosis is associated with high morbidity and mortality [11–13]
Modified Ivor-Lewis transthoracic esophagectomy	Tumors of the gastroesophageal junction	Left thoracoabdominal incision with a gastric pull-up and an esophagogastric anastomosis in the left side of the chest	High incidence of complications [14]
Tri-incisional esophagectomy		Transthoracic total esophagectomy, a lymphadenectomy, and cervical esophagogastric anastomosis [15, 16]	
Esophagogastric junction resection	Esophageal cancers at the esophagogastric junction or intra-abdominal esophagus	An esophagectomy with partial gastrectomy or an extended gastrectomy, with or without thoracotomy [17, 18]	
Minimal invasive approach		Either total endoscopic resection with thoracoscopic or laparoscopic approaches. Advantages are less surgical stress and pain, shorter ICU and hospital stay, decreased incidence of postoperative complications combined with quicker return to working, less intraoperative blood loss	Prolonged surgical time, one-lung ventilation in prone position that may result in impaired oxygenation [19, 20]

Another important anesthesia technique which has influence on postoperative outcome and complication is ventilation during esophagectomy. Esophagectomy often requires one-lung ventilation. It has been demonstrated that lung-protective ventilation with small tidal volume and with the use of moderate PEEP provides sufficient oxygenation during OLV and resulted in reduced inflammatory response after esophagectomy, improved lung function, and earlier extubation [27–29].

9.5 Postoperative Care After Esophagectomy

9.5.1 Timing of Extubation and Supplemental Oxygen Therapy

Timing of extubation is a crucial issue after esophagectomy. Basically there are two concepts of extubation after esophagectomy: prolonged ventilation and early extubation. Before the introduction of thoracic epidural analgesia, studies suggested prolonged postoperative ventilation up to 2 days. However, prolonged ventilation has not been shown to decrease incidence of postoperative pulmonary complications. Moreover, there are disadvantages of this approach: sedation-related side effects, risk of aspiration, and weaning problems.

The use of thoracic epidural and shorter operative time, early extubation has been advocated to reduce mortality, morbidity, and cost after esophagectomy. Early extubation may reduce intensive stay and cost, decreases postoperative respiratory complications, and does not increase the risk of reintubation.

However, there are conditions that could require prolonged ventilation: bleeding, hemodynamic instability, respiratory insufficiency, and neurologic impairment.

After extubation supplemental oxygen administration should be used either by face mask or nasal cannula (1–6 l/min) for maintaining of oxygen saturation above 90 %. Supplemental oxygen has advantages after esophagectomy: decreased incidence of postoperative nausea and vomiting, improved wound healing, maintenance of adequate cardiac and central nervous function, and decreased incidence of arrhythmias. There are data that low oxygen delivery after esophagectomy is associated with the risk of complications [30–32].

9.5.2 Analgesia

Effective analgesia after esophagectomy is a challenging issue in anesthesia. As we noted above, this procedure often requires an abdominal, cervical incision and either thoracotomy as well.

Analgesia for thoracic procedures has been discussed extensively in another chapter of this book. However, it is important to remember that sympathetic activation caused by surgical procedure and pain manifests as tachycardia, hypertension, and increased contractility, all of which result in increased myocardial oxygen consumption. As it has been noted, most of the patients undergoing esophagectomy have cardiovascular coexisting diseases, especially ischemic heart disease (IHD).

These patients' response to surgical stress differs from that of healthy patients. Sympathetic stimulation caused by pain may constrict post-stenotic coronary arteries and reduce blood supply to the subendocardium. The difference in oxygen delivery and demand presents as postoperative myocardial ischemia. The selective sympathectomy using thoracic anesthesia in patients with IHD can dilate constricted coronary vessels, reduce heart rate, and improve cardiac function by reducing preload and afterload and optimizing myocardial oxygen delivery.

The sympathectomy of thoracic epidural analgesia causes vasodilatation in mesenteric vessels and has been shown to improve bowel function by reducing the duration of postoperative ileus, enhancing bowel blood. The increase in bowel motility from unopposed parasympathetic activity is not associated with any significant increase in anastomotic dehiscence.

In patients in whom thoracic epidural analgesia is contraindicated, there are several alternative methods. Using intercostal nerve block a catheter is placed in a paravertebral space just below the level of incision. Effectiveness of this method is mostly similar to epidural analgesia. Intravenous opioids and nonsteroid analgesics can work synergistically and can reduce postoperative pain [33–37].

9.5.3 Fluid Management

Fluid management is also crucial for all thoracic surgeries including esophagectomy and has been discussed extensively in a separate chapter of this book. Anesthesiologists should consider a restrictive fluid administration in the first 24 h (<20 ml/kg, less than 2 L crystalloid and less than 1 L albumin intraoperatively with less than 3 L of total amount of crystalloids in the first 24 h).

Therefore, close monitoring of intravascular volume status is required, along with invasive hemodynamic monitoring (arterial blood pressure, central venous pressure, thermodilution techniques) and urine output [38–41].

9.5.4 Nutrition Considerations

Patients undergoing esophagectomy are frequently malnourished due to several reasons: stenosis of the esophagus by the tumor, systemic effects of the tumor, side effects of the chemotherapy, and surgery.

Most common problem in patients with esophageal cancer is difficult swallowing. These patients eat only soft, easy-to-swallow foods, primarily consume liquids. Therefore, patients with dysphagia are at risk for deficiencies in protein, fat, carbohydrate, vitamins, minerals, and total calorie.

Nutritional assessment helps to identify the nutritional status and risk of malnutrition. Nutritional history and anthropometric parameters can be inaccurate; however, assessment of the metabolically active body cells by bioelectrical impedance may solve as a better marker. Assessment of sarcopenia, defined as loss of skeletal mass and strength, helps to identify high-risk patients who require perioperative nutrition.

Table 9.2 Biomarkers of nutritional status [44]

Biomarker	Normal range	Half-life
Albumin	35–50 g/L	12–20 days
Transferrin	2–3.6 g/L	8–9 days
C-reactive protein	<10 mg/L	2 days
Prealbumin	160–400 mg/L	12 h
Retinol-binding protein	30–80 mg/L	12 h

Biomarkers, such as albumin, transferrin, C-reactive protein, prealbumin, and retinol-binding protein, are also used in assessing nutritional condition (Table 9.2). However, in postoperative period, accuracy of these biomarkers is questionable. Medication, inflammation, changes in fluid shift and vascular permeability, and hepatic and renal function have influence on levels of biomarkers. However, data are showing that patients with hypoalbuminemia are at risk of postoperative complications compared with those who have normal albumin level.

There are several nutritional scoring systems for nutritional assessment. The Subjective Global Assessment (based on patient's history, loss of subcutaneous fat, muscle wasting, and presence of edema or ascites) has high sensitivity and specificity. The prognostic nutritional index is focusing on serum albumin level and current and usual weight. The Nutritional Risk Screening Score is based on the severity of nutritional status. An accurate estimation of energy expenditure is important in patients with nutritional disorders. The traditionally used Harris-Benedict equation is inaccurate, and the indirect calorimetry is the gold standard method to measure caloric requirements.

It is known that malnutrition is associated with increased rate of postoperative complications (including impaired wound healing, loss of muscle tissue, reduced immunocompetence, depression, apathy, immobility, and increased frequency of decubitus and ulcer) and delayed recovery.

Benefits have been found when severely malnourished patients received nutrition support prior to surgery. There are different ways for preoperative nutrition support. Most physiological route is the enteral way. Dysphagic patients should be modifying the consistency of food. It can include normal food with accurate chewing and or soft, pureed and blenderized foods. Patients should learn to eat frequently and smaller portions, because pureed foods have larger volume than normal foods containing same calories.

If these modifications are insufficient, there are options for insertion of a nasogastric or nasojejunal tube, feeding jejunostomy, or percutaneous endoscopic gastrostomy (PEG). Nevertheless, most of the surgeons do not prefer the use of PEG because stomach is most frequently used as conduit that forms the new esophagus.

There are different methods for delivery. Continuous feeding is used if a patient is unable to tolerate large volumes of feed and usually refers to feeding over 16–20 h. In this case, feed is delivered by pump. Continuous feeding usually includes a break of at least 4 h in 24 h to allow the stomach to re-acidify. The second method is the intermittent feeding that involves periods of feeding using the pump with breaks. The third way is the bolus feeding involves the delivery of 100 mls to 300 mls over a period of 10–30 min and can be given four to six times a day depending on patients' individual feeding regime.

There are several type of feeds is available. Standard whole-protein feeds provide 1 kcal/ml, while high-energy feeds provide 1.5 kcal/ml. High-energy feeds are useful when fluid is restricted or to reduce feeding time. Most feeds are lactose-, gluten-, and wheat-free and suitable for vegetarians.

There is no need to change the regime in diabetic patients, but blood glucose level should be monitored frequently.

Feeding tubes should be flushed with water before and after administration of feed and medication and in between medications.

It is known that enteral nutrition is cheaper than parenteral nutrition, and it is comfortable, because patients can be fed at home. Nevertheless, in severely undernourished patients who cannot be fed adequately orally or enterally, preoperative parenteral nutrition is indicated. Moreover, parenteral nutrition requires hospitalization and sophisticated nursing.

Surgical stress leads to insulin resistance and increases blood glucose levels. In diabetic patients, blood glucose should be monitored every 4–6 h. Guidelines suggest that blood glucose be maintained between 5.5 and 11 mmol/l in stressed patients and then tightened to 5.5–8.5 mmol/l once control is established.

Good oral hygiene is essential for patients receiving nutritional support or nil by mouth. Saliva is normally produced when eating and keeps the mouth clean. However, saliva production is often reduced during nutritional support and the oral mucosa can develop sores. Patients should be encouraged to brush their teeth regularly and use a suitable mouth rinse [42–52].

9.5.5 Blood Administration

Regardless of the specific approach (transthoracic versus transhiatal), esophagectomy with lymphadenectomy represents a major operation with a mean operative blood loss of 3–500 ml approximately. The use of neoadjuvant chemotherapy can cause bone marrow suppression and anemia in patients undergoing esophagectomy. All of these factors require consideration of administration of blood transfusion in the perioperative period. Nevertheless, there are evidences that blood transfusion may worsen the oncologic outcome, though these reports were uncontrolled. Patients who received blood transfusion have had larger tumors, more sever medical conditions. Therefore, the relationship between cancer recurrence and death has not been clearly proven.

The ideal perioperative hemoglobin level is not clear. Keeping the hemoglobin level above 100 g/l is poorly supported with evidences. Recently, in hemodynamically stable patients, the transfusion trigger is 70 g/l.

There are evidences that the use of allogenic blood transfusion decreases survival and increases the incidence of cancer recurrence, compared with the use of autologous transfusion [53, 54].

9.5.6 Deep Vein Thrombosis Prophylaxis

Postoperatively, a majority of thoracic surgery patients are not able to move because of pain, respiratory distress, and age. The lack of ambulation can result in a blood stasis in lower extremities; this increases the contact time between blood and vein wall irregularities, helping a blood clot formation. The incidence of deep venous thrombosis in patients in medical and surgical intensive care units is about 10 % to 30 %. Prophylaxis with mechanical (compression stockings are applied to both lower extremities) and pharmacological methods (heparin shots are given subcutaneously twice a day) has been shown to be effective and safe in most types of surgery and should be routinely implemented. Both subcutaneous, low-dose unfractionated heparin (LDUH) and low-molecular-weight heparin (LMWH) have been shown to reduce the risk of venous thrombosis. Low-dose unfractionated heparin use does not interfere with epidural catheter placement or removal. However, LMWH should be held for 12–24 h before epidural placement or removal, to decrease the risk of hematoma formation. The use of LMWH for 2–3 weeks after hospital discharge in patients undergoing major cancer surgery may reduce the incidence of asymptomatic deep venous thrombosis.

Until patients are ambulating independently, they should keep the stockings on when in bed. Encourage early ambulation as well as leg and ankle exercises. Early mobilization of patients includes getting them out of bed to a chair the first postoperative day and three times each day thereafter [54, 55].

9.5.7 Management of Drainage Tubes

Chest tubes are indwelling catheters placed into the pleural space to evacuate air and fluids and maintain a physiological negative pleural pressure. Air collects at the less dependent part (apically or retrosternal, depending on patient's position), and fluid collects at the lower part of the chest cavity. That's why most guideline recommends the use of two chest tubes.

In the absence of air leak (50 ml/min in 12 h or less than 20 ml/min in 8 h), most postoperative chest tube removal protocol is based on quantity and quality of secretions. If bleeding, chylothorax, or empyema does not exist, the normal daily pleural secretion is about 350 ml. Most surgeons remove chest drains if the daily secretion is less than 300 ml.

If an air leak exists, a digital drainage system with continuous suction with (minus15 cmH2O) is recommended. If air leak reach less than 50 ml/min in 12 or 20 ml/min in 8 h, chest tubes are removable.

As chest tubes are playing major role in postoperative pain, their early removal appears to accelerate postoperative recovery [56, 57].

9.5.8 Physiotherapy

Respiratory complications are frequent after esophagectomy. The benefits of physiotherapy in the perioperative period have been shown by numerous studies.

It has been showed that preoperative physiotherapy (e.g., inspiratory muscle training) for two or more weeks before cardiac surgery reduced the incidence of pulmonary complications. Preoperative physiotherapy is also feasible for patients undergoing esophagectomy to preserve respiratory muscle strength.

There are two main types of breathing exercises: active cycles of breathing and using incentive spirometry. Both techniques aim to re-expand the lung with maximum sustained and fractional inspiration and clear airways with assisted cough.

For both types of exercises, patients must be in upright position either in bed or chair. During active cycle of breathing, patients must place hand over upper abdomen and take slow deep breaths and hold for 3–5 s and repeat four to five times. After this cycle, the patient has to huff as this maneuver helps move phlegm to clear.

Using incentive spirometer, patient inhales from the spirometer and holds breath as long as it is possible. This should be practiced up to ten breaths per hour. It is important to mobilize patients as soon as possible after esophagectomy to prevent postoperative complications such as pneumonia and deep vein thrombosis. At the first day, the aim is to sit in chair that can help to improve lungs by increasing the depth of each breath. By the second postoperative day, patients should aim to walk with assistance on the ward and increase gradually the exercise tolerance.

Due to the wound and chest drains, patients may be reluctant to move arm on the operated side. It is important to practice shoulder mobility to prevent joint stiffness [24, 58–61].

9.6 Management of Complications After Esophagectomy

Complications after esophagectomy include pulmonary complications (including pleural effusions, atelectasis, chylothorax, pneumonia, respiratory failure, and pulmonary embolism) as well as wound infection, empyema, bronchopleural fistula, recurrent laryngeal nerve injury, cardiac complications such as arrhythmias and atrial fibrillation, and complications of the conduit.

9.6.1 Anastomotic Leak

Esophageal anastomotic leak is a serious complication after esophageal surgery. Incidence is about 14 %, and the associated mortality is between 5 % and 35 %. Anastomotic leak or perforation occurs because of several conditions (ischemia or distention of conduit, poor nutrition, low serum albumin level, pressure at suture lines and anastomotic tension, intraoperative bleeding, tumor at resection margin, use of colon as conduit, drain contacts with the anastomosis). Leakage of digestive fluids, saliva, overgrowth of bacteria, and fungi in the perianastomotic tissues can lead to severe inflammation.

Clinical presentation of the anastomosis insufficiency depends on the size and location of the dehiscence. Symptoms of the thoracic leak could be fever, leukocytosis, chest pain, arrhythmia and hypotension, fulminant sepsis, and increased output through the drains, while cervical leak can be present as a simple neck infection.

Integrity of the anastomosis can be evaluated with swallowing methylene blue or using water-soluble contrast agent.

Although most of the anastomotic leakage can be managed conservatively with drainage and broad-spectrum antibiotics, in severe cases surgical approach may be required.

Treatment is determined by the location and size of the leak. If the leak is at the cervical anastomosis, the neck wound is opened to allow drainage and healing over time. This can lead to stricture which requires dilation, but that is usually not incapacitating. The patient should generally be kept nothing per os to reduce the pressure and fluid draining past the hole. Administration of antibiotics that provide coverage for aerobes and anaerobes (ampicillin/sulbactam 3 g every 6 h or piperacillin/tazobactam 3.375 g every 6 h or a carbapenem) must be initiated along with adequate drainage. In case of beta lactam hypersensitivity, administration of clindamycin (900 mg every 8 h) with ciprofloxacin (400 mg every 12 h) is appropriate. Antifungal coverage (400 mg fluconazole in a single dose) is recommended in selected cases. Swallow test with methylene blue is repeated 1 week after the initial test. If the leak is smaller, the nasogastric tube can be removed and the patient can drink clear fluid. As the leak healed, the patient's diet is advanced to a normal diet. If the leak is more than a quarter of the circumference of the anastomosis, surgical intervention should be considered.

In case of intrathoracic anastomotic leakage, contamination of pleural cavity or mediastinum may occur. A leak into the pleural cavity should be drained with chest tubes. Fasting by mouth is necessary. Intravenous antibiotics should be administered unless the patient has no signs of infection (fever, leukocytosis, decrease of procalcitonin, and CRP level). Leakage of mediastinal anastomosis and resulted mediastinitis may remain undetected for prolonged time and can be fatal if it is not evacuated [62–65].

9.6.2 Anastomotic Stricture

Stricture after esophageal resection can occur at different places: at the anastomosis, at the diaphragmatic hiatus, or at the pylorus. Stricture may be secondary to technical problems, ischemia, leak, ulceration, or reflux, and it may be multifactorial. Most strictures can be treated with either balloon or bougie dilation [66, 67].

9.6.3 Conduit Ischemia

The viability and function of the esophageal conduit are the most important factors affecting postoperative outcome and quality of life. It can be difficult to diagnose the conduit ischemia in the postoperative period after esophagectomy. Average rates of ischemic complications for stomach, colon, and jejunum are 3.2 %, 5.1 %, and 4.2 %, respectively. Signs of infection, elevated level inflammatory markers (C-reactive protein, procalcitonin), and symptoms (tachycardia, respiratory failure, fever, leukocytosis, or any evidence for graft or anastomotic leak) should suggest problems due to insufficient blood supply of the conduit. The diagnostic tools include contrast esophagography, endoscopy, or direct operative inspection. Without treatment conduit ischemia can lead to further morbidity or mortality. Treatment for mild cases may be supportive, with or without management of anastomotic leak. In more severe cases of necrosis debridement, takedown of the anastomosis and creation of an esophagostomy are recommended [68, 69].

9.6.4 Functional Conduit Disorders

9.6.4.1 Postgastrectomy Syndrome

Postgastrectomy syndromes include small capacity, early and late dumping syndrome, postvagotomy diarrhea, afferent loop syndrome, efferent loop syndrome, alkaline reflux gastritis, roux stasis syndrome, anemia, and metabolic bone disease (impaired absorption of calcium, vitamin D, vitamin B, iron, copper).

Dumping syndrome may occur due to the loss of pyloric regulation and receptive relaxation. This can lead to rapid emptying of stomach contents into proximal bowel. Early dumping is initiated 10–30 min after ingestion. Symptoms are nausea, vomiting, feeling of postprandial epigastric, fullness, crampy pain, and belching, explosive diarrhea. Dumping syndrome can be accompanied or followed by cardiovascular symptoms (tachycardia, palpitations, diaphoresis, light-headedness).

Pathophysiologic mechanism of early dumping syndrome is that rapid entry of hyperosmolar chyme into the small bowel triggers rapid fluid shifts from the intravascular space to the gut lumen to maintain isotonicity and this leads to gut distention. This fluid shifts can cause hypotension, triggering autonomic catecholamine surge. Early dumping syndrome can be diagnosed with oral administration of 50 g glucose as a provocative test. Therapy of early dumping syndrome is based on control of feeding that includes frequent small meals, separation of solid foods and liquids, and avoiding high-carb meals.

Late dumping syndrome usually occurs 2–3 h after meals and much less common than early dumping syndrome. Pathophysiology of this syndrome is different from the pathophysiology of the early dumping syndrome. In this case rapid delivery of sugars into small bowel causes hyperglycemia and increase in insulin release, inducing a marked hypoglycemia. Concomitant insulin shock causes catecholamine release with tachycardia, tachypnea, diaphoresis, palpitation sensations, and confusion. Medical management is dietary modification or surgery in refractory cases.

The postvagotomy diarrhea for the vast majority is not severe and resolves after several months. In severe form, it may be 10–20 episodes per day which are often explosive, and often there is no temporal relationship with food. It may occur at all times (during sleep) and may result in weight loss, malnutrition, and weakness. Explanation of the syndrome is that vagal denervation leads to intestinal dysmotility and rapid gastric emptying of liquids. Postvagotomy diarrhea is much less common after highly selective vagotomy. Complications could be hypoacidity, malabsorption of bile acids, and bacterial overgrowth in the proximal bowel. Therapy contains more fiber intake, frequent small meals, decreased carbohydrate intake, oral administration of neomycin to treat bacterial overgrowth, and administration of antidiarrheal agents such as loperamide.

Afferent and efferent limb syndrome may be acute, completely obstructed or chronic, and partially obstructed. The syndrome can manifest at any time from the first postoperative day to many years after surgery. The acute form usually occurs in the early postoperative period (first to second week), but it has been described to occur 30–40 years after surgery [70–72].

9.6.4.2 Reflux

Gastroesophageal reflux is a common phenomenon in patients after esophagectomy. Loss of the lower esophageal sphincter plays a key role in the emergence of reflux. The lower portion of the stomach remains in the abdomen under positive intraperitoneal pressure, while the upper portion of the stomach is in the thoracic cavity under negative intrathoracic pressure. Patients after esophagectomy need to be counseled to eat and drink in the upright position and remain upright for at least 2 h after eating. The head of the bed should be elevated 30°, or they should sleep on a foam wedge to avoid regurgitation and aspiration. Avoiding damage to the recurrent laryngeal nerves helps to prevent from aspiration when reflux occurs [73, 74].

9.7 Summary

Due to the prolonged and complex surgical procedure and poor preoperative condition of the patients, esophagectomy leads to significant mortality and morbidity. Surgical technique, adequate analgesia, careful anesthesia, strictly controlled fluid management, and optimal timing of extubation may decrease the incidence of complications (respiratory, cardiac complications, and problems of the conduit). Inadequate preoperative diet also contributes in increased mortality and morbidity. Adequate nutrition is a crucial issue after esophagectomy.

References

1. Mariette C, Piessen G, Triboulet JP (2007) Therapeutic strategies in oesophageal carcinoma: role of surgery and other modalities. Lancet Oncol 8(6):545–553
2. Holmes RS, Vaughan TL (2007) Epidemiology and pathogenesis of esophageal cancer. Semin Radiat Oncol 17(1):2–9
3. Hirst J, Smithers BM, Gotley DC, Thomas J, Barbour A (2011) Defining cure for esophageal cancer: analysis of actual 5-year survivors following esophagectomy. Ann Surg Oncol 18(6):1766–1774
4. Miyata H, Yamasaki M, Kurokawa Y et al (2011) Multimodal treatment for resectable esophageal cancer. Gen Thorac Cardiovasc Surg 59(7):461–466
5. Narsule CK, Montgomery MM, Fernando HC (2012) Evidence-based review of the management of cancers of the gastroesophageal junction. Thorac Surg Clin 22(1):109–121
6. Lagarde SM, Vrouenraets BC, Stassen LP, van Lanschot JJ (2010) Evidence-based surgical treatment of esophageal cancer: overview of high-quality studies. Ann Thorac Surg 89(4):1319–1326

7. Daiko H, Hayashi R, Saikawa M et al (2007) Surgical management of carcinoma of the cervical esophagus. J Surg Oncol 96(2):166–172
8. Peracchia A, Bonavina L, Botturi M, Pagani M, Via A, Saino G (2001) Current status of surgery for carcinoma of the hypopharynx and cervical esophagus. Dis Esophagus 14(2):95–97
9. Macha M, Whyte RI (2000) The current role of transhiatal esophagectomy. Chest Surg Clin N Am 10(3):499–518
10. Hulscher JB, Tijssen JG, Obertop H, van Lanschot JJ (2001) Transthoracic versus transhiatal resection for carcinoma of the esophagus: a meta-analysis. Ann Thorac Surg 72(1):306–313
11. Müller JM, Erasmi H, Stelzner M, Zieren U, Pichlmaier H (1990) Surgical therapy of oesophageal carcinoma. Br J Surg 77(8):845–857
12. Mathisen DJ, Grillo HC, Wilkins EW Jr, Moncure AC, Hilgenberg AD (1988) Transthoracic esophagectomy: a safe approach to carcinoma of the esophagus. Ann Thorac Surg 45(2):137–143
13. Visbal AL, Allen MS, Miller DL, Deschamps C, Trastek VF, Pairolero PC (2001) Ivor Lewis esophagogastrectomy for esophageal cancer. Ann Thorac Surg 71(6):1803–1808
14. Krasna MJ (1995) Left transthoracic esophagectomy. Chest Surg Clin N Am 5(3):543–554
15. Swanson SJ, Sugarbaker DJ (2000) The three-hole esophagectomy. The Brigham and Women's hospital approach (modified McKeown technique). Chest Surg Clin N Am 10(3):531–552
16. Swanson SJ, Batirel HF, Bueno R et al (2001) Transthoracic esophagectomy with radical mediastinal and abdominal lymph node dissection and cervical esophagogastrostomy for esophageal carcinoma. Ann Thorac Surg 72(6):1918–1924
17. Ito H, Clancy TE, Osteen RT, Swanson RS et al (2004) Adenocarcinoma of the gastric cardia: what is the optimal surgical approach? J Am Coll Surg 199(6):880–886
18. Schiesser M, Schneider PM (2010) Surgical strategies for adenocarcinoma of the esophagogastric junction. Recent Results Cancer Res 182:93–106
19. Santillan AA, Farma JM, Meredith KL, Shah NR, Kelley ST (2008) Minimally invasive surgery for esophageal cancer. J Natl Compr Canc Netw 6(9):879–884
20. Biere SS, van Berge Henegouwen MI, Maas KW et al (2012) Minimally invasive versus open oesophagectomy for patients with oesophageal cancer: a multicentre, open-label, randomised controlled trial. Lancet 379(9829):1887–1892
21. Davis PA, Law S, Wong J (2003) Colonic interposition after esophagectomy for cancer. Arch Surg 138(3):303–308
22. Akiyama H, Miyazono H, Tsurumaru M, Hashimoto C, Kawamura T (1978) Use of the stomach as an esophageal substitute. Ann Surg 188(5):606–610
23. Foker JE, Ring WS, Varco RL (1982) Technique of jejunal interposition for esophageal replacement. J Thorac Cardiovasc Surg 83(6):928–933
24. Akutsu Y, Matsubara H (2009) Perioperative management for the prevention of postoperative pneumonia with esophageal surgery. Ann Thorac Cardiovasc Surg 15(5):280–285
25. Donington JS (2005) Preoperative preparation for esophageal surgery. Thorac Surg Clin 15(2):277–285
26. Herbella FAM, Zamuner M, Patti MG (2014) Esophagectomy perianesthetic care from a surgeon's point of view SOJ. Anesthesiol Pain Manag 1(1):1–7
27. Ng JM (2011) Update on anesthetic management for esophagectomy. Curr Opin Anaesthesiol 24(1):37–43
28. Pennefather SH (2007) Anaesthesia for oesophagectomy. Curr Opin Anaesthesiol 20(1):15–20
29. Jaeger JM, Collins SR, Blank RS (2012) Anesthetic management for esophageal resection. Anesthesiol Clin 30(4):731–747
30. Shackford SR, Virgilio RW, Peters RM (1981) Early extubation versus prophylactic ventilation in the high risk patient: a comparison of postoperative management in the prevention of respiratory complications. Anesth Analg 60(2):76–80
31. Caldwell MT, Murphy PG, Page R, Walsh TN, Hennessy TP (1993) Timing of extubation after oesophagectomy. Br J Surg 80(12):1537–1539
32. Robertson SA, Skipworth RJ, Clarke DL, Crofts TJ, Lee A, de Beaux AC, Paterson-Brown S (2006) Ventilatory and intensive care requirements following oesophageal resection. Ann R Coll Surg Engl 88(4):354–357

33. Clemente A, Carli F (2008) The physiological effects of thoracic epidural anesthesia and analgesia on the cardiovascular, respiratory and gastrointestinal systems. Minerva Anestesiol 74(10):549–563
34. Freise H, Van Aken HK (2011) Risks and benefits of thoracic epidural anaesthesia. Br J Anaesth 107(6):859–868
35. Sentürk M, Ozcan PE, Talu GK et al (2002) The effects of three different analgesia techniques on long-term postthoracotomy pain. Anesth Analg 94(1):11–15
36. Komatsu R, Makarova N, Dalton JE et al (2015) Association of thoracic epidural analgesia with risk of atrial arrhythmias after pulmonary resection: a retrospective cohort study. J Anesth 29(1):47–55
37. Hanna MN, Murphy JD, Kumar K, Wu CL (2009) Postoperative pain management in the elderly undergoing thoracic surgery. Thorac Surg Clin 19(3):353–361
38. Ashes C, Slinger P (2014) Volume management and resuscitation in thoracic surgery. Curr Anesthesiol Rep 4:386–396
39. Chau EH, Slinger P (2014) Perioperative fluid management for pulmonary resection surgery and esophagectomy. Semin Cardiothorac Vasc Anesth 18(1):36–44
40. Kita T, Mammoto T, Kishi Y (2002) Fluid management and postoperative respiratory disturbances in patients with transthoracic esophagectomy for carcinoma. J Clin Anesth 14(4):252–256
41. Casado D, López F, Martí R (2010) Perioperative fluid management and major respiratory complications in patients undergoing esophagectomy. Dis Esophagus 23(7):523–528
42. Kight CE (2008) Nutrition considerations in esophagectomy patients. Nutr Clin Pract 23(5):521–528
43. Baker A, Wooten LA, Malloy M (2011) Nutritional considerations after gastrectomy and esophagectomy for malignancy. Curr Treat Options Oncol 12(1):85–95
44. Mahanna E, Crimi E, White P, Mann DS, Fahy BG (2015) Nutrition and metabolic support for critically ill patients. Curr Opin Anaesthesiol 28(2):131–138
45. Preiser JC, van Zanten AR, Berger MM et al (2015) Metabolic and nutritional support of critically ill patients: consensus and controversies. Crit Care 19(1):35
46. Braga M, Ljungqvist O, Soeters P et al (2009) ESPEN guidelines on parenteral nutrition: surgery. Clin Nutr 28(4):378–386
47. Daryaei P, Vaghef Davari F, Mir M, Harirchi I, Salmasian H (2009) Omission of nasogastric tube application in postoperative care of esophagectomy. World J Surg 33(4):773–777
48. Kobayashi K, Koyama Y, Kosugi S et al (2013) Is early enteral nutrition better for postoperative course in esophageal cancer patients? Nutrients 5(9):3461–3469
49. Weijs TJ, Berkelmans GH, Nieuwenhuijzen GA et al (2015) Routes for early enteral nutrition after esophagectomy. A systematic review. Clin Nutr 34(1):1–6
50. Seres DS, Valcarcel M, Guillaume A (2013) Advantages of enteral nutrition over parenteral nutrition. Therap Adv Gastroenterol 6(2):157–167
51. Shils ME, Gilat T (1966) The effect of esophagectomy on absorption in man: clinical and metabolic observations. Gastroenterology 50(3):347–357
52. Motoyama S, Okuyama M, Kitamura M et al (2004) Use of autologous instead of allogeneic blood transfusion during esophagectomy prolongs disease-free survival among patients with recurrent esophageal cancer. J Surg Oncol 87(1):26–31
53. Hébert PC, Wells G, Blajchman MA (1999) A multicenter, randomized, controlled clinical trial of transfusion requirements in critical care. Transfusion Requirements in Critical Care Investigators, Canadian Critical Care Trials Group. N Engl J Med 340(6):409–417
54. Rollins KE, Peters CJ, Safranek PM, Ford H, Baglin TP, Hardwick RH (2011) Venous thromboembolism in oesophago-gastric carcinoma: incidence of symptomatic and asymptomatic events following chemotherapy and surgery. Eur J Surg Oncol 37(12):1072–1077
55. Thodiyil PA, Walsh DC, Kakkar AK (2001) Thromboprophylaxis in the cancer patient. Acta Haematol 106(1–2):73–80
56. Zardo P, Busk H, Kutschka I (2015) Chest tube management: state of the art. Curr Opin Anaesthesiol 28(1):45–49

57. Coughlin SM, Emmerton-Coughlin HM (2012) Malthaner. Management of chest tubes after pulmonary resection: a systematic review and meta-analysis. Can J Surg 55(4):264–270
58. Nakatsuchi T, Otani M, Osugi H, Ito Y, Koike T (2005) The necessity of chest physical therapy for thoracoscopic oesophagectomy. J Int Med Res 33(4):434–441
59. Lunardi AC, Cecconello I, Carvalho CR (2011) Postoperative chest physical therapy prevents respiratory complications in patients undergoing esophagectomy. Rev Bras Fisioter 15(2):160–165
60. Overend TJ, Anderson CM, Lucy SD, Bhatia C, Jonsson BI, Timmermans C (2001) The effect of incentive spirometry on postoperative pulmonary complications: a systematic review. Chest 120(3):971–978
61. Avendano CE, Flume PA, Silvestri GA, King LB, Reed CE (2002) Pulmonary complications after esophagectomy. Ann Thorac Surg 73(3):922–926
62. Lerut T, Coosemans W, Decker G, De Leyn P, Nafteux P, van Raemdonck D (2002) Anastomotic complications after esophagectomy. Dig Surg 19(2):92–98
63. Briel JW, Tamhankar AP, Hagen JA et al (2004) Prevalence and risk factors for ischemia, leak, and stricture of esophageal anastomosis: gastric pull-up versus colon interposition. J Am Coll Surg 198(4):536–541
64. Turkyilmaz A, Eroglu A, Aydin Y, Tekinbas C, Muharrem Erol M, Karaoglanoglu N (2009) The management of esophagogastric anastomotic leak after esophagectomy for esophageal carcinoma. Dis Esophagus 22(2):119–126
65. Blewett CJ, Miller JD, Young JE, Bennett WF, Urschel JD (2001) Anastomotic leaks after esophagectomy for esophageal cancer: a comparison of thoracic and cervical anastomoses. Ann Thorac Cardiovasc Surg 7(2):75–88
66. Rice TW (2006) Anastomotic stricture complicating esophagectomy. Thorac Surg Clin 16(1):63–73
67. Park JY, Song HY, Kim JH et al (2012) Benign anastomotic strictures after esophagectomy: long-term effectiveness of balloon dilation and factors affecting recurrence in 155 patients. Am J Roentgenol 198(5):1208–1213
68. Wormuth JK, Heitmiller RF (2006) Esophageal conduit necrosis. Thorac Surg Clin 16(1):11–22
69. Meyerson SL, Mehta CK (2014) Managing complications II: conduit failure and conduit airway fistulas. J Thorac Dis 6(Suppl 3):S364–S371
70. Donington JS (2006) Functional conduit disorders after esophagectomy. Thorac Surg Clin 16(1):53–62
71. Lerut TE, van Lanschot JJ (2004) Chronic symptoms after subtotal or partial oesophagectomy: diagnosis and treatment. Best Pract Res Clin Gastroenterol 18(5):901–915
72. Burrows WM (2004) Gastrointestinal function and related problems following esophagectomy. Semin Thorac Cardiovasc Surg 16(2):142–151
73. Aly A, Jamieson GG (2004) Reflux after oesophagectomy. Br J Surg 91(2):137–141
74. Yuasa N, Sasaki E, Ikeyama T, Miyake H, Nimura Y (2005) Acid and duodenogastroesophageal reflux after esophagectomy with gastric tube reconstruction. Am J Gastroenterol 100(5):1021–1027

Do the New Hemodynamic Monitoring Devices Make Sense Compared to the "Classical" Ones?

10

Giorgio Della Roca

10.1 Introduction

Postoperative hemodynamic monitoring of high-risk patients, including those who undergone thoracic surgery, should be inside the modern concept that insufficient tissue perfusion and cellular oxygenation due to hypovolemia and/or heart dysfunction is one of the leading causes of perioperative complications in terms of morbidity and mortality. The modern and new various available hemodynamic monitoring systems should be used to guide cardiovascular and fluid management in the perioperative period in high-risk surgical patients [1–5].

The risk of perioperative complications is related to patient status and comorbidities (Table 10.1), the type of surgery performed and its duration, the degree of urgency, the skills and experience of the operating and anesthetic teams, and the postoperative management. Insufficient tissue perfusion and cellular oxygenation due to hypovolemia and/or heart dysfunction is one of the leading causes of perioperative complications and poor outcomes [6–9]. Effective fluid management to prevent and treat hypo-/hypervolemia and titration of vasoactive drugs for heart dysfunction is thus crucial to maintain adequate oxygen delivery (DO_2) and prevent fluid overload and its consequences [10–12]. Selecting the most appropriate hemodynamic monitoring device (for diagnosis and to guide therapies) may, therefore, be an important first step in reducing the risk of complications.

G. Della Roca
Medical University of Udine, Department of Anesthesia and Intensive Care Medicine of the University of Udine, Udine, Italy
e-mail: giorgio.dellarocca@uniud.it

© Springer International Publishing Switzerland 2017

M. Şentürk, M.O. Sungur (eds.), *Postoperative Care in Thoracic Surgery*,
DOI 10.1007/978-3-319-19908-5_10

Table 10.1 High-risk surgical patient definition

Cardiac pt	1. Severe cardiac or respiratory illness resulting in severe functional limitation (acute myocardial infarction, coronaropathy, dilatative cardiomiopathy, EF<40 %)
	2. Extensive surgery planned for carcinoma involving bowel anastomosis
Bleeding	3. Acute massive blood loss (>2.5 L)
Elderly	4. Age>70 years with moderate functional limitation of one or more organ systems
Sepsis	5. Septicemia (positive blood cultures or septic focus)
Respiratory pt	6. Respiratory failure (PaO_2/FiO_2 <285 mmHg, $PaCO_2$>45 mmHg, Fev1< 60 % of predicted value)
Fluids shift	7. Acute abdominal catastrophe (i.e. pancreatitis, perforated viscous, gastro-intestinal bleed)
Renal pt	8. Acute renal failure (urea >45 mg/dL, creatinine >2.9 mg/dL)
Diabetes	9. Diabetes (preoperative glycemia>150 mg/dL)
ESLD	10. Chronic hepatopathy (Child B or C)
	11. Surgery for abdominal aortic aneurysm

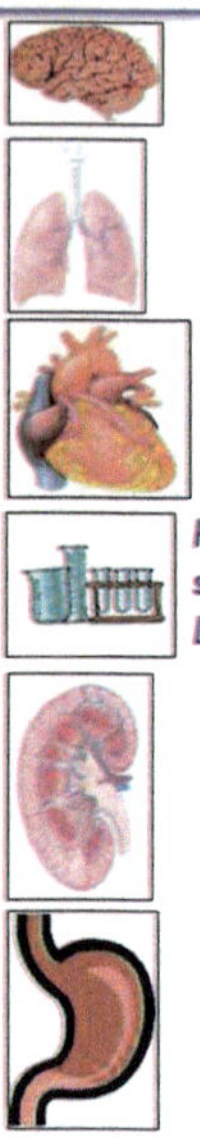

10.2 Basic Hemodynamic Monitoring

Blood pressure is a variable influenced by both cardiac output (CO) and vascular tone; hence, blood pressure can remain within the normal range in the presence of low-flow states, including hypovolemia, as a result of increased peripheral vascular resistance. Similarly, heart rate may fail to reflect the development of hypovolemia under anesthesia [13].

Combining and integrating parameters from various hemodynamic monitoring systems may help improve our understanding of hemodynamic status [14].

Continuous arterial pressure invasive measurement helps identify the rapid fluctuations in arterial pressure that may occur in high-risk patients. Artifacts (over- or under-damping) should be carefully identified and eliminated, especially when systolic-diastolic components and waveform have to be analyzed. Noninvasive techniques for continuous measurement of blood pressure are usually performed in peripheral arteries and may become unreliable in case of vasoconstriction or low peripheral flow.

Changes in central venous pressure (CVP) with concomitant CO variations can give an indication of RV function and potential peripheral venous congestion, an important factor for organ perfusion [15]. In addition, careful checking of the CVP wave may help to diagnose tricuspid regurgitation with a "v" wave during systole. When the CVP is low with a concomitant low CO, there is some degree of hypovolemia, although changes in CVP correlate poorly with changes in CO [16].

10.3 Cardiac Output Monitoring

The perioperative period is characterized by large variations in whole body oxygen consumption (VO_2). The main goal in this period is to maintain an adequate DO_2 to meet the fluctuating tissue oxygen requirements. Global DO_2 is determined by CO and the oxygen content of arterial blood (CaO_2) so, after correction of hypoxemia and anemia (topics that will not be treated here), maintenance of an adequate CO is the next logical step to improve DO_2. There are various methods available for monitoring CO: calibrated and not calibrated [17–21].

10.3.1 Pulmonary Artery Catheter: The "Classical" One

Although criticized during the recent years for its intrinsic invasiveness and no clear evidence of improved outcomes [22–25], the pulmonary artery catheter (PAC) is the only tool that provides continuous monitoring of pulmonary artery (PA) pressure, right-sided and left-sided filling pressures, and CO and mixed venous oxygen saturation (SvO_2). While the PAC can now be replaced by less invasive hemodynamic monitoring techniques in some cases, in some complex clinical situations, for example, cardiac surgery, organ transplant surgery, and surgery associated with major fluid shifts, high risk of respiratory failure, or in patients with compromised right ventricle (RV) function, the PAC still represents a valuable tool when used by physicians adequately trained to correctly interpret and apply the data provided [26, 27]. In such patients, the PAC can be inserted for limited periods of time and removed when no longer necessary.

10.3.2 Other Cardiac Output Monitoring Devices: The "New" Ones

10.3.2.1 Pulse Contour Analysis

Stroke volume (SV) can be estimated continuously by analysis of the arterial pressure waveform, usually derived from an indwelling arterial catheter or by a noninvasive finger pressure cuff. To calculate SV from a pressure trace, the algorithms used by these devices have to compensate for the overall impedance of the system, based on the estimation of compliance and resistance of the cardiovascular tree. In this regard, optimization of the input signal is imperative, and severe distortions of the arterial waveform (e.g., severe arrhythmias, multiple ectopic beats) and inadequate response of fluid-filled transducer systems (i.e., over- and under-damping) [28] can result in unreliable CO measurement.

Calibrated Devices

- The PiCCOplus™/PiCCO$_2$™ system (Pulsion Medical Systems, Munich, Germany) consists of a thermistor-tipped catheter which is usually placed in the

femoral artery, although catheters for radial, axillary, or brachial applications are also available. The PiCCO™ device measures CO by transpulmonary thermodilution, which additionally provides the computation of volumetric preload parameters (global end-diastolic volume [GEDV], intrathoracic blood volume [ITBV]), and extravascular lung water (EVLW). The CO measured by the Stewart-Hamilton principle from the thermodilution curve is used to calibrate a pulse contour algorithm, which measures the area under the systolic pulse pressure curve and calculates the SV in order to provide beat-by-beat CO measurement. The system has to be frequently recalibrated, at least every eight hours in hemodynamically stable patients and more often if changes in vasoactive support are provided [29]. The system has been validated in a variety of clinical settings [30].
- The EV1000™/VolumeView™ system (Edwards Lifesciences, Irvine, California) has been more recently introduced, but is analogous to the PiCCO™ monitor, using pulse wave analysis to calculate CO. A proprietary thermistor-tipped femoral artery catheter and a separate sensor are the main components of the system. This system requires calibration by transpulmonary thermodilution. It has been validated off-line against the PiCCO™ and transpulmonary thermodilution in critically ill patients [31].
- The LiDCO™plus system (LiDCO Ltd, Cambridge, UK) uses pulse power analysis to calculate SV and is therefore not technically a pulse contour device. The algorithm is based on the principle of conservation of mass (power), assuming a linear relationship between the net power change and the net flow in the vascular system. This system requires correction for vascular compliance, with calibration using a transpulmonary lithium indicator dilution technique performed via an indwelling arterial catheter. It has been validated in critically ill patients [32, 33].

Uncalibrated Devices (with No External Calibration)

- The PulsioFlex™ system (Pulsion Medical Systems) displays trends of estimated CO by using the patient's anthropometric and demographic characteristics (necessary for internal calibration), analysis of the arterial pressure tracing, and a proprietary algorithm for data analysis. The system requires a dedicated additional sensor, which can be connected to a regular arterial pressure catheter. Based on the same pulse contour algorithm used by the PiCCO™, the device can be calibrated by entering a CO obtained from an external source (e.g., Doppler echocardiography) or by the system's own internal algorithm.
- The LiDCO™*rapid* (LiDCO Ltd) device uses the same algorithm as the LiDCO™plus system, but instead of lithium dilution, nomograms based on the patient's age, weight, and height are used to estimate SV and CO (the so-called "nominal" SV and CO). An externally estimated CO can be used to calibrate the device.
- The FloTrac™/Vigileo™ system (Edwards Lifesciences) consists of a proprietary transducer (FloTrac™) connected to a standard (radial or femoral) arterial catheter. Individual demographic variables (age, sex, height, and weight) and a

database containing CO variables derived using the PAC are used to calculate impedance and a "normal" SV against which the standard deviation of the pulse pressure sampled during a 20-s interval is correlated to estimate CO. Arterial waveform analysis is used to calculate vascular resistance and compliance. The algorithm used by the Vigileo™ device has been modified over time, and recent studies evaluating the device in the perioperative setting have shown an improved performance and a significant reduction in the time needed to adapt to vascular dynamics. In the ICU setting, concerns remain regarding the accuracy in situations of acute hemodynamic instability as well as hyperdynamic conditions, although recent software modifications seem to improve the reliability of CO measurements. The FloTrac™/Vigileo™ system has been shown to be suitable for integration into perioperative optimization protocols, resulting in improved clinical outcomes [34, 35].

10.3.2.2 Pitfalls in the Interpretation of Cardiac Output

Although CO can be measured with reasonable accuracy and precision with some of these systems, it is difficult to assess the optimal CO for an individual patient. A "normal" or even high CO does not preclude the presence of inadequate regional and microcirculatory flow, and a low CO may be adequate in a context of low metabolic demand, especially during surgery under general anesthesia. Moreover, simple identification of a low CO does not tell us what to do about it. Data acquired can be correctly interpreted by any of the described devices, but we need to combine/integrate several variables to help decide whether the CO/SV is adequate and how it can be optimized in the most effective manner [36–39].

10.3.2.3 How to Select the Best System?

All monitoring systems have unique characteristics in terms of accuracy, precision, validity, stability, and reliability [18]. Not all monitoring devices have been evaluated against the same set of criteria, and uncertainty remains regarding acceptance thresholds for the performance of CO monitors and the used reference techniques [54–57]. Clinicians must consider the technical limitations of each monitoring system and the potential trade-off between more invasive but highly accurate measurements of CO and less invasive but also less accurate modalities.

Many questions can be raised when considering the choice of CO monitoring in the perioperative period [40]:

1. Are we ready to accept a less accurate measurement in order to limit invasiveness? (Fig. 10.1). A less accurate measurement may be acceptable if the trend analysis is reliable. Cost may also be an important issue.
2. Do we need continuous, semicontinuous, or intermittent measurements? Most complications after surgery do not have a sudden onset (except sudden cardiac failure due, e.g., to myocardial infarction or pulmonary embolism) or an obvious cause (e.g., massive bleeding during surgery), but develop slowly; therefore, semicontinuous or intermittent measurements may be acceptable. However, it should be noted that only beat-by-beat measurement of SV allows assessment of

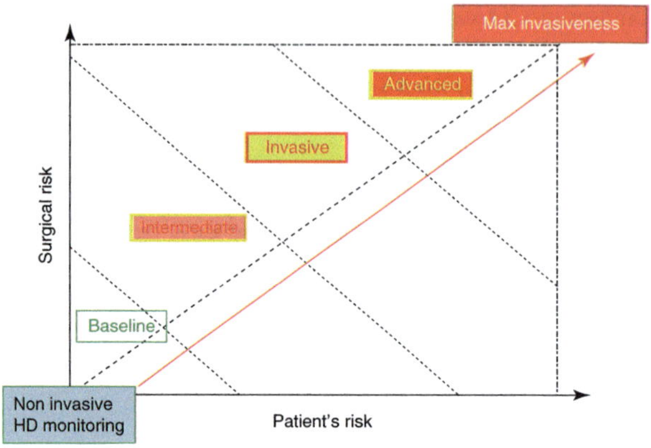

Fig. 10.1 Perioperative HD monitoring

the response to preload-modifying maneuvers, such as a fluid challenge or passive leg raising (PLR) test.

3. Are calibrated or uncalibrated systems preferable? Non-calibrated systems are acceptable for the operating room (OR) or the post-anesthesia care unit (PACU) but may not be suitable for more complex cases, especially in the ICU. In unstable patients, there is a necessity to "recalibrate" more often because of frequent changes in vascular tone and also because derived variables (e.g., EVLW, GEDV) need to be recalculated. A practical option may be to use an uncalibrated system in the OR/PACU and replace it with a calibrated system in the ICU.
4. What alarms do we need? A major problem for patient surveillance by telemetric monitoring is artifact robustness. Any system with too many false alarms is prone to failure as personnel become desensitized.
5. What kind of monitoring for what kind of patient? This decision is not a "one size fits all"; rather, the optimal monitoring technique for each patient will vary depending on the degree of risk and the extent of the surgical procedure (Fig. 10.1).

10.4 Echocardiography

Although difficult to use as a continuous monitor of CO with conventional probes, transthoracic (TTE) or transesophageal (TEE) echocardiography can provide immediate point-of-care assessment of acute hemodynamic changes in selected patients. Echo techniques can also help to visualize the lungs, but this is beyond the scope of this review. Obviously, it is not possible to use TEE in all types of surgery. In addition to the estimation of CO (usually easier with TEE than with TTE), Doppler echocardiographic examination can provide an indication of cardiac function, because it allows visualization of the cardiac chambers, valves, and pericardium [20]. It also allows measurement of the ejected stroke volume (SV) and derived left ventricular (LV) function parameters.

TEE provides several views, including:

- The LV short-axis view, which can be used to evaluate LV function. Calculation of the LV fractional area contraction, or the simpler "eyeballing method," informs about the kinetic (contractile) state and the shape (volume) of the heart. Poor contractility may indicate that inotropic support could help, and "kissing" of the papillary muscle may indicate the need for fluids if the right heart is functioning normally. The short-axis view may also be used to identify septal dyskinesia. The finding of a right ventricle *D*-shape may suggest the presence of RV dysfunction/failure, indicating a non-adaptation to an acute increase in RV afterload (pulmonary embolism) or RV myocardial ischemia.
- The four-chamber view, which can help in assessing LV and RV function by evaluation of the right-to-left size ratio (normal <0.6).

In more advanced echocardiographic evaluation, fluid status and fluid responsiveness can also be assessed in mechanically ventilated patients by means of the superior vena cava collapsibility index (TEE bicaval view) or inferior vena cava distensibility index (TTE subcostal view). In addition, echocardiography allows the rapid and reliable estimation of SV. Finally, there are particular and specific conditions in which diagnosis and treatment are strictly related to the echocardiographic examination (e.g., pericardial effusion, valve disruptions, aortic dissection, and systolic anterior motion of the mitral valve).

A miniaturized, disposable monoplane TEE probe that can be left in place for up to 72 h (ClariTEE™, ImaCor Inc., Garden City, NY) has recently been introduced and has the potential to provide ongoing qualitative cardiac assessment.

We believe that where expert echocardiography skills are not available, then training programs should be developed to ensure that clinicians taking care of the high-risk patient are familiar with at least the basic applications of TTE and TEE.

Echocardiography has become an indispensable tool in the evaluation of medical and surgical patients. As ultrasound (US) machines have become more widely available and significantly more compact, there has been an exponential growth in the use of transthoracic echocardiography (TTE), transesophageal echocardiography (TEE), and other devices in the perioperative setting. Here, we review recent findings relevant to the use of perioperative US, with a special focus on the hemodynamic management of the surgical patient.

In an attempt to make hemodynamic monitoring less invasive and to acquire additional relevant information not obtained with other monitoring approaches, ultrasound (US) devices are increasingly being used in perioperative medicine [1]. The field is rapidly evolving as technology advances. Here, we describe the basic principles of ultrasonography and how it can be used for hemodynamic monitoring in the perioperative setting.

TTE and TEE allow the differentiation between noncardiac and cardiac causes of hemodynamic instability. Valvular pathologies and abnormalities in ventricular function can be assessed. During noncardiac surgery, the American Heart Association (AHA) and the American College of Cardiology (ACC) recommend the use of echocardiography in the "evaluation of acute, persistent and life-threatening haemodynamic disturbances in which ventricular function and its determinants are uncertain and have not responded to treatment" [41].

10.4.1 Ventricular Function

Global, systolic LV function can be visually estimated. According to current SCA recommendations, this basic qualitative assessment is not precise, but sufficient for the identification of patients who might benefit from inotropic therapy [12]. The SCA recommends using the transgastric (TG) mid-papillary short-axis (SAX) view, as well as the mid-esophageal (ME) four-chamber, the ME two-chamber, and the MOE long-axis (LAX) views for the monitoring of LV function.

10.4.2 Intravascular Volume Status

Hypovolemia is a common cause of cardiocirculatory instability in the operating theater and the intensive care unit. A central concept in the care of critically ill patients and patients undergoing surgery is to predict fluid responsiveness: Will a patient's hemodynamic situation improve (i.e., increase in SV and CI) with fluid administration or not? If certain preconditions are met (closed chest, controlled ventilation with sufficiently high tidal volumes, regular heart rhythm, and normal intra-abdominal pressure), systolic pressure variation (SPV), arterial pulse pressure variation (PPV), and stroke volume variation (SVV) represent "dynamic" parameters that more reliably predict fluid responsiveness. CVP and LV end-diastolic area (EDA) do not predict fluid responsiveness, as they are static parameters that are dependent not only on volume status. Other variables impacting CVP and LV-EDA include cardiac compliance (i.e., diastolic ventricular function) as well as intrathoracic pressure. Consequently, LV-EDAI (LV-EDA indexed to the body surface area) does not correlate with fluid responsiveness. Other studies confirmed the inferiority of LV-EDA in predicting fluid responsiveness in comparison to dynamic parameters. Different systematic reviews also concluded that LV-EDA is inferior compared to dynamic parameters such as PPV.

10.4.3 Valvular Function

For a basic assessment of valvular regurgitation, visual inspection of the regurgitant jet area, vena contracta width, as well as flow reversal in receiving or originating cardiovascular chambers can be used among other criteria. Stenotic lesions can be grossly evaluated by continuous-wave Doppler using an imaging plane parallel to blood flow (see the Doppler section above). An orienting assessment of valvular function should be part of every basic echocardiographic examination.

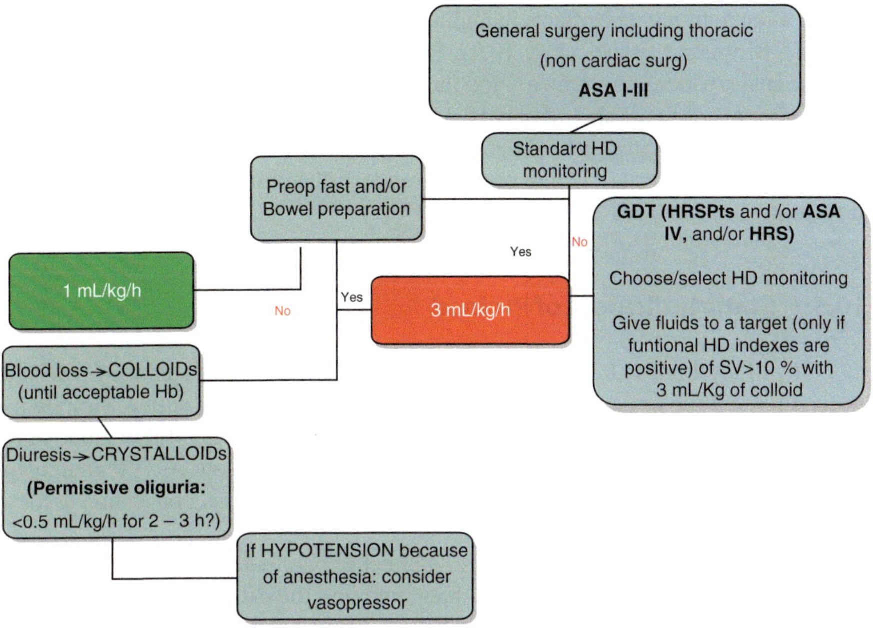

Fig. 10.2 Periop fluid and HD management. *HSR* high risk surgery, *Pts* patients, *HD* hemodynamic, *Hb* hemoglobin

10.4.4 Pulmonary Embolism, Pericardial Effusion, and Thoracic Trauma

Hemodynamically relevant pulmonary embolism (PE) is one reason of cardiocirculatory compromise. In the intraoperative or emergency setting, TOE might be the only feasible yet reliable tool to detect the presence of hemodynamically relevant emboli. Signs of RV failure and motion abnormalities of the RV free wall permit the diagnosis of PE in patients with hypotension or shock.

The modern approach to the hemodynamic evaluation including the TTE/TEE evaluation is a part of the anesthetist skill [42].

10.5 Fluid Management and Functional Hemodynamic Monitoring

Inadequate fluid management may lead to reduced CO and DO_2 to injured tissues, which is associated with an increased incidence of postoperative complications [43]. Moreover, the systemic inflammatory response associated with tissue injury results in capillary leak and tissue edema (Fig. 10.2). Fluid restriction and diuresis may decrease edema in patients with poor ventricular function but may also increase the incidence of acute kidney injury. Meanwhile, excessive fluid administration may lead to a range of adverse effects including coagulopathies and edema of the lungs, gut, and peripheral tissues (Fig. 10.2). Retention of sodium and water following surgery may reduce requirements for fluids. Once the patient is stabilized, additional amounts of fluids should only be given to correct deficit or continuing losses. Unfortunately, estimates of fluid deficit based on traditional physiological parameters, such as heart rate, blood pressure, and cardiac filling pressures, are not sufficient.

10.5.1 Static Indicators of Preload

- CVP: Many high-risk surgical patients have a CVC in place and a CVC is a requirement for some devices needing calibration by thermodilution. Despite its limitations (vide supra), changes in CVP over time may be helpful to guide fluid therapy, especially when it is low and associated with low flow. A CVP >8 mmHg might also be considered as an "alarm" for potential venous congestion associated or not with fluid overload [15].
- GEDV/ITBV and EVLW: These are volumetric parameters derived from transpulmonary thermodilution and are integrated into the PiCCO™*plus*, $PiCCO_2$™, and EV1000™ monitors. EVLW can help in the identification of (cardiogenic or non-cardiogenic) pulmonary edema and has the potential to increase the safety of fluid therapy in patients with structural lung disease, ARDS, or congestive heart failure.
- The end-diastolic area of the left ventricle may be the most reliable static parameter of preload, but is largely dependent on LV diastolic compliance. Its ability to accurately predict fluid responsiveness is limited.

10.5.2 Functional Hemodynamic Parameters

Positive pressure ventilation induces cyclical changes in intrathoracic pressure, which affect preload by decreasing venous return to the right heart and increasing venous return to the left ventricle. The degree of the resulting changes in LV SV (SVV) and pulse pressure (PPV) better predict fluid responsiveness than do static parameters, when RV function is not a limitation and for a fixed tidal volume. Most devices using pulse contour analysis, including the current version of the noninvasive ClearSight monitor, display SVV and PPV. Despite the numerous validity criteria required to interpret such variations, these variables may help predict fluid responsiveness at different thresholds and have been integrated into hemodynamic optimization protocols [44].

Respiratory variations in the pulse oximeter plethysmographic waveform (ΔPOP) have been shown to predict fluid responsiveness in mechanically ventilated patients, similar to changes in the arterial pressure waveform [45]. The Masimo™

(Masimo Corp., Irvine, California, USA) device provides automated calculation of the pleth variability index (PVI) by measuring changes in perfusion index over a time interval including at least one complete respiratory cycle. The PVI has been shown to predict fluid responsiveness in various perioperative settings and has been integrated into fluid optimization algorithms. However, the PVI has the same limitations as the other dynamic parameters and has limited accuracy in the presence of vasoconstriction with or without the use of vasopressors [46–48].

Today, *we can recommend that dynamic parameters be used as an integral part of GDT protocols*. The limitations of each dynamic index must be taken into consideration as well as the concept of a gray zone. Dynamic parameters neither provide a measure of fluid bolus effectiveness nor should they be used as an indication to give fluids. The final decision to administer fluids must be supported by the apparent need for hemodynamic improvement, the presence of fluid responsiveness, and by the lack of associated risk.

We recommend crystalloid solutions for routine surgery of short duration. However, in major surgery, the use of a goal-directed fluid regimen containing colloid and balanced salt solutions is recommended. Though a black box warning for the use of starch solutions exists within the United States, there is limited data relative to their harm in the perioperative space. Careful consideration should occur in patients with known renal dysfunction and/or sepsis prior to administering starch solutions [43].

10.5.3 Limitations

It is important to note that all the dynamic variables have significant confounding factors [44]. The reliability of these indices is affected by spontaneous breathing activity, arrhythmias, right heart failure, decreased chest wall compliance, and increased intra-abdominal pressure, although most of these limitations are uncommon in the OR. Nevertheless, in the ICU a relatively small proportion of patients present suitable criteria for these indices [49]. Another major limitation of dynamic parameters is that they are dependent on the size of the tidal volume. Some authors have suggested that they require a tidal volume of at least 8 ml/kg body weight [50], although they have been successfully used with tidal volumes of 6–8 ml/kg body weight [47, 48]. A recent study and meta-analysis have indicated a decreased rate of postoperative complications when low tidal volumes are applied during anesthesia [51, 52], and increased use of protective ventilation (lower tidal volumes) in the OR may reduce the usefulness of dynamic parameters or at least require new interpretation rules. Finally, within a range of PPV values of 9–13 %, fluid responsiveness cannot always be reliably predicted; there is a "gray zone" in which prediction of fluid responsiveness is difficult. One study [53] indicated that fluid responsiveness could not be reliably predicted using dynamic measures in as many as 25 % of anesthetized patients.

A passive leg raising (PLR) test has been suggested to overcome some of these limitations in dynamic evaluation, but should be performed rigorously with simultaneous analysis of continuous CO monitoring. It is obviously impractical during most operative conditions [54]. In addition, the blood volume shift from the leg to the central compartment is non-predictable. In a hypovolemic state, it is reasonable to consider a volume shift less than that generated in "normal" volemic conditions.

Despite these limitations and confounding factors, whenever possible, one is advised to assess fluid responsiveness using the available functional hemodynamic parameters before attempting to increase CO with fluid administration. This approach can indicate if and when CO can be further increased by fluids, and identify when the flat portion of the cardiac function curve has been reached, thus preventing unnecessary fluid loading [44]. It is also important to remember that, generally speaking, fluid responsiveness is not an (absolute) indication to give fluids. Decisions about fluid administration should not be based only on dynamic parameters but also on the likely risk associated with fluid administration. During surgery, systematic fluid administration in the presence of fluid responsiveness may improve postoperative outcomes [55].

10.6 Venous Oxygen Saturation

Changes in SvO_2 may reflect important pathophysiological changes in the relationship between DO_2 and VO_2, both of which may fluctuate significantly during the perioperative period.

Reorganization of the Fick equation shows that

$$SvO_2 = SaO_2 - \left(VO_2 / [CO \times Hb \times C]\right)$$

From this equation, it is clear that SvO_2 will decrease in the presence of hypoxemia, hypermetabolic states (increased VO_2), a decrease in CO, or anemia. Changes in SvO_2 are therefore directly proportional to those in CO, only when SaO_2, VO_2, and hemoglobin concentration remain constant. The normal SvO_2 in health is around 75 %, but it is closer to 70 % in acutely ill patients who have a somewhat lower hemoglobin concentration.

Central venous oxygen saturation ($ScvO_2$) from a central venous catheter is used as a surrogate for SvO_2 when a PAC is not in situ, with some limitations. Although the determinants of $ScvO_2$ and SvO_2 are similar, they cannot be used interchangeably [56]. Regional variations in the balance between DO_2 and VO_2 result in differences in the hemoglobin saturation of blood in the superior and inferior vena cava. $ScvO_2$ is affected disproportionately by changes in the upper body and does not reflect the SvO_2 of coronary sinus blood. In healthy individuals, $ScvO_2$ may be slightly less than SvO_2, because of the high oxygen content of effluent venous blood from the kidneys, but this relationship is reversed during periods of hemodynamic instability as blood is redistributed to the upper body at the expense of the splanchnic and renal circulations. In shock states, therefore, $ScvO_2$ may exceed SvO_2 by up to 20 %. This lack of equivalence has been demonstrated in various groups of acutely ill patients including not only those with shock but also in patients undergoing general anesthesia for cardiac and noncardiac surgery. Even trends in $ScvO_2$ do not closely reflect those of SvO_2 [57–59].

Lower values of $ScvO_2$ have been associated with more complications in patients undergoing cardiothoracic surgery. Some authors have proposed to maintain SvO_2 or $ScvO_2$ above a cutoff value. In patients undergoing elective cardiac surgery, administration of intravenous fluid and inotropic therapy to attain a target $SvO_2 \geq 70\,\%$ in the first eight hours after surgery was associated with fewer complications and a shorter hospital stay. In patients undergoing major abdominal (including aortic) surgery, achieving an oxygen extraction ratio of less than 27 % (from intermittent measurements of $ScvO_2$) was associated with a shorter hospital stay [57, 58].

During surgery this measurement is less informative: Firstly, hypoxemia is generally corrected; secondly, under anesthesia, especially with neuromuscular paralysis, oxygen use decreases in all tissues, so that reductions in $ScvO_2$ are uncommon. Nevertheless, low $ScvO_2$ values imply first and foremost that CO may be inadequate. At the same time, very high $ScvO_2$ values may imply that oxygen extraction is low, purporting a worse prognosis, at least during cardiac surgery [59].

10.7 Blood Lactate Concentrations

Lactate is a physiological substrate (carbohydrate) produced from pyruvate reduction during cytosolic glycolysis. In stable conditions, lactate production and elimination are equivalent, i.e., 1200–1500 mmol per day, leading to a stable blood lactate concentration of 0.8–1.2 mmol/L. The net flux of lactate depends on the difference between release and uptake and varies among organs and with their energetic conditions [60]. Hyperlactatemia is associated with increased morbidity and mortality in critically ill patients [61–64]. Persistent hyperlactatemia is a more relevant indicator of poor outcome than an isolated elevated lactate value. Hyperlactatemia is not always a consequence of tissue hypoxia, but also of an accelerated "aerobic" glycolysis resulting from cytokine influence and catecholamine stimulation, a situation termed "stress hyperlactatemia." In practice, irrespective of the different metabolic modifications, an elevated lactate level indicates the presence of shock, and a decrease in lactate levels over time is a good indicator of effective treatment. Accordingly, repeated blood lactate measurements are recommended to monitor lactate production and clearance over time during surgery in high-risk patients.

10.8 Management Strategies Based on Perioperative Monitoring

There is good evidence that the use of flow-based hemodynamic monitoring combined with hemodynamic manipulation in the perioperative period can reduce morbidity and sometimes mortality [65–71]. For a variety of reasons, however, this approach has not been adopted everywhere and has even been challenged [72]. Indeed, there have been some important problems with many clinical trials in the field, such as lack of blinding and suboptimal management of the control group.

There are basically two options to optimize perioperative cardiovascular management, both of which aim to increase SV/CO by means of fluid loading (increase in cardiac preload) and/or inotrope administration (increase in contractility):

(a) One is *reactive*, by applying a rapid intervention only when a hemodynamic change occurs. One should then individualize treatment with fluid challenge techniques. The response to the rapid administration of a fluid bolus (e.g., 150 ml) can be evaluated during surgery (especially in the presence of signs of fluid responsiveness). The response can be monitored by evaluating the blood pressure or heart rate but the CO/SV response is much more accurate. Inotropic agents are added in the absence of an adequate response. Reactive approach includes:
  - Correct hypotension and tachycardia.
  - Give fluids in the presence of suspected hypovolemia with increased pulse pressure variation (PPV), systolic pressure variation (SPV), stroke volume variation (SVV), or pleth variability index (PVI).
  - Identify a reduction in cardiac output (CO) and react promptly with fluid challenge.
  - Identify a reduction in central venous oxygen saturation ($ScvO_2$) and react promptly with fluid challenge.

(b) The other chance is *proactive*, based on a strategy of hemodynamic manipulation targeting supranormal CO or DO_2 values to minimize the risk of tissue hypoperfusion. Adequate fluid administration is the first element of this strategy. Several studies have indicated that fluid management based on PPV, SVV, and SV optimization may decrease postoperative wound infections and possibly postoperative organ dysfunction [73, 74]. Inotropic agents may be added if fluids alone are not sufficient for this purpose. There is a risk of overtreatment as excessive use of dobutamine has been associated with increased rates of complications [75]. The use of dopexamine as an alternative has given controversial results [76, 77]. Proactive approach includes:
  - Maintain arterial pressure and heart rate within acceptable ranges.
  - Maximize stroke volume (SV).
  - Maintain PPV or SVV $<12\,\%$ or PVI $<14\,\%$.

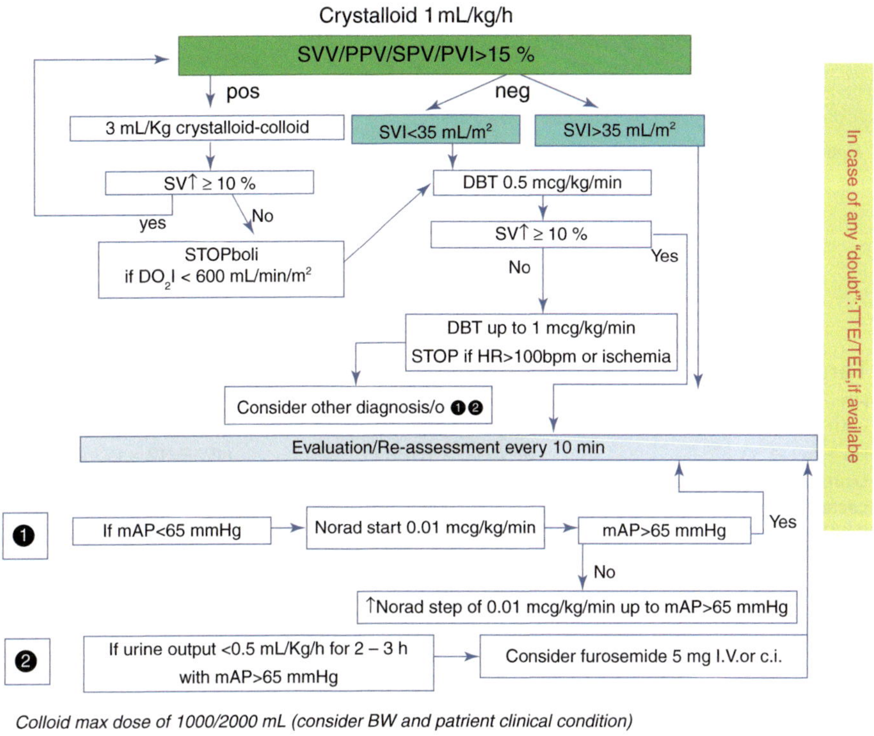

Fig. 10.3 Perioperative fluids and GDT "tailored"

- Maintain cardiac index (CI) or oxygen delivery (DO_2) in a desired range (e.g., CI>4.5 L/min.M^2, DO_2>600 mL/min).
- Maintain $ScvO_2$>65 %.

The algorithms should be used as part of the perioperative fluid plan. These should be available and easily accessible within all operating rooms, PACU, and ICU (Fig. 10.3). Clinical needs, invasiveness, accuracy, and precision of available technologies should be considered when selecting monitoring devices.

While the benefits of perioperative goal-directed fluid therapy have yet to be proven, the bulk of clinical research supports the *implementation of a step-by-step GDT plan and an appropriate HD monitoring* (*Fig.* 10.4) *which is to begin in high-risk surgical patients immediately after induction of anesthesia until the first post-operative hours*. First, determine if the patient requires hemodynamic support or augmentation of cardiovascular function. Second, if the need is apparent *and* the patient is fluid responsive, fluid bolus therapy should be considered and guided by continual, and if available continuous, assessment of fluid responsiveness as described below and to continue for the first six postoperative hours.

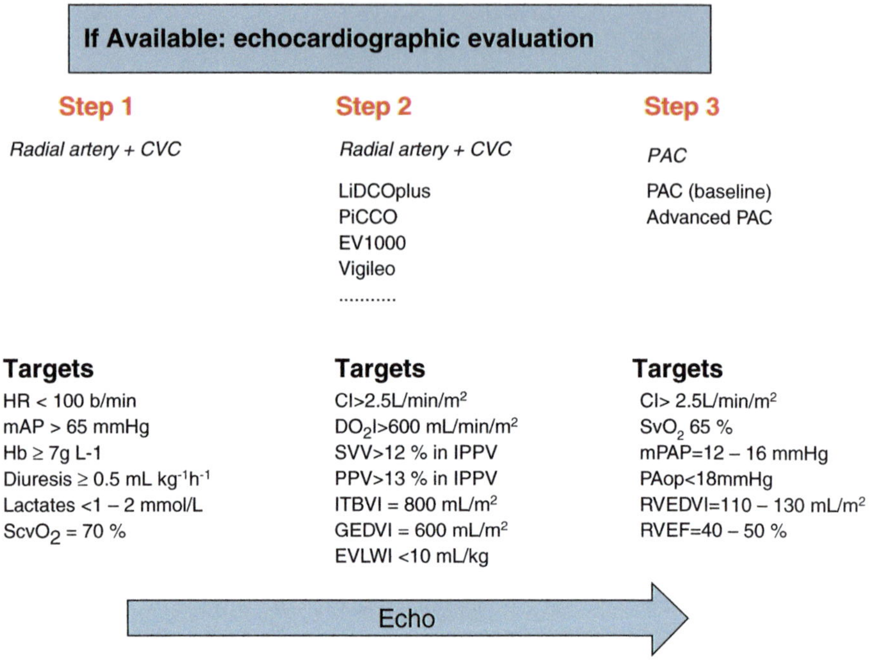

Fig. 10.4 A step-by-step approach to the appropriate HD monitoring

Bolus therapy rather than continuous infusion when the goal is to improve pressure, perfusion, and oxygen delivery is recommended. Standardization of the fluid bolus relative to fluid composition, volume, infusion rate, and time to post-bolus assessment should be implemented. The variables used for assessing the effectiveness of the fluid bolus should include appropriate changes in cardiac output or stroke volume (Fig. 10.3, 4).

Conclusions

Hemodynamic monitoring systems play an important role in optimizing perioperative hemodynamic management.

The new HD monitoring devices implement the classical one, but the use of hemodynamic monitoring devices per se in the perioperative setting has not been shown to be associated with improved outcomes. However, appropriate measurement and interpretation of cardiovascular variables may help guide therapeutic interventions, which could improve patient outcomes. The most appropriate system must be selected for the individual patient prior to surgery, taking into consideration the individual risks of the patient and the procedure. Appropriate interpretation of the information offered by hemodynamic monitoring requires the integration of several variables. The PAC still represents the goal standard for the PA pressure monitoring and for all the very critically ill patients. The mini-invasive CO monitoring systems are very useful tools in the OR and in all those intermediate-risk patients undergoing major surgery.

Echocardiography is increasingly used as a first tool to identify a problem and help select initial treatment. To improve patient management and outcome, the clinician must understand the advantages and the limitations of the various tools and parameters used during perioperative care.

Although perioperative fluid management remains a highly debated subject, data suggests that goal-directed fluid therapy with the objective of hemodynamic optimization can reduce complications after major surgery. Specific hemodynamic goals include maintaining adequate circulating volume, perfusion pressure, and oxygen delivery.

In summary, fluids should be treated as any other intravenous drug therapy; thus, careful consideration of its timing and dose is mandatory. A perioperative fluid plan should be developed which is easily understood and used by all anesthesiologists within a group, facility, or healthcare system. Determining both the need for augmented perfusion and fluid responsiveness is fundamental when making fluid therapy decisions to avoid unjustified fluid administration. The use of algorithms as part of the perioperative fluid plan is recommended.

References

1. Weiser TG, Regenbogen SE, Thompson KD, Haynes AB, Lipsitz SR, Berry WR, Gawande AA (2008) An estimation of the global volume of surgery: a modelling strategy based on available data. Lancet 372:139–144
2. Jhanji S, Thomas B, Ely A, Watson D, Hinds CJ, Pearse RM (2008) Mortality and utilisation of critical care resources amongst high-risk surgical patients in a large NHS trust. Anaesthesia 63:695–700
3. Pearse RM, Harrison DA, James P, Watson D, Hinds C, Rhodes A, Grounds RM, Bennett ED (2006) Identification and characterisation of the high-risk surgical population in the United Kingdom. Crit Care 10:R81
4. Lobo SM, de Oliveira NE (2013) Clinical review: what are the best hemodynamic targets for noncardiac surgical patients? Crit Care 17:210
5. Khuri SF, Henderson WG, DePalma RG, Mosca C, Healey NA, Kumbhani DJ (2005) Determinants of long-term survival after major surgery and the adverse effect of postoperative complications. Ann Surg 242:326–341
6. Hamilton MA, Cecconi M, Rhodes A (2011) A systematic review and meta-analysis on the use of preemptive hemodynamic intervention to improve postoperative outcomes in moderate and high-risk surgical patients. Anesth Analg 112:1392–1402
7. Gurgel ST, do Nascimento P Jr (2011) Maintaining tissue perfusion in high-risk surgical patients: a systematic review of randomized clinical trials. Anesth Analg 112:1384–1391
8. Cecconi M, Corredor C, Arulkumaran N, Abuella G, Ball J, Grounds RM, Hamilton M, Rhodes A (2013) Clinical review: goal-directed therapy-what is the evidence in surgical patients? The effect on different risk groups. Crit Care 17:209
9. Jhanji S, Lee C, Watson D, Hinds C, Pearse RM (2009) Microvascular flow and tissue oxygenation after major abdominal surgery: association with post-operative complications. Intensive Care Med 35:671–677
10. Marjanovic G, Villain C, Juettner E, Zur Hausen A, Hoeppner J, Hopt UT, Drognitz O, Obermaier R (2009) Impact of different crystalloid volume regimes on intestinal anastomotic stability. Ann Surg 249:181–185
11. Kulemann B, Timme S, Seifert G, Holzner PA, Glatz T, Sick O, Chikhladze S, Bronsert P, Hoeppner J, Werner M, Hopt UT, Marjanovic G (2013) Intraoperative crystalloid overload

leads to substantial inflammatory infiltration of intestinal anastomoses-a histomorphological analysis. Surgery 154:596–603
12. Nessim C, Sideris L, Turcotte S, Vafiadis P, Lapostole AC, Simard S, Koch P, Fortier LP, Dube P (2013) The effect of fluid overload in the presence of an epidural on the strength of colonic anastomoses. J Surg Res 183:567–573
13. Pizov R, Eden A, Bystritski D, Kalina E, Tamir A, Gelman S (2012) Hypotension during gradual blood loss: waveform variables response and absence of tachycardia. Br J Anaesth 109:911–918
14. Vincent JL, Rhodes A, Perel A, Martin GS, Della Rocca G, Vallet B, Pinsky MR, Hofer CK, Teboul JL, de Boode WP, Scolletta S, Vieillard-Baron A, De Backer D, Walley KR, Maggiorini M, Singer M (2011) Clinical review: update on hemodynamic monitoring–a consensus of 16. Crit Care 15:229
15. Legrand M, Dupuis C, Simon C, Gayat E, Mateo J, Lukaszewicz AC, Payen D (2013) Association between systemic hemodynamics and septic acute kidney injury in critically ill patients: a retrospective observational study. Crit Care 17:R278
16. Marik PE, Baram M, Vahid B (2008) Does central venous pressure predict fluid responsiveness? A systematic review of the literature and the tale of seven mares. Chest 134:172–178
17. Vincent JL, Weil MH (2006) Fluid challenge revisited. Crit Care Med 34:1333–1337
18. Thiele RH, Bartels K, Gan TJ (2015) Cardiac output monitoring: a contemporary assessment and review. Crit Care Med 43:177–185
19. Cannesson M, Pestel G, Ricks C, Hoeft A, Perel A (2011) Hemodynamic monitoring and management in patients undergoing high risk surgery: a survey among North American and European anesthesiologists. Crit Care 15:R197
20. Repesse X, Bodson L, Vieillard-Baron A (2013) Doppler echocardiography in shocked patients. Curr Opin Crit Care 19:221–227
21. Maltais S, Costello WT, Billings FT, Bick JS, Byrne JG, Ahmad RM, Wagner CE (2013) Episodic monoplane transesophageal echocardiography impacts postoperative management of the cardiac surgery patient. J Cardiothorac Vasc Anesth 27:665–669
22. Rhodes A, Cusack RJ, Newman PJ, Grounds RM, Bennett ED (2002) A randomised, controlled trial of the pulmonary artery catheter in critically ill patients. Intensive Care Med 28:256–264
23. Harvey S, Harrison DA, Singer M, Ashcroft J, Jones CM, Elbourne D, Brampton W, Williams D, Young D, Rowan K (2005) Assessment of the clinical effectiveness of pulmonary artery catheters in management of patients in intensive care (PAC-Man): a randomised controlled trial. Lancet 366:472–477
24. Harvey S, Young D, Brampton W, Cooper AB, Doig G, Sibbald W, Rowan K (2006) Pulmonary artery catheters for adult patients in intensive care. Cochrane Database Syst Rev 28: CD003408
25. Shah MR, Hasselblad V, Stevenson LW, Binanay C, O'Connor CM, Sopko G, Califf RM (2005) Impact of the pulmonary artery catheter in critically ill patients: meta-analysis of randomized clinical trials. JAMA 294:1664–1670
26. Vincent JL, Pinsky MR, Sprung CL, Levy M, Marini JJ, Payen D, Rhodes A, Takala J (2008) The pulmonary artery catheter: in medio virtus. Crit Care Med 36:3093–3096
27. Vincent JL (2012) The pulmonary artery catheter. J Clin Monit Comput 26:341–345
28. Gardner RM (1981) Direct blood pressure measurement – dynamic response requirements. Anesthesiology 54:227–236
29. Hamzaoui O, Monnet X, Richard C, Osman D, Chemla D, Teboul JL (2008) Effects of changes in vascular tone on the agreement between pulse contour and transpulmonary thermodilution cardiac output measurements within an up to 6-hour calibration-free period. Crit Care Med 36:434–440
30. Oren-Grinberg A (2010) The PiCCO monitor. Int Anesthesiol Clin 48:57–85
31. Bendjelid K, Marx G, Kiefer N, Simon TP, Geisen M, Hoeft A, Siegenthaler N, Hofer CK (2013) Performance of a new pulse contour method for continuous cardiac output monitoring: validation in critically ill patients. Br J Anaesth 111:573–579

32. Cecconi M, Fawcett J, Grounds RM, Rhodes A (2008) A prospective study to evaluate the accuracy of pulse power analysis to monitor cardiac output in critically ill patients. BMC Anesthesiol 8:3
33. Cecconi M, Dawson D, Grounds RM, Rhodes A (2009) Lithium dilution cardiac output measurement in the critically ill patient: determination of precision of the technique. Intensive Care Med 35:498–504
34. Senn A, Button D, Zollinger A, Hofer CK (2009) Assessment of cardiac output changes using a modified FloTrac/Vigileo algorithm in cardiac surgery patients. Crit Care 13:R32
35. Cecconi M, Fasano N, Langiano N, Divella M, Costa MG, Rhodes A, Della Rocca G (2011) Goal-directed haemodynamic therapy during elective total hip arthroplasty under regional anaesthesia. Crit Care 15:R132
36. Critchley LA, Critchley JA (1999) A meta-analysis of studies using bias and precision statistics to compare cardiac output measurement techniques. J Clin Monit Comput 15:85–91
37. Cecconi M, Rhodes A, Poloniecki J, Della Rocca G, Grounds RM (2009) Bench-to-bedside review: the importance of the precision of the reference technique in method comparison studies – with specific reference to the measurement of cardiac output. Crit Care 13:201
38. Squara P, Cecconi M, Rhodes A, Singer M, Chiche JD (2009) Tracking changes in cardiac output: methodological considerations for the validation of monitoring devices. Intensive Care Med 35:1801–1808
39. Critchley LA, Lee A, Ho AM (2010) A critical review of the ability of continuous cardiac output monitors to measure trends in cardiac output. Anesth Analg 111:1180–1192
40. Vincent JL, Pelosi P, Pearse R, Payen D, Perel A, Hoeft A, Romagnoli S, Ranieri VM, Ichai C, Forget P, Rocca GD, Rhodes A (2015) Perioperative cardiovascular monitoring of high-risk patients: a consensus of 12. Crit Care 19(1):224
41. Reeves ST, Finley AC, Skubas NJ et al (2013) Basic perioperative transesophageal echocardiography examination: a consensus statement of the American Society of Echocardiography and the Society of Cardiovascular Anesthesiologists. Anesth Analg 117(3):543e58
42. Poth JM, Beck DR, Bartels K (2014) Ultrasonography for haemodynamic monitoring. Best Pract Res Clin Anaesthesiol 28:337e351
43. Navarro LH, Bloomstone JA, Auler JO Jr, Cannesson M, Rocca GD, Gan TJ, Kinsky M, Magder S, Miller TE, Mythen M, Perel A, Reuter DA, Pinsky MR, Kramer GC (2015) Perioperative fluid therapy: a statement from the international fluid optimization group. Perioper Med (Lond) 4:3
44. Perel A, Habicher M, Sander M (2013) Bench-to-bedside review: functional hemodynamics during surgery – should it be used for all high-risk cases? Crit Care 17:203
45. Desebbe O, Cannesson M (2008) Using ventilation-induced plethysmographic variations to optimize patient fluid status. Curr Opin Anaesthesiol 21:772–778
46. Sandroni C, Cavallaro F, Marano C, Falcone C, De Santis P, Antonelli M (2012) Accuracy of plethysmographic indices as predictors of fluid responsiveness in mechanically ventilated adults: a systematic review and meta-analysis. Intensive Care Med 38:1429–1437
47. Forget P, Lois F, de Kock M (2010) Goal-directed fluid management based on the pulse oximeter-derived pleth variability index reduces lactate levels and improves fluid management. Anesth Analg 111:910–914
48. Forget P, Lois F, Kartheuser A, Leonard D, Remue C, de Kock M (2013) The concept of titration can be transposed to fluid management. But does is change the volumes? Randomised trial on pleth variability index during fast-track colonic surgery. Curr Clin Pharmacol 8:110–114
49. Mahjoub Y, Lejeune V, Muller L, Perbet S, Zieleskiewicz L, Bart F, Veber B, Paugam-Burtz C, Jaber S, Ayham A, Zogheib E, Lasocki S, Vieillard-Baron A, Quintard H, Joannes-Boyau O, Plantefeve G, Montravers P, Duperret S, Lakhdari M, Ammenouche N, Lorne E, Slama M, Dupont H (2014) Evaluation of pulse pressure variation validity criteria in critically ill patients: a prospective observational multicentre point-prevalence study. Br J Anaesth 112:681–685
50. Marik PE, Cavallazzi R, Vasu T, Hirani A (2009) Dynamic changes in arterial waveform derived variables and fluid responsiveness in mechanically ventilated patients: a systematic review of the literature. Crit Care Med 37:2642–2647

51. Futier E, Constantin JM, Paugam-Burtz C, Pascal J, Eurin M, Neuschwander A, Marret E, Beaussier M, Gutton C, Lefrant JY, Allaouchiche B, Verzilli D, Leone M, De Jong A, Bazin JE, Pereira B, Jaber S (2013) A trial of intraoperative low-tidal-volume ventilation in abdominal surgery. N Engl J Med 369:428–437
52. Serpa Neto A, Cardoso SO, Manetta JA, Pereira VG, Esposito DC, Pasqualucci Mde O, Damasceno MC, Schultz MJ (2012) Association between use of lung-protective ventilation with lower tidal volumes and clinical outcomes among patients without acute respiratory distress syndrome: a meta-analysis. JAMA 308:1651–1659
53. Cannesson M, Le Manach Y, Hofer CK, Goarin JP, Lehot JJ, Vallet B, Tavernier B (2011) Assessing the diagnostic accuracy of pulse pressure variations for the prediction of fluid responsiveness: a "gray zone" approach. Anesthesiology 115:231–241
54. Monnet X, Teboul JL (2008) Passive leg raising. Intensive Care Med 34:659–663
55. Michard F (2014) Long live dynamic parameters! Crit Care 18:413
56. Dueck MH, Klimek M, Appenrodt S, Weigand C, Boerner U (2005) Trends but not individual values of central venous oxygen saturation agree with mixed venous oxygen saturation during varying hemodynamic conditions. Anesthesiology 103:249–257
57. Ho KM, Harding R, Chamberlain J, Bulsara M (2010) A comparison of central and mixed venous oxygen saturation in circulatory failure. J Cardiothorac Vasc Anesth 24:434–439
58. Collaborative Study Group on Perioperative ScvO2 Monitoring (2006) Multicentre study on peri- and postoperative central venous oxygen saturation in high-risk surgical patients. Crit Care 10:R158
59. Perz S, Uhlig T, Kohl M, Bredle DL, Reinhart K, Bauer M, Kortgen A (2011) Low and "supranormal" central venous oxygen saturation and markers of tissue hypoxia in cardiac surgery patients: a prospective observational study. Intensive Care Med 37:52–59
60. Fuller BM, Dellinger RP (2012) Lactate as a hemodynamic marker in the critically ill. Curr Opin Crit Care 18:267–272
61. Meregalli A, Oliveira RP, Friedman G (2004) Occult hypoperfusion is associated with increased mortality in hemodynamically stable, high-risk, surgical patients. Crit Care 8:R60–R65
62. Bakker J, Coffernils M, Leon M, Gris P, Vincent JL (1991) Blood lactate levels are superior to oxygen-derived variables in predicting outcome in human septic shock. Chest 99:956–962
63. Jansen TC, van Bommel J, Schoonderbeek FJ, Sleeswijk Visser SJ, van der Klooster JM, Lima AP, Willemsen SP, Bakker J (2010) Early lactate-guided therapy in intensive care unit patients: a multicenter, open-label, randomized controlled trial. Am J Respir Crit Care Med 182:752–761
64. Jansen TC, van Bommel J, Woodward R, Mulder PG, Bakker J (2009) Association between blood lactate levels, sequential organ failure assessment subscores, and 28-day mortality during early and late intensive care unit stay: a retrospective observational study. Crit Care Med 37:2369–2374
65. McKendry M, McGloin H, Saberi D, Caudwell L, Brady AR, Singer M (2004) Randomised controlled trial assessing the impact of a nurse delivered, flow monitored protocol for optimisation of circulatory status after cardiac surgery. BMJ 329:258
66. Pearse R, Dawson D, Fawcett J, Rhodes A, Grounds RM, Bennett ED (2005) Early goal-directed therapy after major surgery reduces complications and duration of hospital stay. A randomised, controlled trial [ISRCTN38797445]. Crit Care 9:R687–R693
67. Bundgaard-Nielsen M, Holte K, Secher NH, Kehlet H (2007) Monitoring of peri-operative fluid administration by individualized goal-directed therapy. Acta Anaesthesiol Scand 51:331–340
68. Wilson J, Woods I, Fawcett J, Whall R, Dibb W, Morris C, McManus E (1999) Reducing the risk of major elective surgery: randomised controlled trial of preoperative optimisation of oxygen delivery. BMJ 318:1099–1103
69. Lobo SM, Salgado PF, Castillo VG, Borim AA, Polachini CA, Palchetti JC, Brienzi SL, de Oliveira GG (2000) Effects of maximizing oxygen delivery on morbidity and mortality in high-risk surgical patients. Crit Care Med 28:3396–3404

70. Lopes MR, Oliveira MA, Pereira VO, Lemos IP, Auler JO Jr, Michard F (2007) Goal-directed fluid management based on pulse pressure variation monitoring during high-risk surgery: a pilot randomized controlled trial. Crit Care 11:R100
71. Pearse RM, Harrison DA, MacDonald N, Gillies MA, Blunt M, Ackland G, Grocott MP, Ahern A, Griggs K, Scott R, Hinds C, Rowan K (2014) Effect of a perioperative, cardiac output-guided hemodynamic therapy algorithm on outcomes following major gastrointestinal surgery: a randomized clinical trial and systematic review. JAMA 311:2181–2190
72. Morris C (2013) Oesophageal Doppler monitoring, doubt and equipoise: evidence based medicine means change. Anaesthesia 68:684–688
73. Scheeren TW, Wiesenack C, Gerlach H, Marx G (2013) Goal-directed intraoperative fluid therapy guided by stroke volume and its variation in high-risk surgical patients: a prospective randomized multicentre study. J Clin Monit Comput 27:225–233
74. Goepfert MS, Richter HP, Zu EC, Gruetzmacher J, Rafflenbeul E, Roeher K, von Sandersleben A, Diedrichs S, Reichenspurner H, Goetz AE, Reuter DA (2013) Individually optimized hemodynamic therapy reduces complications and length of stay in the intensive care unit: a prospective, randomized controlled trial. Anesthesiology 119:824–836
75. Fellahi JL, Parienti JJ, Hanouz JL, Plaud B, Riou B, Ouattara A (2008) Perioperative use of dobutamine in cardiac surgery and adverse cardiac outcome: propensity-adjusted analyses. Anesthesiology 108:979–987
76. Pearse RM, Belsey JD, Cole JN, Bennett ED (2008) Effect of dopexamine infusion on mortality following major surgery: individual patient data meta-regression analysis of published clinical trials. Crit Care Med 36:1323–1329
77. Takala J, Meier-Hellmann A, Eddleston J, Hulstaert P, Sramek V (2000) Effect of dopexamine on outcome after major abdominal surgery: a prospective, randomized, controlled multicenter study. European Multicenter Study Group on Dopexamine in Major Abdominal Surgery. Crit Care Med 28:3417–3423

What Are the Specific Challenges in the Postoperative Mechanical Ventilation After Thoracic Surgery?

11

Edmond Cohen, Peter Biro, and Mert Şentürk

11.1 Introduction

The incidence of mechanical ventilation for more than 48 h after thoracic surgery has been reported to be necessary in up to 9.3 % [1]. It is also well known that the requirement and also the duration of mechanical ventilation after thoracic surgery are significantly correlated to postoperative morbidity [2, 3]. Although these figures in older publications appear to be unrealistically high for current practice, it has to be kept in mind that thoracic surgery and anesthesia deal with patients with more morbidities than 20 years ago. Moreover, even if the incidence of problems might not be higher, the intensity of the challenge remains the same. In a recent meta-analysis, it has been demonstrated that the incidence of postoperative "acute lung injury" (ALI) after thoracic surgery was 4.3 %. Although this rate was similar to the one of the abdominal surgery (3.4 %), the attributable mortality of postoperative lung injury was higher in patients after thoracic interventions (26.5 % vs 12.2 %) [4].

Other chapters in this book cover some topics of this chapter too, such as the ICU indications after thoracic surgery, how to predict and protect postoperative respiratory failure, as well as noninvasive ventilation and extracorporeal lung assist. This chapter will focus therefore on some specific challenges of mechanical ventilation in postthoracotomy patients.

E. Cohen
Departments of Anesthesiology and Thoracic Surgery, The Icahn School of Medicine at Mount Sinai, New York, NY, USA

P. Biro
Institute of Anesthesiology, University Hospital Zurich, Zurich, Switzerland

M. Şentürk (✉)
Department of Anesthesiology and Intensive Care Medicine, Istanbul University, Istanbul Faculty of Medicine, Istanbul, Turkey
e-mail: senturkm@istanbul.edu.tr

© Springer International Publishing Switzerland 2017

M. Şentürk, M.O. Sungur (eds.), *Postoperative Care in Thoracic Surgery*,
DOI 10.1007/978-3-319-19908-5_11

11.2 Ventilatory Support After Thoracic Surgery

Thoracic surgery is unique in the sense that the target organ of both the surgery and of mechanical ventilation is the same. Not only may surgeons remove large parts of the lungs, they often traumatize parts of the remaining healthy lung tissue, and they also may damage the respiratory muscles. Moreover, thoracotomy is one of the most painful incisions which can further impair ventilation. One can assume that the postoperative lung injury would be more likely due to the surgical trauma. However, it has been shown that the degree of radiological density increase was significantly greater in the nonoperative lung compared to operative lung after lobectomy [5].

Almost all complications (both respiratory and non-respiratory) after thoracic surgery result in respiratory failure (Fig. 11.1). The clinical picture is usually a mixed one rather than pure hypoxemic or pure hypocapnic:

- A reduced functional lung volume may result from resection of parenchyma, atelectasis, lung edema, and thoracic restriction from postoperative pain.
- Decreased functional residual and volume capacities, dysfunction of the diaphragm and intercostal muscles, and increased airway resistance may cause impaired ventilation.
- Ventilation-perfusion mismatch and decreased minute ventilation may lead to impaired gas exchange [6].

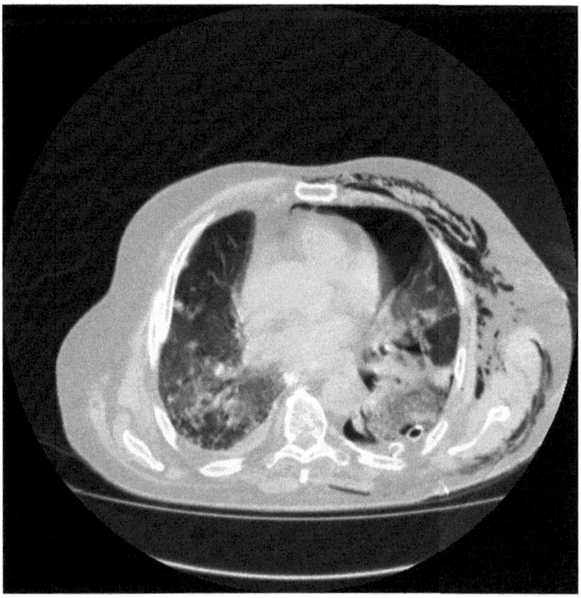

Fig. 11.1 CT scan of a patient who developed adult respiratory distress syndrome after thoracotomy. CT scan of a patient following thoracotomy for left upper lobectomy who subsequently developed adult respiratory distress syndrome: There is space where the lung tissue was resected, atelectatic areas in the remaining lung tissue, infiltrations in both lungs without any clinical signs of infection, and subcutaneous emphysema

In addition, excessive intravenous fluid infusion and blood transfusion can directly harm or exacerbate harm to the lungs.

Actually, mechanical ventilation in the PACU or ICU should be avoided if possible, since it can cause a "ventilator-associated or ventilator-related lung injury" or worsen it. Every attempt of invasive mechanical ventilation is associated with a risk of making things worse while trying to improve the patient's condition. This risk is higher in patients after thoracotomy because the lungs (both the operated and the ventilated lung) have already been exposed to a "first hit" during the operation. In addition, clinical experience would suggest that positive pressure ventilation can injure fresh anastomoses or bronchial stump, although there is no evidence for this plausible assumption.

11.3 Practical Hints

Pragmatic rules that would help to decrease the possibility of having unwarranted events when deciding to continue mechanical ventilation after thoracic operations:

- On the one hand, anesthesiologists, surgeons, and intensivists have to avoid post-thoracotomy mechanical ventilation. On the other hand, the longer the patient has to deliver an increased work of breathing, the later he will recover from respiratory failure.
- Spontaneous breathing is better than mechanical ventilation, and assisted ventilation is better than controlled one. However, the need for tracheal re-intubation can be considered as a worst case scenario.
- The decision to ventilate should be made intraoperatively, and preoperative predictions should be continuously reevaluated.
- If mechanical ventilation needs to be continued, the intraoperative double-lumen tube (DLT) should be replaced at the end of surgery with a normal single-lumen tracheal tube. However, in patients who are intended to be extubated within two hours postoperatively, the DLT may remain in place with a deflated bronchial lumen cuff.
- Transition to a single-lumen tube should be performed via a tube exchanger of sufficient length (caveat: DLTs are longer than single-lumen tubes). It should be kept in mind that an "easy" intubation at the start of the operation may later become "difficult" due to various reasons such as airway edema.
- In a patient, in whom postoperative ventilation is planned, the use of a bronchial blocker (BB) can be indicated because this avoids the transition from the double- to a single-lumen tube. Thus, the BB has to be removed only.
- A Univent® tube (LMA North America Inc, San Diego, CA) can remain in place for postoperative ventilation, but the blocker should be pulled back into the main lumen.
- Finally, weaning from mechanical ventilation is a process that should start on admission of a patient to ICU whose trachea is intubated.

11.4 Protective Lung Ventilation

Actually, the concept of "protective lung ventilation" (PLV) was defined and determined in ARDS patients [7], but this approach becomes even more important in the vulnerable lungs of patients after thoracic surgery. PLV includes:

- Low tidal volumes (TV) of 6–8 ml/kg
- Appropriate positive end-expiratory pressure (PEEP)
- Recruitment maneuvers (RM)

Meta-analyses have found PLV to be effective and protective in both ARDS in the ICU and in OLV [8–10]. An intraoperative TV of 6–8 ml/kg has been associated with a decreased frequency of postoperative pulmonary failure [11]. Although there is no evidence that the same argument is also valid for the postoperative period, there is clear evidence for using these guidelines in general ICU patients. Moreover, this circumstance means to have a reduction of functional lung tissue that is similar to the "baby lung" in ARDS [12].

The details of this strategy are extensively discussed elsewhere in this book; the authors will only focus on some recent dilemmas:

1. Is any particular component "more" important than the other? Recently, it has been reported that the driving pressure (defined as TV/respiratory system compliance) (DP) is the ventilation variable that best classifies as a risk of ALI in ARDS patients [13]. Changes in DP play a much more important role as compared to PEEP or peak inspiratory pressure (PIP). It is questionable, whether it is more appropriate to define the PLV with "low DP" (of less than approximately 20 cmH_2O) rather than "low TV."
2. Is a TV of 6 mL/kg protective enough? Considering that thoracic surgery is usually associated with a reduction in lung volume, e.g., in a patient after pneumonectomy, 6 mL/kg would mean again to be too high and maybe not protective anymore. In an animal study, applying the same TV to one lung compared with two lungs has resulted in significantly greater lung injury shown in histologically assessed "diffuse alveolar damage" score [14]. On the other hand, halving the TV to 3–4 mL/kg, its size would decrease below dead space ventilation. Empirically, a TV of 4–6 mL/kg seems rational, but needs to be proven and checked on an individual basis.
3. What if the DP is still high even if TV is kept low? In cases of severely decreased lung compliance and/or severe reduction effective lung volume, very high driving pressures can be necessary even for low TVs. Although it is a very rare condition, the so-called ultraprotective ventilation (application of extracorporeal lung assist (ECLA) systems) might become necessary. It has been shown in two studies (an animal study [15] and a clinical study [16]) that ECLA helps to decrease the TV to very low amounts to avoid high pressures during ALI in the postoperative period. The resulting survival rate was much higher than in the conventional setting (100 % in the animal study and 86 % (six of seven patients) in humans). ECLA is discussed in another chapter in this book.

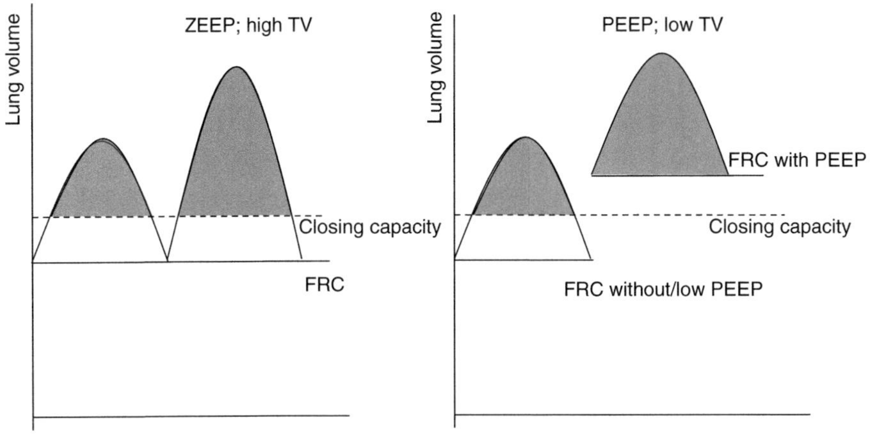

Fig. 11.2 Relationship of *FRC* (functional residual capacity) and *CC* (closing capacity) in different ventilatory settings. *Right*: FRC falls below CC during mechanical ventilation; a larger tidal volume (TV) can obtain a better gas exchange (note the larger area above the CC line); however, a cyclic recruitment cannot be avoided. *Left*: Applying PEEP during keeping the TV low: PEEP obtains an FRC above the CC. Cyclic recruitment is avoided; and the ventilation (now the area above the "new" FRC) is still better than the one without PEEP (Adapted from [17] (with permission))

4. "How to apply 'PEEP'?" PEEP is "good" not only for the improvement of oxygenation but also (and maybe more importantly) for the improvement of the V/Q relationship in the dependent lung and for prevention of alveolar collapse at end expiration by increasing the functional residual capacity (Fig. 11.2) [17]. However, excessive PEEP can also lead to an unnecessary and harmful rightward shift of the ventilation in pressure-volume curve (Fig. 11.3). Moreover, although it is not evidence based and may even sound irrational, "clinical experience" would suggest that positive pressure ventilation can injure fresh anastomoses or bronchial stumps. An approach to keep PEEP "as high as necessary" and "as low as possible" can help to overcome both atelectasis and alveolar overdistension [18]; but practically, this issue is more complicated than at first sight. A "decremental trial" following a recruitment maneuver (RM) (stepwise decline of PEEP from 20 cm H_2O) to adjust the best compliance appears to be appropriate [19].
5. How to recruit? While PEEP can keep the lung open, it is not capable of opening an atelectatic lung. To open collapsed regions, a recruitment maneuver (RM) is necessary [20]. However, in patients with air leak, RM is contraindicated; moreover, in patients without an air leak (or with a small one), there is a common "fear" of the high pressure generated by RM, and PEEP may disrupt bronchial stumps and anastomoses. RM after thoracic surgery is an issue, of which pros and cons have to be examined in the individual clinical setting.

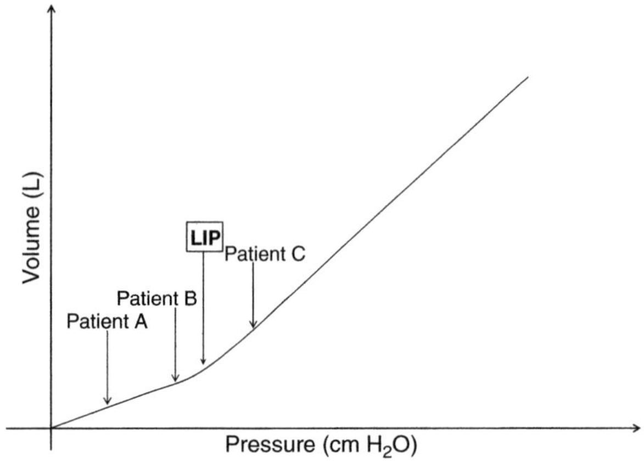

Fig. 11.3 Relationship of PEEP and *LIP* (lower inflection point). Note that LIP can differ in each individual and can sometimes be zero. *A*, *B*, and *C* are possible points for total (intrinsic + external) end-expiratory pressure. The level of external PEEP should be adjusted to get closer to LIP, e.g., if the external PEEP brings the total PEEP from *A* to *B*, oxygenation gets better, but if the external PEEP brings the total PEEP from *B* to *C*, oxygenation gets impaired; if the LIP is 0, the best oxygenation is obtained by *A* (Adapted from [17] (with permission))

11.5 Permissive Hypercapnia

Clinicians tend to compensate the reductions in TV by an increase in frequency to maintain the minute ventilation volume. However, this might be wrong:

1. The price of shorter inspiration can be a higher airway pressures, and the consequence of shorter expiration can be air trapping and auto-PEEP.
2. Physically, it is the "power" that plays a role in the lung injury (rather than "work"), and therefore "the number of the hammer hits per time" is also important (quote of Luciano Gattinoni). Increasing the respiratory rate (=hits with the hammer) increases the energy that causes the lung injury.
3. More importantly, mild hypercapnia is not only something that can be permitted in many cases [21], it can also be even therapeutic for several hours [22]. Permissive hypercapnia may protect the lung and improve the tissue oxygenation as a result of the increased cardiac output and the resulting right shift of the oxygen (O_2) saturation curve [23].
4. On the other hand, it should be kept in mind that hypercapnia exacerbates hypoxic pulmonary vasoconstriction, and therefore, it is contraindicated in pulmonary hypertension, which is more frequent in patients after thoracotomy. In the remaining population, permissive hypercapnia can be considered as a standard procedure of protective lung ventilation.

11.6 Inspired Oxygen Fraction

Increased O_2 consumption in postoperative patients has led to a routine administration of supplemental O_2. However, it has been shown that this approach could be more harmful than beneficial [24]. Although this study was performed in medical emergencies, the mechanism of the damage from high FiO_2 can be viewed as valid for patients after thoracic surgery. These are the postulated pathways of possible damages caused by hyperoxia:

1. Coronary and systemic vasoconstriction leading to a decreased stroke volume.
2. Even a short period of preoxygenation with an FiO_2 of 1.0 can lead to atelectasis as a result of collapsed alveoli because of the replacement of nitrogen [25].

Obviously, hypoxemia of the postoperative patient should be treated, but one still has to avoid hyperoxia: Hypoxemia should be treated with stepwise increases in FiO_2 as high as necessary to avoid hyperoxia [24].

Recently, increasing the FiO_2 prior to application of the bundle of "low TV-PEEP-RM" has been advocated: the so-called permissive atelectasis. Although this suggestion was limited to mechanical ventilation during anesthesia of the "healthy" lungs, the extrapolation to postthoracotomy patients should be examined [18].

11.7 Ventilation Mode

Considering that it is the "driving pressure" (DP) that is the principle reason for lung injury, it appears to have less or even no meaning whether to apply the same DP with pressure-controlled (PCV) or volume-controlled way (VCV). Previous studies advocating PCV because of its "descending flow pattern" that resembles more to physiologic spontaneous breathing in OLV [26] have not been confirmed in more recent studies with similar settings [27]. The effects during postoperative period can be considered to be similar.

The only difference between these ventilation modes is probably the lower peak (not the plateau) airway pressures, which contributes less (if any) to ALI. Recently it has been shown in OLV that PCV was more associated with an improvement in right ventricular function than VCV.[28] Right ventricular function is crucial for patients after thoracic surgery; however, whether the reported advantage can also be extrapolated for the postoperative period also remains to be examined.

Physiological breathing is irregular in all its components (TV, frequency, sighs, etc.). It has been shown in an experimental ALI study that a so-called "noisy" pressure support ventilation was associated with an improvement in oxygenation and also a redistribution of pulmonary blood flow [29].

11.8 Patients Requiring Mechanical Ventilation, but Having a Leak

The most "specific" challenge of postthoracotomy mechanical ventilation appears to be the patients with a persisting air leak and a need of mechanical ventilation. Both conditions deteriorate each other: persisting air leak aggravates the respiratory failure and increases the need for mechanical ventilation, and positive pressure ventilation sustains and aggravates the air leak. In these patients, noninvasive ventilation can be tried (which is discussed in another chapter). In some cases, application of high-frequency jet ventilation or differential lung ventilation can be necessary.

11.9 High-Frequency Jet Ventilation (HFJV) After Thoracic Surgery

High-frequency jet ventilation (HFJV) plays a marginal role in the postoperative ventilation after thoracic surgery since it has only one rational indication: the presence of a bronchopleural fistula [30]. It's a basic characteristic of jet ventilation in general that it usually produces lower positive airway pressure than conventional ventilation. This is due to the circumstance that HFJV is only possible if the airway is kept open to the atmosphere to enable free air egress. This way, a positive airway pressure cannot build up, except when the exhalation pathway is blocked. In the case of a bronchopleural fistula, there are even two separate openings that permit the efflux of gas: (1) the proximally open upper airway (e.g., via a tracheal or bronchial tube) and (2) via the fistula. Air egress through the fistula is nevertheless an undesired effect, since it prevents closure and healing of the pathology. Therefore, it is the goal of the therapy that this pathway should occlude as soon as possible by minimizing the gas flow. This might be facilitated by a lower airway pressure, than it would occur during conventional ventilation. Additionally, a large amount of gas loss through the fistula would even impede the application of positive pressure ventilation. These circumstances lead to the consideration of HFJV as a better means to ventilate the affected lung if a unilateral single-lung ventilation of the dependent lung is considered insufficient to maintain gas exchange. Usually, the bronchopleural fistula is unilateral and may occur on the side of the preceding lung surgery. If the leak caused by the fistula is small, spontaneous breathing should be maintained, since this way the airway pressure is also very low. However, if ventilator support is considered necessary, a differential ventilation of the two lungs should be considered.

During the operation, the airway was intubated with a double-lumen tube. If the fistula becomes apparent after extubation, and it attains a magnitude that requires ventilator support, the most feasible interface to apply ventilation would be again a double-lumen tracheal tube in order to separate the two lungs. The primary scope of lung separation is to permit conventional ventilation of the healthy lung, while the affected one will receive HFJV [31, 32].

The settings of HFJV for the affected lung may be adjusted according to the metabolic needs of the patient. The goal is to apply as much HFJV as necessary (to maintain an adequate gas exchange) and to reduce it to the lowest possible extent (to obtain the lowest possible gas loss through the fistula). The main determinant of the amount of HFJV is driving pressure (DP), which leads to resulting parameters such as gas flow, tidal volume, and airway pressure. It's absolutely necessary to titrate the DP stepwise to the magnitude which is optimal in the mentioned sense. This setting has to be readjusted regularly to changes in the size of the gas leak. Other settings are oxygen concentration, inspiration duration, and frequency. Oxygen concentration should be set according to the resulting oxygenation parameters; the inspiration duration is of secondary importance and should be set at 40 or 50 %, while the ventilation frequency may be variated between 120 and 300 cycles per minute. The choice of the frequency should allow for the lowest possible airway pressure by choosing a high frequency, while an eventually necessary contribution to carbon dioxide elimination might require a low frequency; in this respect an ideal balance between these two interests should be found. In most cases one would begin HFJV with 100 % oxygen, a DP at 1.5 bar, inspiration duration of 40 %, and a frequency of 150 cycles per minute. The resulting blood gases may indicate the moment when the DP may be stepwise lowered as well as the frequency may be increased. This development would represent the desired healing of the underlying pathology. As soon as one arrives at a DP < 0.8 bar and a frequency of 300 cycles per minute, the contribution of HFJV to oxygenation and carbon dioxide elimination becomes small and might be discontinued. This also would allow abrogating lung separation and ventilator support.

11.10 Differential Lung Ventilation

For a thoracic anesthetist, differential lung ventilation (DLV) appears to be familiar as a variant of OLV. For patients after thoracic surgery, DLV has two major indications: unilateral lung processes and air leaks [33]. The rationale is to ventilate both lungs – synchronized or not – with different TVs and/or PEEPs. In ARDS, this method has been used primarily in unilateral pathologies; however, it can be used also successfully in bilateral ARDS in lateral decubitus position, where the heterogeneous distribution of ventilation can be divided to both lungs via the decubitus position; in this manner, DLV enables the titration and application of "selective optimal PEEPs" to both lungs [34].

The aim of DLV in a patient with air leak/fistula is to promote healing in the sick lung with a very modest DP while compromising less severely oxygenation and gas exchange. It can also protect the healthy lung against the pathologic processes of the other lung including massive unilateral hemoptysis, bronchiectasis, and lung abscesses.

During DLV, two coupled ventilators ("master" and "slave") with synchronized inspiration and expiration can be used. Two ventilators can also be used in an asynchronized manner, but this may cause a mediastinal shift. The "healthy" lung is ventilated with conventional setting (to take over the gas exchange); the lung with the leak is ventilated with very less TV, lower or no PEEP, and never recruitment maneuvers.

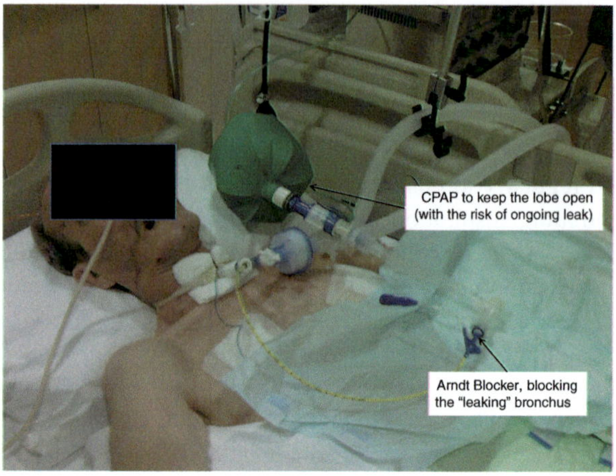

Fig. 11.4 In a patient with persistent bronchopleural fistula requiring mechanical ventilation, the lung (or the lobe) with the fistula can be blocked with a bronchial blocker. The remaining lung can be mechanically ventilated, and in the blocked part lung, a low level of continuous positive airway pressure can be applied to prevent a full collapse without exacerbating a fistula

An easier solution is to ventilate one lung (the "healthy" one) with the conventional setting, while continuous positive airway pressure (CPAP) or high-frequency ventilation (HFV) can be applied to the "sick" lung (Fig. 11.4).

Obviously, the use of DLV in the ICU for a prolonged time can be associated with several problems (such as possible tube disposition, obligatory muscle relaxation, etc.). Therefore, the use of DLV in postthoracotomy patients is still limited to patients, in whom mechanical ventilation is necessary, but the air leak persists.

11.11 Weaning

An essential rule of mechanical ventilation is (or should be) that the weaning should start – at least in the mind of the physician – when the mechanical ventilation starts. Weaning from mechanical ventilation should be performed as quickly as possible but not so fast as to be unsuccessful. Some criteria should be fulfilled to obtain an uncomplicated extubation, no matter how long was the duration of mechanical ventilation:

- Normothermia
- Cooperation
- Sufficient coughing
- Reliable spontaneous breathing and acceptable levels of pH, $PaCO_2$, and PaO_2

One of the key points of a successful weaning is to follow a well-defined protocol [35]. The weaning protocols should clearly define patients in whom weaning should be tried, the methods and strategies of weaning, and what is successful weaning (Fig. 11.5).

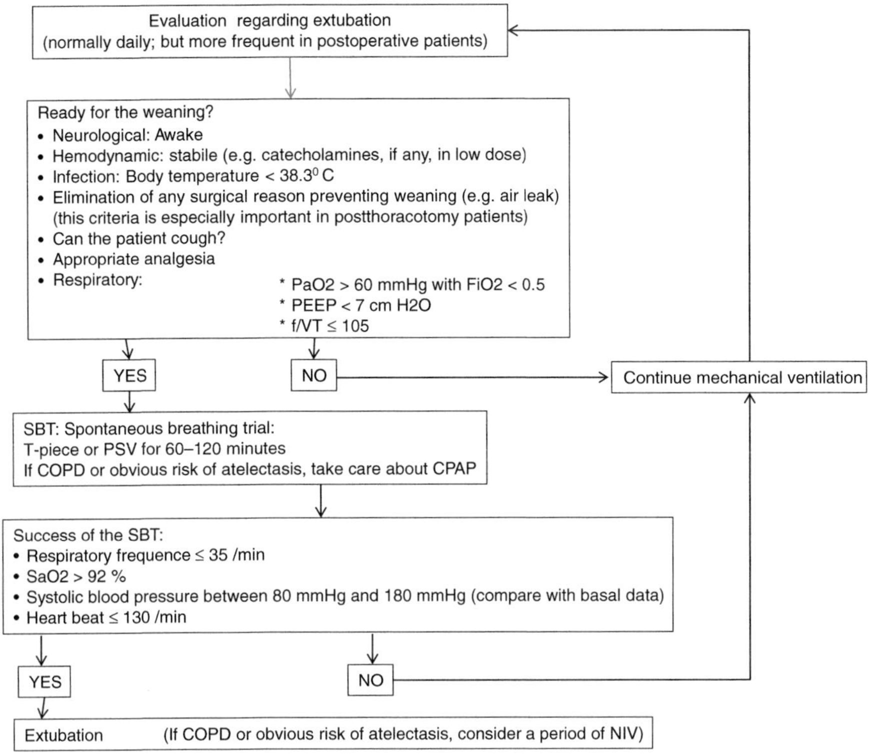

Fig. 11.5 Weaning protocol. A weaning protocol for patients with delayed tracheal extubation following surgery including thoracotomy, which is used in the Istanbul Medical Faculty. Note that protocols can differ between centers, but an institutional protocol should exist and be followed

Some rules for the successful weaning include:

- Daily trials of spontaneous breathing: should be performed in every patient who is mechanically ventilated more than 24 h to prevent remaining "unrecognized"
- Search and treatment of the reason of a failing trial
- An algorithmic protocol that directs from controlled to supported ventilation and from invasive ventilation to NIV
- Prevention of oversedation (and also undersedation)

11.12 Tracheostomy

In cases of prolonged mechanical ventilation, or even a prediction of prolonged mechanical ventilation of more than 7 days along with unsuccessful weaning trials, tracheostomy should be considered. Even removing the tube and associated tapes obtains reduced doses of sedatives. Moreover, and more importantly, it eases mobilization and facilitates removal of tracheal secretions. The patient may be able to eat, drink, and even speak. In spite of some contrary studies, it is generally considered that early tracheostomy is associated with easier weaning and a decrease in infections.

For postthoracotomy patients, surgeons tend to perform a surgical tracheotomy, but as a routine practice of ICU, percutaneous tracheostomy is easier, safer, and cheaper, at least in uncomplicated cases.

11.13 Management of Chest Tubes

For thoracic surgery, chest tube placement is a routine and almost mandatory procedure. Therefore, the physician responsible for the postoperative care should also be familiar with the management of the drainage of the thorax including diagnosis and treatment of its complications. Chest tubes allow drainage of air (ventral or cranial placement) and/or fluid (dorsal or caudal placement). Therefore, the physician's goal is to monitor, prevent, or treat air leaks and excessive pleural drainage [36]. Via the classical three-bottle chest tube drainage system (Fig. 11.6), the air from the pleura can be aspirated passively with a water seal or actively by attaching

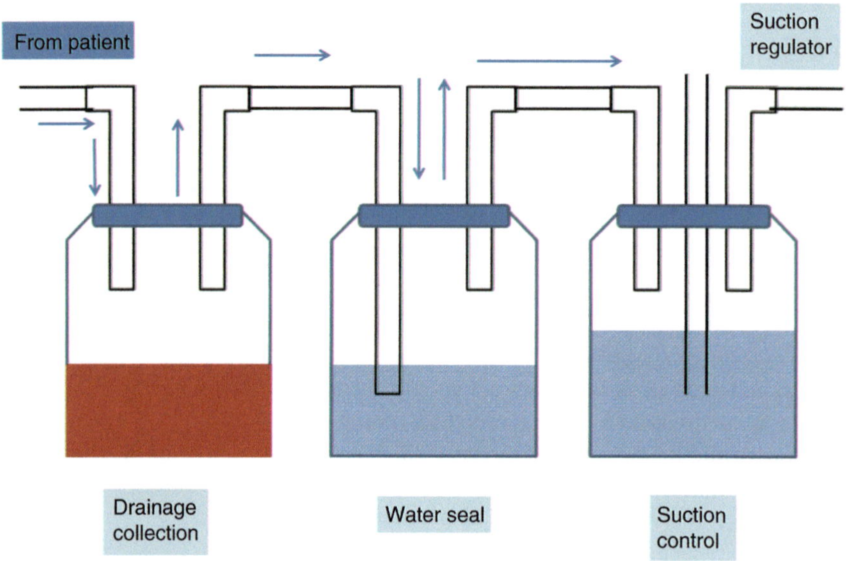

Fig. 11.6 Three-bottle chest drainage system. Using the *first* (drainage collection) *bottle* only would cause an increased resistance to drainage as a result of rising fluid/blood level and/or the foamy mixture of blood and air in the bottle. Adding a *second bottle* (water seal) allows fluid to drain into the first bottle only and the air into the second, also preventing the foam from forming. However, the added length of the tubing can increase the dead space and add further resistance, causing a reversal of flow back up into the tube and back into the pleural space. Therefore, a *third bottle* (suction control) allows for active suction to be exerted on the system, preventing the chest tube effluent from going back toward the patient (Adapted from [40] (with permission))

a piped source of vacuum. There are controversial reports regarding the effects of passive and active (or alternating) suction [37, 38]. A balanced chest drainage system may be the most rational strategy to maintain the mediastinum in a neutral position. If active aspiration is chosen, the negative pressure should not exceed 15–20 cm H_2O. Negative pressure should be avoided after pneumonectomy, because it can cause mediastinal shift. Tubes should never be clamped, for example, during patient transport, because of the risk of tension pneumothorax.

The volume of blood draining from chest tubes should be monitored, especially during the early phase after the operation. Excessive blood drainage should signal an emergency alarm to recall the surgeons. In later phases, chest tubes are commonly left in situ when drainage was more than 250 ml per day. However, this unproven measure was refuted in a recent study which found that the chest tubes may be removed if the drainage is less than 450 ml per day as long as there is no air leak, and the drainage fluid does not contain cerebrospinal fluid, chyle, or blood [39]. Chest X-ray and chest tube status should be evaluated simultaneously, and any discrepancy between them may indicate failing thorax drainage because of tube blockage from kinking or clot or suction failure.

Conclusion

Today, only a few of the patients after thoracic surgery require – prolonged – mechanical ventilation in ICU settings. However, it should be always kept in mind that the postoperative mechanical ventilation can lead to additional complications. In these cases, problems of other systems, such as cardiac arrhythmias, fluid overload, etc., can worsen the conditions of the patient. Mechanical ventilation should be considered only if necessary, but if necessary, then as early as possible. During the mechanical ventilation, the recently traumatized lung tissue should be protected; an aggravation of air leaks and fistula should be prevented, with a least compromise of gas exchange. Weaning should be considered as early as possible.

References

1. Harpole DH Jr, DeCamp MM, Daley J et al (1999) Prognostic models of thirty day mortality and morbidity after major pulmonary resection. J Thorac Cardiovasc Surg 5:969–979
2. Wada H, Nakamura T, Nakamoto K et al (1998) Thirty-day operative mortality for thoracotomy in lung cancer. J Thorac Cardiovasc Surg 1:70–73
3. Stephan F, Boucheseiche S, Hollande J et al (2000) Pulmonary complications following lung resection, a comprehensive analysis of incidence and possible risk factors. Chest 5:1263–1270
4. Serpa Neto A, Hemmes SN, Barbas CS, et al; PROVE Network Investigators (2014) Incidence of mortality and morbidity related to postoperative lung injury in patients who have undergone abdominal or thoracic surgery: a systematic review and meta-analysis. Lancet Respir Med 2:1007–15
5. Padley SP, Jordan SJ, Goldstraw P et al (2002) Asymmetric ARDS following pulmonary resection: CT findings initial observations. Radiology 223:468–473
6. Jordan S, Evans TW (2008) Predicting the need for intensive care following lung resection. Thorac Surg Clin 18:61–69

7. The acute respiratory distress syndrome network: ventilation with lower tidal volumes as compared with traditional tidal volumes for acute lung injury and the acute respiratory distress syndrome (2000) N Engl J Med 342:1301–1308
8. Petrucci N, Iacovelli W (2007) Lung protective ventilation strategy for the acute respiratory distress syndrome. Cochrane Database Syst Rev (3):CD003844.
9. Verbrugge SJ, Lachmann B, Kesecioglu J (2007) Lung protective ventilatory strategies in acute lung injury and acute respiratory distress syndrome: from experimental findings to clinical application. Clin Physiol Funct Imaging 27:67–90
10. Kozian A, Schilling T, Schütze H, Senturk M, Hachenberg T, Hedenstierna G (2011) Ventilatory protective strategies during thoracic surgery: effects of alveolar recruitment maneuver and low-tidal volume ventilation on lung density distribution. Anesthesiology 114:1025–1035
11. Fernández-Pérez ER, Keegan MT, Brown DR, Hubmayr RD, Gajic O (2006) Intraoperative tidal volume as a risk factor for respiratory failure after pneumonectomy. Anesthesiology 105:14–18
12. Sentürk M (2006) New concepts of the management of one-lung ventilation. Curr Opin Anaesthesiol 19:1–4
13. Amato MB, Meade MO, Slutsky AS et al (2015) Driving pressure and survival in the acute respiratory distress syndrome. N Engl J Med 372:747–755
14. Kozian A, Schilling T, Röcken C et al (2010) Increased alveolar damage after mechanical ventilation in a porcine model of thoracic surgery. J Cardiothorac Vasc Anesth 24: 617–623
15. Iglesias M, Jungebluth P, Petit C et al (2008) Extracorporeal lung membrane provides better lung protection than conventional treatment for severe postpneumonectomy noncardiogenic acute respiratory distress syndrome. J Thorac Cardiovasc Surg 135:1362–1371
16. Iglesias M, Martinez E, Badia JR, Macchiarini P (2008) Extrapulmonary ventilation for unresponsive severe acute respiratory distress syndrome after pulmonary resection. Ann Thorac Surg 85:237–244
17. Şentürk M, Slinger P, Cohen E. (2015) Intraoperative mechanical ventilation strategies for one-lung ventilation. Best Pract Res Clin Anaesthesiol 29:357–369.
18. Güldner A, Kiss T, Serpa Neto A et al (2015) Intraoperative protective mechanical ventilation for prevention of postoperative pulmonary complications: a comprehensive review of the role of tidal volume, positive end-expiratory pressure, and lung recruitment maneuvers. Anesthesiology 123:692–713
19. Ferrando C, Mugarra A, Gutierrez A et al (2014) Setting individualized positive end-expiratory pressure level with a positive end-expiratory pressure decrement trial after a recruitment maneuver improves oxygenation and lung mechanics during one-lung ventilation. Anesth Analg 118:657–665
20. Tusman G, Bohm SH, Sipmann FS, Maisch S (2004) Lung recruitment improves the efficiency of ventilation and gas exchange during one-lung ventilation anesthesia. Anesth Analg 98:1604–1609
21. Hickling KG, Walsh J, Henderson S, Jackson R (1994) Low mortality rate in adult respiratory distress syndrome using low-volume, pressure-limited ventilation with permissive hypercapnia: a prospective study. Crit Care Med 22:1568–1578
22. Kavanagh BP, Laffey JG (2006) Hypercapnia: permissive and therapeutic. Minerva Anestesiol 72:567–576
23. Akça O (2008) Carbon dioxide and tissue oxygenation: is there sufficient evidence to support application of hypercapnia for hemodynamic stability and better tissue perfusion in sepsis? Intensive Care Med 34:1752–1754
24. Akça O (2016) Supplemental oxygen, hyperoxia, and perioperative period. Turk J Anaesthesiol Reanim; accepted for publication
25. Magnusson L, Spahn DR (2003) New concepts of atelectasis during general anaesthesia. Br J Anaesth 91:61–72
26. Tuğrul M, Camci E, Karadeniz H, Sentürk M, Pembeci K, Akpir K (1997) Comparison of volume controlled with pressure controlled ventilation during one-lung anaesthesia. Br J Anaesth 79:306–310

27. Unzueta MC, Casas JI, Moral MV (2007) Pressure-controlled versus volume-controlled ventilation during one-lung ventilation for thoracic surgery. Anesth Analg 104:1029–1033
28. Al Shehri AM, El-Tahan MR, Al Metwally R et al (2014) Right ventricular function during one-lung ventilation: effects of pressure-controlled and volume-controlled ventilation. J Cardiothorac Vasc Anesth 28:892–896
29. Carvalho AR, Spieth PM, Güldner A et al (2011) Distribution of regional lung aeration and perfusion during conventional and noisy pressure support ventilation in experimental lung injury. J Appl Physiol (1985) 110:1083–1092
30. Spinale FG, Linker RW, Crawford FA, Reines HD (1989) Conventional versus high frequency jet ventilation with a bronchopleural fistula. J Surg Res 46:147–151
31. Roustan JP (1995) High frequency jet ventilation combined with conventional mechanical ventilation in the treatment of adult respiratory distress syndrome. Ann Fr Anesth Reanim 14:276–288
32. Ford JM, Shields JA (2012) Selective bilateral bronchial intubation for large, acquired tracheo-esophageal fistula. AANA J 80:49–53
33. Anantham D, Jagadesan R, Tiew PE (2005) Clinical review: independent lung ventilation in critical care. Crit Care 9:594–600
34. Borges JB, Senturk M, Ahlgren O, Hedenstierna G, Larsson A. (2015) Open Lung in Lateral Decubitus With Differential Selective Positive End-Expiratory Pressure in an Experimental Model of Early Acute Respiratory Distress Syndrome. Crit Care Med 43:e404–e411
35. Caroleo S, Agnello F, Abdallah K, Santangelo E, Amantea B. (2007) Weaning from mechanical ventilation: an open issue. Minerva Anestesiol 73:417–427
36. Cerfolio RJ, Bryant AS. (2010) The management of chest tubes after pulmonary resection. Thorac Surg Clin 20:399–405
37. Cerfolio RJ, Bass C, Katholi CR. (2001) Prospective randomized trial compares suction versus water seal for air leaks. Ann Thorac Surg 71:1613–1617
38. Brunelli A, Monteverde M, Borri A, et al. (2004) Comparison of water seal and suction after pulmonary lobectomy: a prospective, randomized trial. Ann Thorac Surg 77:1932–1937
39. Cerfolio RJ, Bryant AS. (2008) Results of a prospective algorithm to remove chest tubes after pulmonary resection with high output. J Thorac Cardiovasc Surg 135:269–273
40. Şentürk M, Slinger P, Cohen E. (2015) Intraoperative mechanical ventilation strategies for one-lung ventilation. Best Pract Res Clin Anaesthesiol. 29:357–369

12 Pros and Cons of Non-invasive Ventilation After Thoracic Surgery

Lorenzo Ball, Maddalena Dameri, and Paolo Pelosi

12.1 Introduction

Thoracic surgical procedures have a significant impact on respiratory function, mediated by multiple surgery-related and patient-related factors [1]. Thus, thoracic surgery is at high risk for developing postoperative pulmonary complications (PPCs), and attributable mortality due to postoperative lung injury is higher compared to abdominal surgery [2]. Concerning patient-related factors, most of the patients undergoing lung resection procedures have a history of smoking and chronic obstructive pulmonary disease (COPD), contributing to this increased postoperative risk [1]. Among procedure-related factors, general anaesthesia, chest pain, phrenic nerve irritation, obliteration of distal airways and loss of aerated parenchyma play a major role in determining postoperative lung function impairment [3]. The lung and chest wall modifications that follow thoracic surgery may determine the onset of hypoxemia, atelectasis and pneumonia, potentially leading to acute respiratory failure (ARF) [4]. Thoracic surgery has also been included as a specific risk factor in predictive scores aimed at identifying patients at high risk of development of PPCs [5].

Non-invasive positive pressure ventilation (NPPV) can relieve dyspnoea and improve respiratory function in the postoperative patient and has been proposed for both preventing [6] and treating respiratory failure following thoracic surgery. The aim of this chapter is to briefly describe the most commonly used methods for delivering NPPV and their applications in the postoperative care of the patient undergoing thoracic surgical procedures.

L. Ball • M. Dameri • P. Pelosi (✉)
IRCCS AOU San Martino-IST, Department of Surgical Sciences and Integrated Diagnostics, University of Genoa, Genoa, Italy
e-mail: ppelosi@hotmail.com

© Springer International Publishing Switzerland 2017

M. Şentürk, M.O. Sungur (eds.), *Postoperative Care in Thoracic Surgery*,
DOI 10.1007/978-3-319-19908-5_12

12.2 Non-invasive Positive Pressure Ventilation

Non-invasive ventilation (NIV) is a technique of ventilator support consisting in the provision of mechanical ventilation without the need of an invasive artificial airway [7]. Among the various non-invasive approaches, NPPV (non-invasive positive pressure ventilation) delivered using different interfaces has become the predominant technique, because of its effectiveness and convenience. Initially used only for long-term assistance of patients with chronic diseases, NPPV is being used increasingly in the last decades in selected cases of ARF, where it has shown several advantages compared to intubation.

In fact, invasive mechanical ventilation is highly effective in supporting alveolar ventilation, but endotracheal intubation carries several risks which can be related to intubation and extubation manoeuvres, mechanical ventilation itself and loss of airway defence mechanisms. NPPV can avoid many of these complications because, since the upper airways are preserved, it reduces the incidence of respiratory infections [8] and allows patients to expectorate secretions spontaneously, verbalize and with some interfaces even drink and eat. Despite the advantages of NIV, the lack of a direct connection to lower airways poses several issues. The main absolute contraindications to NIV administration are expectoration inability and airway obstruction at any level.

NPPV can improve the respiratory function in several ways. The main mechanism of action through which NPPV relieves dyspnoea and restores respiratory function is mediated by the reduction of the work of breathing [9]. This reduction in the work of breathing is the result of the intermittent application of a positive pressure to the airways, increasing lung inflation and tidal volumes while unloading inspiratory muscles. In the patient, this reduction of energy consumption to maintain an adequate ventilation translates in a reduced respiratory rate, use of accessory inspiratory muscles, dyspnoea and CO_2 retention in the alveoli [10]. NPPV can also guarantee an enhancement of ventilation-perfusion ratio and a reduction of pulmonary shunt by increasing functional residual capacity and thereby opening collapsed alveoli. Among the other beneficial effects, NPPV produces an increase in intrathoracic pressure which allows reducing both preload and afterload. The afterload reduction, which is the greatest haemodynamic effect especially in patients with dilated cardiomyopathy, leads to a trans-myocardial pressure reduction, thereby potentially enhancing myocardial output. Several studies were focused on the use of NIPPV to treat acute cardiogenic pulmonary oedema: patients treated with non-invasive ventilation have shown a lower intubation rate and a more rapid improvement of blood oxygenation [11].

NIV is most commonly employed to treat patients with chronic respiratory failure: in these patients, long-term NIPPV is often administered night time during sleep, in order to obtain a greater daytime gas exchange. The beneficial effect of NIV on the respiratory function of these patients can be mainly explained by an improvement of respiratory muscle function. NIV administration during sleep allows fatigued respiratory muscles to rest, improving daytime respiratory function [12], reducing respiratory work [13] and modifying the respiratory centre set point for CO_2 [12].

More recently NPPV has been introduced also for acute care application, including the postoperative period. Several studies have been conducted to compare traditional techniques and NPPV in critically ill patient's management. The greater advantage of this technique is the possibility to assist ventilation without the need to invade the airways, which reduces the incidence of infections. First of all, NPPV has been used to treat patients with acute exacerbation of COPD. The most important registered effects are a reduction of respiratory rate, a quick decrease of $PaCO_2$ and a significant reduction of intubation rate compared to standard care [7]. Another possible application for NPPV is represented by the treatment of respiratory failure related to severe pneumonia; patients treated with non-invasive ventilation have shown a lower intubation rate [14], a shorter ICU length of stay and a significantly better short-term survival. The use of NPPV as treatment for ARDS is considered controversial. A recent multicenter randomized trial showed that, when used at an early stage in mild ARDS, NPPV can reduce the intubation rate compared to standard oxygen therapy [15]. Caution in this field is mandatory: patients should be carefully selected in order to discriminate cases in which NPPV can be a treatment option, from those where NPPV only represents a delay to a necessary and unavoidable intubation.

12.2.1 NPPV in the Perioperative Period

Concerning the postoperative period, the interest towards NPPV is increasing in the last decades. Several studies suggested a role for NPPV in treating postoperative respiratory failure. Among others, a randomized, controlled, unblinded study held on 209 patients that developed severe hypoxemia after elective major abdominal surgery found that NPPV, compared to oxygen therapy, reduced intubation rate and occurrence of postoperative pneumonia and sepsis [16]. Nasal continuous positive airway pressure was proposed in a cohort of 56 patients undergoing elective prosthetic replacement of the thoracoabdominal aorta, as a prophylactic measure to reduce the incidence of postoperative respiratory failure: this approach leads to a reduction of incidence of PPCs, as well as a reduction of hospital length of stay [17]. Most of the studies agree in supporting the rationale of the use of NPPV as both a preventive and therapeutic measure for postoperative pulmonary complications and respiratory failure, especially in high-risk surgery.

12.2.2 Modes of NPPV

Virtually, any ventilation mode can be delivered through a non-invasive interface instead of a conventional artificial airway [18]. Nonetheless, NPPV cannot be simply considered interchangeable with conventional mechanical ventilation, for the intrinsic non-hermetic nature of the system, resulting in a variable degree of unavoidable air leaks, and for the variable resistance opposed by the upper respiratory tract. In this paragraph the authors will briefly describe only the ventilation modes that play a role in the postoperative period.

NPPV can be delivered with dedicated ventilators or with conventional ICU ventilators. The formers are usually smaller and simpler to set up than the latters, also because they are often designed also for home use in chronic patients. Their ease of use might raise interest in the perioperative period, for the possibility of initiating NPPV in the surgical ward where ICU ventilators are not promptly available. These small ventilators can have a two-limb respiratory circuit, similar to that of an ICU ventilator with a true expiratory valve allowing CO_2 washout or a single-limb circuit that permits exhalation and carbon dioxide removal through a calibrated leak port [18].

12.2.2.1 Continuous Positive Airway Pressure

Continuous positive airway pressure (CPAP) is the provision of a constant pressure to the non-invasive interface. It can be considered the simpler NPPV mode, and it can be delivered with a ventilator or with high-flow systems, consisting in a gas blender delivering a high flow to the patient, with the pressure being set by means of a calibrated or adjustable PEEP valve. The benefits of CPAP have been described initially in the treatment of acute cardiogenic pulmonary oedema, subsequently in ARF, including in the postoperative period. In CPAP, the patient fully controls respiration, deciding frequency and duration of the respiratory cycle. Few studies investigated this NPPV mode in patients that underwent lung resection [19].

12.2.2.2 Pressure Support Ventilation and Related Ventilation Modes

Several modern dedicated ventilators and all ICU ventilators offer pressure support ventilation (PSV) as an option. In this ventilation mode, the patient controls directly the beginning of inspiration and indirectly the cycling into the expiratory phase. Inspiratory trigger can be a fixed negative flow, typically between −2 and −5 L/m, and, in ICU ventilators and several dedicated NPPV ventilators, can be adjusted manually by the operator. Another common inspiratory trigger is based on the detection of a decrease of pressure. Some sophisticated ventilators especially designed for NPPV administration offer algorithm-based flow-time curve analysis software that helps the ventilator to distinguish genuine inspiratory efforts from artefacts due to air leaks.

Once the breath is triggered by the patient, the ventilator maintains a constant desired pressure level. This pressure level can be maintained for a preset duration (time-cycled ventilation) or until inspiratory flow decelerates until a specific value (flow-cycled ventilation). In some home NPPV ventilator, this flow value is fixed, but in most of the ventilators intended for in-hospital use, this threshold can be set as an adjustable percent of the inspiratory peak flow. In case of relevant air leaks, the flow delivered by the ventilator might never reach this threshold value, leading to patient asynchrony. A recent benchtop study showed that many ICU ventilators are not suitable for delivering NPPV in case of large air leaks [20].

This ventilation mode is referred to with different names depending on the ventilator manufacturer. PSV is the mode that was most extensively investigated in the postoperative period after thoracic surgery.

12.2.2.3 Other Ventilation Modes

In some ICU ventilators, several ventilation modes are available that cycle between two levels of constant pressure, allowing spontaneous unassisted breaths at any pressure level. In most cases these ventilation modes are not specifically designed for delivery through non-invasive interfaces; therefore, the lack of air leak compensation can lead to an undesired loss of pressurization [20].

Recently, humidified high-flow nasal cannulas (HHFNC) are under extensive investigation for patients in ARF, also in the perioperative period. Their mechanism of action is unclear and seems mediated by a flow-dependent CPAP effect. Their role after thoracic surgery is still to be determined [21].

12.2.2.4 Interfaces

NPPV can be delivered through several types of interfaces: nasal masks, oronasal masks, full-face masks and helmets [7]. Air leaks are a common problem in the administration of NPPV; therefore, choosing the right interface, tailoring it on the patient's needs, is one of the most important aspects of a good non-invasive respiratory support [22]. Choosing the optimal device allows to reduce complications and discomfort, thereby optimizing patient compliance and beneficial effects of the therapy [23].

Several models of interface are available on the market. Nasal interfaces include nasal mask and nasal pillows: the former is a plastic mask with a soft silicone pad which covers the nose, while the latter are soft rubber caps inserted directly into the nostrils. Oronasal masks can be classified in facial masks, covering the nose and mouth, and full-face masks, covering also the eyes. Helmets are transparent PVC cylinder which includes the neck avoiding contact with the face skin; these devices are usually equipped with anti-suffocation valves, and the adhesion to the neck is guaranteed by an elastic collar attached to padded straps. Each of these devices has advantages and disadvantages. A simpler interface, the mouthpiece, allows to avoid several problems related to the use of nasal or oronasal masks like skin lesion or claustrophobia [24], but the need to a high level of patient cooperativeness [22] limits the interest of this interface in the postoperative period. Nasal masks are usually well tolerated. These devices allow the patient to eat, drink, expectorate and verbalize. Compared to other interfaces, nasal masks have a lower dead space and tend to cause less frequently claustrophobia, but they need a greater collaboration from the patient and can cause skin breakdown as well as conjunctivitis or ocular lesions due to the air leaks. Nasal pillows reduce decubitus and risk of skin ulcers, but they are often associated with nasal irritation and lower seal at high pressure [22].

Facial masks have a greater stability if compared with nasal masks and allow a clearer monitoring of the air leaks. Because of their size, covering a larger part of the face, they can cause claustrophobia, emesis and pressure sore, therefore reducing patient compliance. Full-face masks are usually well tolerated because they adhere on the perimeter of the face where the sensibility is lower. The size of this device is larger than the others; they tend to reduce air leaks, therefore determining a lower incidence of conjunctivitis. On the other hand, when the mask is blurred the patient has a reduced visibility. Furthermore, a recent study found out that these devices may be difficult to adapt to ICU ventilators [20].

The helmet is one of the most recently introduced interfaces. This device completely eliminates the contact with the patient's face and minimizes the risk of skin breakdowns; therefore, the helmet can ensure greater comfort to the patient also for prolonged NPPV administration [25, 26]. Conversely, this interface presents several problems like excessive overall dimensions, positioning difficulties and necessity of ventilators capable of delivering a high airflow. The helmet hampers communication and increases respiratory dead space. Moreover, helmets are not available in several countries where healthcare authorities expressed concerns regarding the risk of CO_2 rebreather through these high-volume devices. In a randomized trial in patients developing hypoxemic respiratory failure after surgery for aortic dissection, helmets were found to be more rapid in improving gas exchange and better tolerated compared to facial masks [27]. Similar results were found in a small matched-control study in patients developing ARF after major abdominal surgery [28], while another study showed slower $PaCO_2$ decrease in COPD exacerbations treated with helmets as compared to full-face masks [29].

Larger randomized trials are warranted to identify advantages of a specific interface over the others, but the intrinsic necessity to tailor the interface on the patient's comfort should also be considered.

12.2.2.5 Humidification

When breathing in normal condition, the air is heated and humidified as it goes through the airways. This obviously does not happen when the airflow is generated by a machine, which produces cold and dry air. That's why, although it is often overlooked, humidification assumes an important role in NPPV. Compared to invasive ventilation, NPPV respects the anatomy of the airways and allows ventilation through natural ways.

Especially in case of a prolonged administration, the absence of humidification can lead to several complications such as sore throat, reactive cough, dry mouth, runny nose, nosebleeds, hoarseness and nasal congestion [30]. Although apparently trivial, these complications can be considered a leading cause of reduced patient compliance, even in short-term administration, like the case of postoperative NPPV. All these issues can be effectively reduced by adding a humidification device to the circuit of NPPV [31].

We can distinguish two main categories of humidifiers: heated humidifiers (HHs) and heat and moisture exchangers (HMEs). The formers are constituted by a heating plate warming a water jar, to which the respiratory circuit is connected. An adjustable thermostat allows the operator to set the temperature of the water contained in the bell. The HME, frequently improperly referred to as "filters", can be distinguished in hygroscopic and hydrophobic filters. The hydrophobic filters contain a ceramic fibre membrane that acts as a filter for viruses and bacteria but allows only partial humidification. Therefore, hydrophobic filters are generally placed at the proximal end of the circuit with the main purpose of protecting the patient from contamination. The hygroscopic filters are formed by a membrane filter of propylene with condensation surface, usually made of paper and soaked with hygroscopic salts which guarantee humidification. The newer HME filters combine the two types of membrane, thus allowing both humidification and bacterial filtration. HHs are active humidifiers, while HMEs are passive systems, only maintaining humidification by retaining water vapour exhaled by the patient. The choice between HH and HME filters requires a specific case-by-case trade-off analysis. HME filters are easier to use and generally have a lower unitary cost. Among their main limitations, it must be mentioned the increase of dead space during NPPV, which results in an increased breathing effort and higher $PaCO_2$ level when compared to the HH systems [32]. On the other hand, HH filters are more expensive and difficult to use, the circuit is prone to contamination and the optimal temperature can be tricky to reach. In a randomized multicentre study, no differences were observed between HH and HME in terms of reduction of the intubation rate [33]. When CPAP is generated with high-flow systems, HHs have been suggested to be preferable [34].

12.2.3 NPPV After Thoracic Surgery

After lung resection surgery, lung function is more impaired compared to other types of surgery because of the loss of parenchyma, thoracic pain, depression of the respiratory drive due to high-dose systemic or epidural opiate use in the perioperative period as well as closure of distal airways [7, 35]. There is an increasing interest towards potential applications of NPPV after thoracic surgery, and several small-sampled studies investigated its use both as a preventive and curative measure in the postoperative period [4]. NPPV can be considered a preventive measure when used routinely after lung resectional surgery, especially in high-risk patients, to reduce the incidence of postoperative ARF, aimed at reducing morbidity, the need of invasive mechanical ventilation and finally mortality. Conversely, NPPV can be used as a curative intervention when ARF is already established [36]. Even fewer studies investigated the possibility of using NPPV as a preventive measure in the preoperative period [37].

Several authors suggested that, for the complexity of the management of respiratory function after lung resection surgery, often it is not easy to discriminate cases in which NPPV is used with a preventive intent from those in which it is used as a therapeutic measure. In fact, in most cases it is applied in a grey zone in which the aim is both to relief respiratory distress and improve the clinical course of the patient, potentially reversing the pathway towards respiratory failure [4, 6, 36].

12.2.3.1 Pathophysiology of NPPV After Thoracic Surgery

The two most common major procedures in thoracic surgery are oesophageal and lung resection interventions. Both procedures were for a long time considered absolute contraindications for NPPV, for concerns regarding risks for surgical anastomotic leak and for aspiration towards the airways [7]. Recently several authors tried to challenge this assumption, based on pathophysiological considerations, experimental models and clinical trials.

Concerning oesophagectomy, a recent study by Raman and colleagues [38] investigated in a porcine in vivo and ex vivo model the air pressure tolerance of an oesophageal anastomosis. Interestingly, the authors found an in vivo tolerance without air leaks to pressures of 84 ± 38 cmH_2O, much higher than the pressures actually transmitted to the oesophagus during positive pressure ventilation. In a retrospective clinical study on NPPV after oesophagectomy for oesophageal cancer [39], the authors found that NPPV used as a first-line treatment for postoperative ARF, by improving gas exchange, avoided intubation in nearly half of the patients. The authors then concluded that NPPV may be an effective option for ARF following oesophageal surgery.

The use of NPPV after lung resection surgery is mistrusted by surgeons and often also by anaesthesiologists and intensive care physicians, for the concerns that positive pressure ventilation could stress the bronchial suture or anastomosis, increasing airway to pleural space leaks or, even worse, causing anastomotic rupture. With a careful titration of NPPV, these concerns are essentially unfounded and based on an erroneous interpretation of the mechanisms leading to the anastomotic leakage. Indeed, the mechanical stress to which the bronchial suture or anastomosis is subject is not proportional to the airway pressure but rather to the difference between the inner airway pressure (Paw) and the pressure of the space surrounding the anastomosis (Ppl). This trans-anastomotic pressure gradient is responsible for the mechanical stress to which airways are subject and corresponds to the transpulmonary pressure (P_L = Paw-Ppl) [40]. After thoracic surgery, a negative pressure is often applied to chest tubes to promote lung expansion and to compensate parenchymal air leaks. Since this negative pressure might contribute to an increase in transpulmonary pressure, in some studies the temporary suspension of chest tube negative pressure during NPPV administration was proposed as a precautionary measure [19].

In the example shown in Fig. 12.1, NPPV is applied to a dyspnoeic patient in ARF after lung resection surgery. As shown in the left panel, despite the small swings in airway pressure, in spontaneous breathing the huge excursion in negative pleural pressure, due to increased inspiratory effort, leads to a relevant transpulmonary pressure. The application of an NPPV with low PEEP results in an increase in airway pressure, but relieving inspiratory muscles allows a reduction in pleural pressures. The resulting transpulmonary pressure during NPPV has comparable average values and reduced peak.

In a clinical study in 1997, Aguiló et al. [35] investigated the effects of short-term (1 h) NPPV after lung resection surgery in ten subjects, compared to nine controls. The author chose a BiPAP ventilation mode with an inspiratory pressure of 10 cmH_2O and an expiratory pressure of 5 cmH_2O, delivered through a nasal interface. The study concluded that short-term NPPV significantly improved gas exchange without increasing either dead space or pleural air leaks detected from the chest tube. Following this pivotal study, several small- to middle-sampled studies investigated the efficacy of NPPV after thoracic surgery.

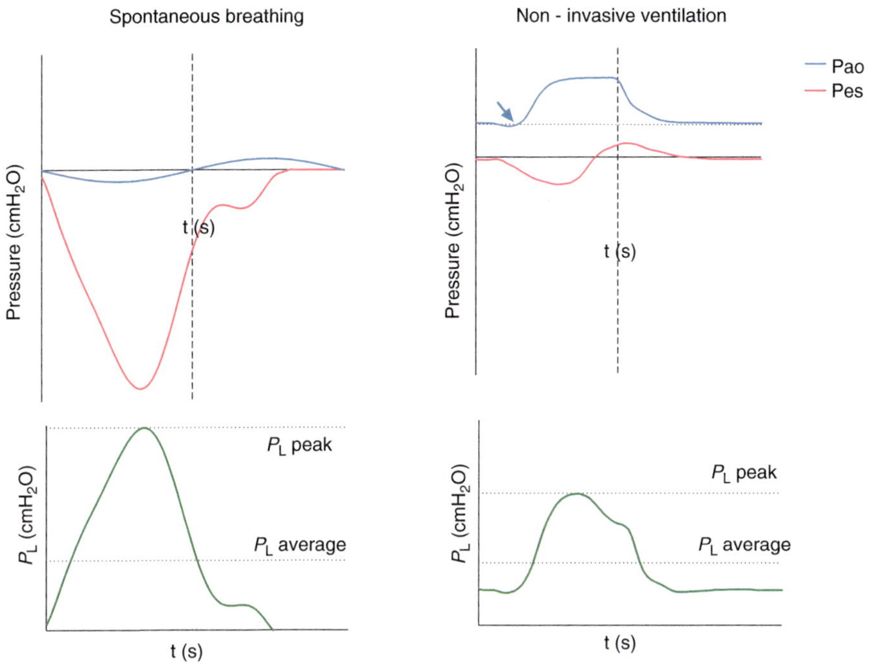

Fig. 12.1 Pathophysiology of respiratory mechanics in a thoracic postoperative patient. The figures illustrate airway (*blue*) and oesophageal (*pink*) pressure-time curves of a patient in respiratory distress in spontaneous breathing (*left*) and during NPPV (*right*). Transpulmonary pressure (P_L), also representing the trans-anastomotic pressure gradient, is plotted in *green*. The vertical dashed line represents the beginning of the expiratory phase

12.2.3.2 Evidence on Preventive Use of NPPV

Several studies investigated the role of NPPV as a preventive measure, namely, routinely administered to all patients after thoracic surgery, in order to decrease the incidence of respiratory events and to improve clinical outcome. Table 12.1 resumes the findings of the most relevant studies.

Several small randomized trials found an improvement in gas exchange [17, 19, 35, 37], and two of them also observed a reduction in hospital length of stay [17, 37]. A single study investigated NPPV also preoperatively [37]. In a randomized trial on 50 patients [41], NPPV improved lung re-expansion, assessed by computed tomography, but no clinical advantage was found; in particular the incidence of PPCs was not lower compared to the control group. In a study using helmets for CPAP delivery [19], the advantages in gas exchange improvement were found to be transient, rapidly returning to the baseline values after the interruption of the CPAP administration.

In the largest randomized trial [42] in 360 COPD patients undergoing major lung resection surgery, NPPV did not reduce the incidence of acute respiratory events nor affected any of the secondary clinical endpoints, including ICU length of stay, intubation rate and mortality. Even if a single middle-sized randomized trial should not be considered definitive, these data suggest that administration of preventive NPPV should not be considered as a standard approach for all patients undergoing lung resectional surgery. It is difficult to aggregate the results from other small studies, due to the heterogeneity of NPPV modes used, interfaces and clinical outcomes. Further studies are necessary to identify subgroups of patients at high risk that could potentially benefit from preventive NPPV.

12.2.3.3 Evidence on Therapeutic Use of NPPV

Several studies investigated the role of NPPV as a therapeutic measure, namely, administered to treat patients which developed ARF postoperatively. Table 12.1 resumes the findings of the most relevant studies. In a pilot study on 20 patients meeting criteria for re-intubation after abdominal and thoracic surgery, nasal CPAP was used as a method to avoid invasive ventilation [43]. In lung transplant recipients, NPPV through face mask avoided intubation in most of the patients that developed ARF postoperatively [44]. NPPV decreased mortality compared to standard oxygen therapy in a randomized trial involving 24 patients in ARF after lung resection [45]. The feasibility of NPPV in ARF following thoracic surgery was further assessed in two prospective observational trials on a larger cohort of patients [46, 47] (Table 12.2).

12.3 Potential Limitations and Pitfalls of NPPV

NPPV should be administered in the right cases in the right time window. Indeed, NPPV should be considered a measure to support the respiratory function while the underlying reversible condition is treated. Further studies are warranted to help the clinician in individuating thresholds and clinical scores to identify patients that can benefit from preventive or curative NPPV.

It is a matter of debate whether postoperative NPPV for ARF should be administered only in the ICU setting [48]. As a general principle, administration of NPPV should be accompanied by adequate respiratory monitoring [49]. In many hospitals ventilators are not available in the medical ward, but this issue could be circumvented by the use of small portable ventilators. In a feasibility study of NPPV in the recovery room of the general surgery, the use of NIV-dedicated small ventilators was proposed and found to be a viable option for relieving ARF in the immediate postoperative period [50]. A recent study in the United States [51] found that most NPPV treatments for ARF were initiated in the ICU or in the emergency department and general wards. NPPV feasibility and efficacy were found to be comparable in different age groups [52].

For the importance of adequately monitoring gas exchange and airway pressures, the authors of this chapter recommend a cautious approach to this very specialized

Table 12.1 Studies investigating the role of preventive NPPV after thoracic surgery

Author	Year	Type of surgery	Study design	Patients	NPPV in the intervention group	Interface	Main results
Aguiló [35]	1997	Pulmonary	Physiological feasibility study	$n=20$ Two groups	PS = 10 cmH_2O PEEP = 5 cmH_2O	Nasal	Feasibility Improved gas exchange
Kindgen-Miles [17]	2005	Thoraco-abdominal	Prospective RCT	$n=50$ Two groups	CPAP = 10 cmH_2O	Nasal	Improved gas exchange Reduced LOS
Perrin [37]	2007	Pulmonary	Prospective RCT (NPPV before and after surgery)	$n=34$ Two groups	PS = 10 cmH_2O PEEP = 5 cmH_2O	Nasal	Improved gas exchange Reduced LOS
Liao [41]	2010	Thoracic	Prospective RCT	$n=50$ Two groups	IPAP = 13 ± 3.2 cmH_2O EPAP = 4 cmH_2O	Nasal or facial	Improved lung re-expansion at CT
Barbagallo [19]	2012	Pulmonary	Prospective RCT	$n=50$ Two groups	High-flow CPAP = 8 cmH_2O	Helmet	Transient improvement in gas exchange
Lorut [42]	2014	Pulmonary	Prospective RCT	$n=360$ Two groups	PS = 10 cmH_2O PEEP = 5 cmH_2O	Facial	No significant difference in acute respiratory events

RCT randomized controlled trial, *PS* pressure support, *CPAP* continuous positive airway pressure, *PEEP* positive end-expiratory pressure, *IPAP* inspiratory positive airway pressure, *EPAP* expiratory positive airway pressure

Table 12.2 Studies investigating the role of curative NPPV for ARF following thoracic surgery

Author	Year	Type of surgery	Study design	Patients	NPPV mode	Interface	Main results
Kindgen-Miles [43]	2000	Thoracic and abdominal	Prospective, observational	$n=20$	CPAP = 10 cmH_2O	Nasal	Improved gas exchange
Rocco [44]	2001	Pulmonary transplant	Prospective, observational	$n=21$	PS = 14 cmH_2O PEEP = 5 cmH_2O	Facial	Feasibility Improved gas exchange
Auriant [45]	2001	Pulmonary	Prospective RCT	$n=48$	PS = 9 cmH_2O PEEP = 4 cmH_2O	Nasal	Intubation rate decrease Mortality decrease
Lefebvre [46]	2009	Pulmonary	Prospective, observational	$n=113$	PS = 14 cmH_2O PEEP = 5 cmH_2O	Facial	Feasibility Success rate of NPPV 85 %
Riviere [47]	2010	Pulmonary or pulmonary thromboendarterectomy	Prospective, observational	$n=135$	PS = 14 cmH_2O PEEP = 5 cmH_2O	Facial	Feasibility Success rate of NPPV 70 %

RCT randomized controlled trial, *PS* pressure support, *CPAP* continuous positive airway pressure, *PEEP* positive end-expiratory pressure

application of NPPV, reserving its use in a clinical setting with an adequate number of trained nurses and respiratory caregivers, with continuous monitoring of SpO_2, blood pressure, respiratory rate and airway pressure. It has been recently shown that the delivery of NPPV by a dedicated trained team can reduce intubation rate and risk of death during non-invasive ventilation [53]. The availability of an intensivist 24 h per day within few minutes from the patient is mandatory: in case of NPPV failure, a rapid intubation and transfer to an ICU for invasive mechanical ventilation should not be delayed.

Conclusions

In the postoperative period after thoracic surgery, NPPV can be a tool to support respiratory function and to avoid unnecessary intubation, potentially reducing morbidity and mortality. Its safety and feasibility have been validated in several trials. There is not enough evidence to support the use of routine administration of NPPV as a preventive measure in all patients undergoing thoracic surgery. Concerning the therapeutic use in postoperative respiratory failure, there is evidence supporting the feasibility, safety and efficacy of NPPV as a treatment for ARF following thoracic surgery.

A compromise between a good gas exchange and an acceptable mechanical stress to the anastomosis must be individuated: the authors suggest using a low PEEP level ($\leq$5 cmH_2O) and the lowest possible pressure support level.

References

1. Miller RD (2010) Miller's anesthesia. Churchill Livingstone/Elsevier, Philadelphia
2. Serpa Neto A, Hemmes SNT, Barbas CSV et al (2014) Incidence of mortality and morbidity related to postoperative lung injury in patients who have undergone abdominal or thoracic surgery: a systematic review and meta-analysis. Lancet Respir Med 2:1007–1015
3. Nunn JF (1987) Applied respiratory physiology. Butterworths, London/Boston
4. Jaber S, Antonelli M (2014) Preventive or curative postoperative noninvasive ventilation after thoracic surgery: still a grey zone? Intensive Care Med 40:280–283
5. Mazo V, Sabaté S, Canet J et al (2014) Prospective external validation of a predictive score for postoperative pulmonary complications. Anesthesiology 121:219–231
6. Jaber S, Chanques G, Jung B (2010) Postoperative noninvasive ventilation. Anesthesiology 112:453–461
7. Tobin MJ (2013) Principles and practice of mechanical ventilation. McGraw-Hill Medical, New York
8. Nourdine K, Combes P, Carton MJ et al (1999) Does noninvasive ventilation reduce the ICU nosocomial infection risk? A prospective clinical survey. Intensive Care Med 25:567–573
9. Girault C, Richard JC, Chevron V et al (1997) Comparative physiologic effects of noninvasive assist-control and pressure support ventilation in acute hypercapnic respiratory failure. Chest 111:1639–1648
10. Carron M, Rossi S, Carollo C, Ori C (2014) Comparison of invasive and noninvasive positive pressure ventilation delivered by means of a helmet for weaning of patients from mechanical ventilation. J Crit Care 29:580–585
11. Masip J, Betbesé AJ, Páez J et al (2000) Non-invasive pressure support ventilation versus conventional oxygen therapy in acute cardiogenic pulmonary oedema: a randomised trial. Lancet 356:2126–2132

12. Roussos C (1985) Function and fatigue of respiratory muscles. Chest 88:124S–132S
13. Bergofsky EH (1979) Respiratory failure in disorders of the thoracic cage. Am Rev Respir Dis 119:643–669
14. Brambilla AM, Aliberti S, Prina E et al (2014) Helmet CPAP vs. oxygen therapy in severe hypoxemic respiratory failure due to pneumonia. Intensive Care Med 40:942–949
15. Zhan Q, Sun B, Liang L et al (2012) Early use of noninvasive positive pressure ventilation for acute lung injury: a multicenter randomized controlled trial. Crit Care Med 40:455–460
16. Squadrone V, Coha M, Cerutti E et al (2005) Continuous positive airway pressure for treatment of postoperative hypoxemia: a randomized controlled trial. JAMA 293:589–595
17. Kindgen-Milles D, Müller E, Buhl R et al (2005) Nasal-continuous positive airway pressure reduces pulmonary morbidity and length of hospital stay following thoracoabdominal aortic surgery. Chest 128:821–828
18. Rabec C, Rodenstein D, Leger P et al (2011) Ventilator modes and settings during non-invasive ventilation: effects on respiratory events and implications for their identification. Thorax 66:170–178
19. Barbagallo M, Ortu A, Spadini E et al (2012) Prophylactic use of helmet CPAP after pulmonary lobectomy: a prospective randomized controlled study. Respir Care 57:1418–1424
20. Nakamura MAM, Costa ELV, Carvalho CRR, Tucci MR (2014) Performance of ICU ventilators during noninvasive ventilation with large leaks in a total face mask: a bench study. J Bras Pneumol Publi-cação Soc Bras Pneumol E Tisilogia 40:294–303
21. Curley GF, Laffy JG, Zhang H, Slutsky AS (2015) Noninvasive respiratory support for acute respiratory failure-high flow nasal cannula oxygen or non-invasive ventilation? J Thorac Dis 7:1092–1097
22. Pisani L, Carlucci A, Nava S (2012) Interfaces for noninvasive mechanical ventilation: technical aspects and efficiency. Minerva Anestesiol 78:1154–1161
23. Sferrazza Papa GF, Di Marco F, Akoumianaki E, Brochard L (2012) Recent advances in interfaces for non-invasive ventilation: from bench studies to practical issues. Minerva Anestesiol 78:1146–1153
24. Garuti G, Nicolini A, Grecchi B et al (2014) Open circuit mouthpiece ventilation: concise clinical review. Rev Port Pneumol 20:211–218
25. Pisani L, Mega C, Vaschetto R et al (2015) Oronasal mask versus helmet in acute hypercapnic respiratory failure. Eur Respir J 45:691–699
26. Redondo Calvo FJ, Madrazo M, Gilsanz F et al (2012) Helmet noninvasive mechanical ventilation in patients with acute postoperative respiratory failure. Respir Care 57:743–752
27. Yang Y, Sun L, Liu N et al (2015) Effects of noninvasive positive-pressure ventilation with different interfaces in patients with hypoxemia after surgery for stanford type A aortic dissection. Med Sci Monit Int Med J Exp Clin Res 21:2294–2304
28. Conti G, Cavaliere F, Costa R et al (2007) Noninvasive positive-pressure ventilation with different interfaces in patients with respiratory failure after abdominal surgery: a matched-control study. Respir Care 52:1463–1471
29. Özlem ÇG, Ali A, Fatma U et al (2015) Comparison of helmet and facial mask during noninvasive ventilation in patients with acute exacerbation of chronic obstructive pulmonary disease: a randomized controlled study. Turk J Med Sci 45:600–606
30. Esquinas Rodriguez AM, Scala R, Soroksky A et al (2012) Clinical review: humidifiers during non-invasive ventilation – key topics and practical implications. Crit Care 16:203
31. Tuggey JM, Delmastro M, Elliott MW (2007) The effect of mouth leak and humidification during nasal non-invasive ventilation. Respir Med 101:1874–1879
32. Lellouche F, Maggiore SM, Deye N et al (2002) Effect of the humidification device on the work of breathing during noninvasive ventilation. Intensive Care Med 28:1582–1589
33. Lellouche F, L'Her E, Abroug F et al (2014) Impact of the humidification device on intubation rate during noninvasive ventilation with ICU ventilators: results of a multicenter randomized controlled trial. Intensive Care Med 40:211–219

34. Chiumello D, Chierichetti M, Tallarini F et al (2008) Effect of a heated humidifier during continuous positive airway pressure delivered by a helmet. Crit Care 12:R55
35. Aguiló R, Togores B, Pons S et al (1997) Noninvasive ventilatory support after lung resectional surgery. Chest 112:117–121
36. Jaber S, De Jong A, Castagnoli A et al (2014) Non-invasive ventilation after surgery. Ann Fr Anesth Reanim 33:487–491
37. Perrin C, Jullien V, Vénissac N et al (2007) Prophylactic use of noninvasive ventilation in patients undergoing lung resectional surgery. Respir Med 101:1572–1578
38. Raman V, MacGlaflin CE, Erkmen CP (2015) Noninvasive positive pressure ventilation following esophagectomy: safety demonstrated in a pig model. Chest 147:356–361
39. Yu K-Y, Zhao L, Chen Z, Yang M (2013) Noninvasive positive pressure ventilation for the treatment of acute respiratory distress syndrome following esophagectomy for esophageal cancer: a clinical comparative study. J Thorac Dis 5:777–782
40. Akoumianaki E, Maggiore SM, Valenza F et al (2014) The application of esophageal pressure measurement in patients with respiratory failure. Am J Respir Crit Care Med 189:520–531
41. Liao G, Chen R, He J (2010) Prophylactic use of noninvasive positive pressure ventilation in post-thoracic surgery patients: a prospective randomized control study. J Thorac Dis 2:205–209
42. Lorut C, Lefebvre A, Planquette B et al (2014) Early postoperative prophylactic noninvasive ventilation after major lung resection in COPD patients: a randomized controlled trial. Intensive Care Med 40:220–227
43. Kindgen-Milles D, Buhl R, Gabriel A et al (2000) Nasal continuous positive airway pressure: a method to avoid endotracheal reintubation in postoperative high-risk patients with severe nonhypercapnic oxygenation failure. Chest 117:1106–1111
44. Rocco M, Conti G, Antonelli M et al (2001) Non-invasive pressure support ventilation in patients with acute respiratory failure after bilateral lung transplantation. Intensive Care Med 27:1622–1626
45. Auriant I, Jallot A, Hervé P et al (2001) Noninvasive ventilation reduces mortality in acute respiratory failure following lung resection. Am J Respir Crit Care Med 164:1231–1235
46. Lefebvre A, Lorut C, Alifano M et al (2009) Noninvasive ventilation for acute respiratory failure after lung resection: an observational study. Intensive Care Med 35:663–670
47. Riviere S, Monconduit J, Zarka V et al (2011) Failure of noninvasive ventilation after lung surgery: a comprehensive analysis of incidence and possible risk factors. Eur J Cardio Thorac Surg Off J Eur Assoc Cardio Thorac Surg 39:769–776
48. Hess DR (2013) Noninvasive ventilation for acute respiratory failure. Respir Care 58:950–972
49. Ball L, Sutherasan Y, Pelosi P (2013) Monitoring respiration: what the clinician needs to know. Best Pract Res Clin Anaesthesiol 27:209–223
50. Battisti A, Michotte J-B, Tassaux D et al (2005) Non-invasive ventilation in the recovery room for postoperative respiratory failure: a feasibility study. Swiss Med Wkly 135:339–343
51. Ozsancak Ugurlu A, Sidhom SS, Khodabandeh A et al (2015) Where is noninvasive ventilation actually delivered for acute respiratory failure? Lung 193(5):779–788
52. Ugurlu AO, Sidhom SS, Khodabandeh A et al (2016) Use and outcomes of noninvasive ventilation for acute respiratory failure in different age groups. Respir Care 61(1):36–43
53. Vaudan S, Ratano D, Beuret P et al (2015) Impact of a dedicated noninvasive ventilation team on intubation and mortality rates in severe COPD exacerbations. Respir Care 60(10): 1404–1408

Lung Surgery and Extracorporeal Oxygenation

13

Edda M. Tschernko and Clemens Aigner

13.1 Introduction

Extracorporeal assist devices, such as extracorporeal membrane oxygenation (ECMO) or heart-lung machine, have been used in selected centers before, during, and after thoracic surgery. Especially the use of ECMO, before (even in awake patients = awake ECMO) [1], during, and after lung transplantation is well established in various centers. Additionally, extracorporeal devices are used in selected patients undergoing extended lung surgery with necessary resection of adjoining vessels or parts of the heart such as the atrium. For complicated tracheobronchial surgery, an extracorporeal device can be of crucial help during the surgical procedure and guarantee for patient safety.

Special considerations for lung transplantation will not be discussed in detail, since it deals with special problems associated with transplant patients and organ selection. In this chapter the use of extracorporeal support during complicated lung surgery and tracheobronchial resection will be dealt with. Nevertheless, lung transplantation will be addressed several times, because extracorporeal devices are commonly used for lung transplant, whereas non-transplant lung surgery with extracorporeal devices is still relatively rare. Advantages and disadvantages as well as indications, complications, and outcome will be critically focused on.

E.M. Tschernko (✉)
Department of Cardiothoracic Anesthesia and Intensive Care Medicine, Vienna General Hospital, University of Vienna, Vienna, Austria
e-mail: edda.tschernko@meduniwien.ac.at

C. Aigner
Department of Thoracic Surgery, Vienna General Hospital, University of Vienna, Vienna, Austria

© Springer International Publishing Switzerland 2017

M. Şentürk, M.O. Sungur (eds.), *Postoperative Care in Thoracic Surgery*,
DOI 10.1007/978-3-319-19908-5_13

13.2 Technology

Various devices are commercially available. Technical considerations like resistance of oxygenator membrane, maximal duration of use, filling volume, and feasibility for transport can play a substantial role in the selection of a specific device.

In general the main components (Fig. 13.1) of extracorporeal devices are an oxygenator, a centrifugal pump, a tube set, and a device for flow measurement. The system is nowadays completely heparin coated. Therefore, heparin has to be administered in relatively low doses [2]. Usually a single shot of heparin 70 IE/kg body weight is administered before the start of the device. The target activated clotting time (ACT) is 160–180 s (measured hourly during surgery). Alternatively aPTT can be used to monitor anticoagulation (aim: aPTT 55–60s). For prolonged use of an extracorporeal device, a heparin bypass is used to avoid clotting of the blood. Advantages and disadvantages of various extracorporeal devices are shown in Table 13.1.

13.2.1 Interventional Lung Assist

This arteriovenous device is driven by the cardiac pump function of the patient because no centrifugal pump is included. Thus, the precondition for the use of

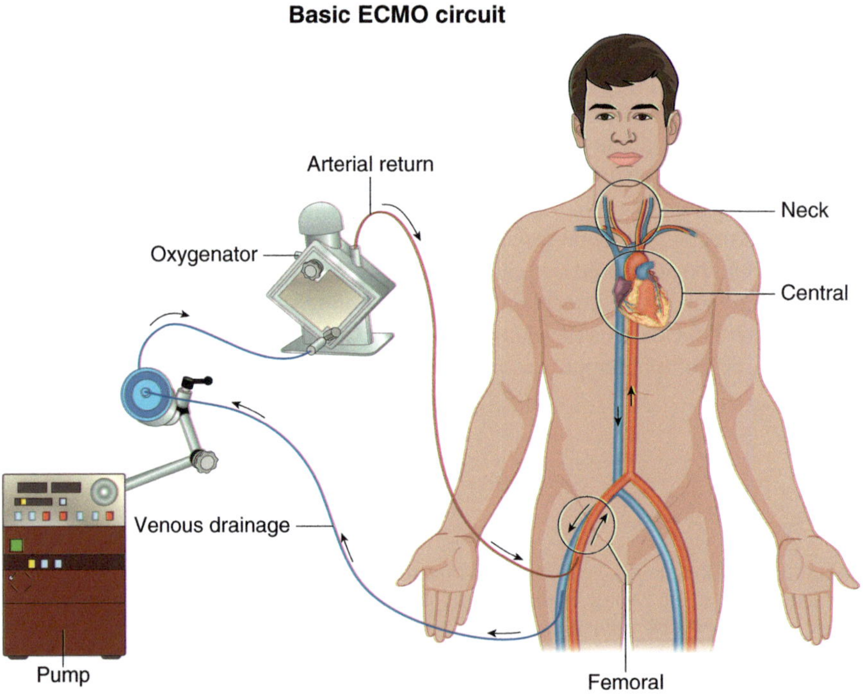

Fig. 13.1 The main components of ECMO are displayed in Fig. 13.1. A venoarterial ECMO is shown in Fig. 13.1. The cannulation site of ECMO is central, via the internal jugular vein and the carotid artery or via the femoral vein and femoral artery. According to the site of cannulation specific complications can occur, e.g., lymphatic fistula in the groin

interventional lung assist (iLA) is a patient with uncompromised cardiac function. Percutaneous cannulation of the tubes is usually performed via the femoral artery and the femoral vein [3]. Central implantation via the pulmonary artery and the left atrium has been described for bridging of patients with pulmonary hypertension [4, 5]. The oxygenator has a low resistance and the priming volume is no more than 200 mL. Only part of the cardiac output is passing through the oxygenator membrane. Therefore, CO2 elimination can be sufficiently provided by an oxygenator flow of no more than 500–1000 mL/min [6]. Oxygenation would require a flow of at least 2000 mL/min. An interventional assist device is shown in Fig. 13.2. The major advantage of this device is the low priming volume. However, this device is mainly used for CO_2 removal.

13.2.2 Venovenous ECMO

The precondition for the insertion of this device is a hemodynamically stable patient with no relevant pulmonary hypertension. Venovenous ECMO can guarantee for

Table 13.1 Comparison of extracorporeal assist devices

	Gas exchange ↓	C	LV ↓	High PAP	Tracheobronchial res.
ILA	CO_2 removal	–	–	–	–
VV-ECMO	CO_2+O_2	–	–	–	+
VA-ECMO	CO_2+O_2	+	+	+	+
HLM	CO_2+O_2	+	+	+	+
Alternative	Ventilation (I/NI)	Inotropes	Inotropes	Prostin/NO	Jet ventilation

ILA interventional lung assist, *VV-ECMO* venovenous ECMO, *VA-ECMO* venoarterial ECMO, *HLM* heart-lung machine, *alternative* alternative therapeutic options, *gas exchange* ↓ impaired gas exchange, *RV* ↓ impaired right ventricular function, *LV* ↓ impaired left ventricular function, *high PAP* high pulmonary artery pressure, *tracheobronchial res.* tracheobronchial resection

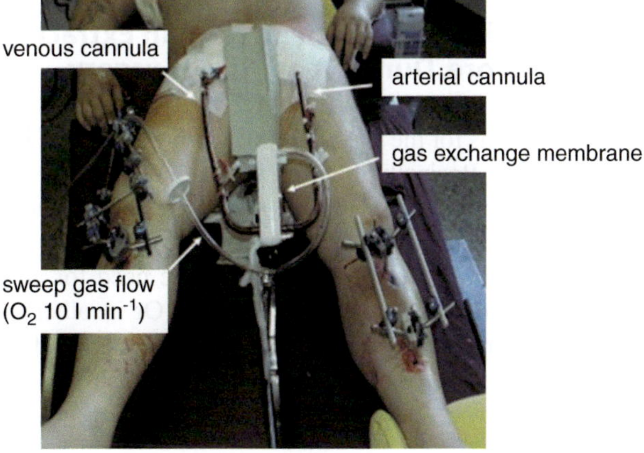

Fig. 13.2 Interventional assist device is displayed in Fig. 13.2

sufficient gas exchange (CO_2 elimination and oxygenation) at flow rates up to 4000 mL/min. Standard cannulation drains the blood via the right femoral vein from the vena cava inferior and recirculates the blood via the right jugular vein to the right atrium. Sufficient distance between the cannulas is essential to avoid recirculation of the blood in the oxygenator.

13.2.3 Venoarterial ECMO

The venoarterial ECMO is a rather invasive form of extracorporeal device. The blood is drained from the right atrium pumped through the oxygenator and recirculated via a large systemic artery (Fig. 13.1). By means of this technique, hemodynamic support is provided and the circulation through the lung is substantially reduced. Cannulation can be performed via the right atrium and the ascending aorta for exclusively intraoperative use and via the femoral vein (drainage of blood from the right atrium) and the femoral artery (recirculation of oxygenated blood) for prolonged postoperative use. The tip of the arterial cannula is situated in the descending aorta. Thus, the cardiac output from the heart (gas exchange through patient's lung) and the recirculated blood from the venoarterial ECMO mix in the descending aorta. This fact may lead to substantially different oxygenation in the upper and lower part of the body. Monitoring of oxygenation has to be performed on the right arm because it is most likely to achieve similar values compared to the cerebral oxygenation.

13.2.4 Heart-Lung Machine

This extracorporeal support is exclusively used during surgery. The patient has to be fully heparinized for the use of this device. Therefore, surgical bleeding is a feared complication associated with the use of the heart-lung machine. Additionally, it should not be used for oncological procedures because systemic spread of tumor cells should be avoided in these patients.

13.3 Indications for the Use of an Extracorporeal Device Before, During, and After Surgery

The indications for the use of an extracorporeal device in lung surgery are displayed in Table 13.2. Basically the pre-, intra-, and postoperative use of an extracorporeal device can be necessary due to pulmonary malfunction (impaired gas exchange), cardiac malfunction (right and/or left ventricular failure), or a mixture of both. The crucial question for all situations with the need for an extracorporeal @device is will the situation improve after surgery? Or in other words: Can medical and/or surgical treatment improve the underlying organ malfunction to an extent that the patient can be successfully weaned from the extracorporeal device after a reasonable time span?

Table 13.2 Advantages of various methods used during tracheobronchial resection

	Cross table Jet ventilation	iLA	ECMO	HLM
Risk for bleeding	+	±	±	–
Hemodynamic stability	–	–	+	+
Gas exchange stability	–	∓	+	+
Surgical sight	–	+	+	+

13.3.1 Impaired Gas Exchange on the Basis of Lung Disease

Several underlying pulmonary diseases result in impaired gas exchange with potential respiratory decompensation. Chronic obstructive pulmonary disease (COPD) is the most frequent indication for lung transplantation in most institutions [6]. In these patients extracorporeal devices are frequently used before, during, and after lung transplantation to guarantee for respiratory and hemodynamic stability. Additionally, acute pulmonary infections in COPD patients occur frequently and lead in some cases to fetal impairment in gas exchange. This situation may occur while a patient is on the waiting list for lung transplant. Especially in young patients an extracorporeal device can be used to overcome the critical time of infection.

However, in this chapter the focus is on patients with severe COPD presenting for non-transplant lung surgery. Malignancies of the lung may create the need for a surgical procedure in these patients. The crucial question is: Does it make sense to use extracorporeal devices during lung surgery because of severe COPD? Only close cooperation of pulmonologists, lung surgeons, anesthesiologists and intensivists can answer this question for the individual patient. Lobectomy or even pneumonectomy can lead to substantial improvement in gas exchange if the removed lung does not participate in ventilation due to occluded bronchial parts. Or the removal of hyperinflated areas (lung volume reduction surgery) may result in substantially improved ventilator mechanics. The blood flow through the lung tissue not participating in gas exchange is redistributed to well-ventilated areas, and thus, intrapulmonary shunt reduced [7]. If the patient´s gas exchange is already severely impaired before surgery extracorporal support can be necessary during a brief intraoperative time span (e.g. during single lung ventilation). Which device chosen will be dependent on considerations including the risk of bleeding, hemodynamic stability, gas exchange and surgical sight (Table 13.1 and 13.2). However, in most cases less invasive measures will be sufficient to overcome the critical time span during surgery, e.g., permissive hypercapnia, FiO_2 of 100 %, jet ventilation, etc. The patient's medical situation and local preferences of the surgical team are usually crucial in the choice of gas exchange support.

13.3.2 Impaired Right Ventricular Function Due to Pulmonary Hypertension

13.3.2.1 Chronic Thromboembolic Pulmonary Hypertension

Impaired right ventricular function is regularly observed in patients with chronic thromboembolic pulmonary disease due to high resistance in the pulmonary circulation. Surgery for chronic thromboembolic pulmonary hypertension (CTEPH) aims at the removal of embolic material in the pulmonary vessels, thus leading to reduced resistance in the pulmonary circulation [8]. It is a well-established procedure with reasonable success rates [7, 9]. This procedure is usually undertaken while the patient is in hypothermic cardiopulmonary arrest. Surgery for CTEPH requires therefore the use of a heart-lung machine (HLM). At our institution about 30–40 cases are performed per year. Appropriate patient selection and standardization of the intraoperative and postoperative care lead to perioperative mortality rates of no more than 5 % [10]. For this very special procedure the HLM is a precondition.

13.3.2.2 Primary Idiopathic Pulmonary Hypertension (PIPH)

The reasons for the development of primary idiopathic pulmonary hypertension (PIPH) are not known to date [11]. However, PIPH frequently develops in young subjects. The medical therapy with prostaglandines, endothelin 1 receptor antagonists or phosphodiesterase 5 inhibitors. can help to a certain extent. As PIPH progresses, a remodeling of the heart occurs. The right ventricle increases in dimension and forms the apex of the heart [12]. Usually a tricuspid insufficiency is present and the septum bulges toward the left ventricle during systolic action. The left ventricle decreases in dimension and its systolic and diastolic function deteriorates [13]. This condition is an indication for lung transplant surgery. During surgery an extracorporeal device (at our institution venoarterial ECMO is used) is necessary for hemodynamic stability and to guarantee for adequate gas exchange. Usually the extracorporeal device will be required for several days after lung transplant to avoid volume overload of the "untrained" left ventricle [14].

If surgery other than transplant becomes necessary in patients suffering from severe PIPH, high attention has to be paid on adequate monitoring of the pulmonary artery pressure and cardiac function. Therefore, a Swan-Ganz catheter in combination with a transesophageal echo may be required for even trivial surgery to avoid any risk of cardiac decompensation during general anesthesia.

13.3.3 Tracheobronchial Surgery and Extended Lung Surgery

For tracheobronchial resections required for the removal of malignancies or benign tracheobronchial diseases, it is a challenge to combine adequate ventilation and proper operative sight [15]. Standard procedures like resection of a small part of the trachea are usually undertaken with cross table ventilation, e.g., sterile ventilator tubing is used close to the operative field [16]. However, this may lead to substantial difficulties for the surgeon to access the surgical field (16). As an alternative, parts of the surgery can be undertaken during apnea or jet ventilation. However, limitation of surgical time during apnea or potential spread of tracheobronchial secretion and/or tumor cells during jet ventilation is undesirable. To avoid this, the use of HLM has been well established for tracheobronchial resections [17–18]. Hemodynamic stability and adequate gas exchange in combination with proper sight on the operative field are guaranteed if HLM is used during complicated tracheobronchial resection or reconstruction. However, the need for anticoagulation may lead to increased frequency of bleeding and transfusion [19]. To avoid the disadvantages of systemic anticoagulation, iLA or ECMO with roller pump can be used. The advantages and disadvantages of the most frequently used approaches are shown in Table 13.2.

13.4 Summary

Various extracorporeal devices are available to support gas exchange and hemodynamic stability before, during, and after lung surgery. The use of these devices changed from being a clinical experiment in a desperate situation to routinely planned procedures for special patients and extended surgery. This development was initiated clearly by the use of extracorporeal devices for lung transplant surgery dealing with severely limited patients for a complicated surgical procedure such as transplant. The improvement of technology of the devices increases which leads to an improved risk/benefit ratio. For patient safety during extended or small procedures in pulmonary and/or circulatory severely limited patients, the use of extracorporeal support becomes more and more common for clinical routine. However, it has to be kept in mind that all of these devices are bridging tools. For surgical success the precondition is that the patient's situation can be substantially improved by surgery and medical therapy within a reasonable time span. Close cooperation of surgeons, pulmonologists, anesthesiologists, and intensivists is necessary for adequate indication of the use of an extracorporeal device before, during, or after lung surgery or complicated lung resection or tracheal resection. The choice of the device is dependent on advantages and disadvantages associated with the device, the patient's morbidities and comorbidities and the experience of the institution. However, the use of extracorporeal devices for lung resection or complicated tracheal resection or reconstruction still has to be called "experimental." Nevertheless, it can be a suitable and lifesaving tool if indications are considered carefully and the procedure is carried out by an experienced team of experts.

References

1. Fuehner T, Kuehn C, Hadem J et al (2012) Extracorporeal membrane oxygenation in awake patients as bridge to lung transplantation in awake patients. Am J Respir Crit Care Med 185:763–768
2. Prat NJ, Meyer AD, Langer T, Montgomery RK, Parida BK, Batchinsky AI, Cap AP (2015) Low dose heparin anti-coagulation during extracorporeal life support for acute respiratory distress syndrome in conscious sheep. Shock 44(6):560–568
3. Fischer S, Simon AR, Welte T et al (2006) Bridge to lung transplantation with the novel pumpless interventional lung assist device Nova Lung. J Thorac Cardiovasc Surg 131:719–723
4. Strueber M, Hoepper MM, Fischer S et al (2009) Bridge to thoracic organ transplantation in patients with pulmonary arterial hypertension using a pumpless lung assist device. Am J Transplant 9:853–857

5. Schmid C, Philipp A, Hilker M et al (2008) Bridge to lung transplantation through a pulmonary artery to left atrial oxygenator circuit. Ann Thorac Surg 85:1202–1205
6. Gattinoni L, Kolobow T, Tomlinson T et al (1978) Control of intermittent positive pressure breathing (IPPV) by extracorporeal removal of carbon dioxide. Br J Anaesth 50:753–758
7. Lang G, Taghavi S, Aigner C et al (2011) Extracorporeal membrane oxygenation support for resection of locally advanced thoracic tumors. Ann Thorac Surg 92:264–270
8. De Perrot M, Granton JT, Mc Rae K et al (2011) Impact of extracorporeal life support on outcome in patients with idiopathic pulmonary artery hypertension awaiting lung transplantation. J Heart Lung Transplant 30:997–1002
9. Wiebe K, Baraki H, Macchiarini P, Haverich A (2006) Extended pulmonary resection of advanced thoracic malignancies with support of cardiopulmonary bypass. Eur J Cardiothorac Surg 29:571–578
10. Baron O, Jouan J, Sagan C, Despines P, Michaud JL, Duveau D (2003) Resection of bronchopulmonary cancers invading the left atrium – benefit of cardiopulmonary bypass. Thorac Cardiovasc Surg 51(3):159–161
11. Hasegawa S, Bando T, Isowa N (2003) The use of cardiopulmonary bypass during extended resection of non-small cell cancer. Interact Cardiovasc Thorac Surg 2:676–679
12. Connolly KM, Mc Guirt WF Jr (2001) Elective extracorporeal membrane oxygenation: an improved perioperative technique in the treatment of tracheal obstruction. Ann Otol Rhinol Laryngol 110(3):205–209
13. Hines MH, Hanesll DR (2003) Elective extracorporeal support for complex tracheal reconstruction in neonates. Ann Thorac Surg 76(1):175–178
14. Byrne JG, Leacche M, Agnihotri HK et al (2004) The use of cardiopulmonary bypass during resection of locally advanced thoracic malignancies. A 10- year two-center experience. Chest 125:1581–1586
15. De Perrot M, Fadel E, Mussot S et al (2005) Resection of locally advanced (T4) non-small cell lung cancer with cardiopulmonary bypass. Ann Thorac Surg 79(5):1691–1696 (discussion 1697)
16. Sehgal S, Chance JC, Steliga MA (2014) Thoracic anesthesia and cross field ventilation for tracheobronchial injuries: a challenge for anesthesiologists. Case Reports in Anesthesiology, Article ID 972762.
17. Woods FM, Neptune WB, Palatchi A (1961)Resection of the carina and main-stem bronchi with the use of extracorporal circulation. N Engl J Med 264:492–494.
18. Naef AP (1969) Extensive tracheal resection and tracheobronchial reconstruction. The Annals of Thoracic Surgery 8 (5):391–401.
19. Smith IJ, Sidebotham DA, McGeorge AD, et al (2009) Use of extracorporal membrane oxygenation during resection of tracheal papillomatosis Anesthesiology 110:427–429.

Pneumonia After Thoracic Surgery

14

Perihan Ergin Özcan and Evren Şentürk

14.1 Introduction

The developments in the field of thoracic surgery and perioperative anesthetic management have extended its patient population; those who were previously inoperable are now undergoing surgery.

Preoperative evaluations by a multidisciplinary team that includes thoracic surgeons, chest physicians, intensive care physicians, and anesthesiologists have benefited patients in terms of reduced postoperative morbidity and mortality.

The causes of postoperative complications can be divided into three categories: infectious, surgery related, and cardiovascular. The most frequent and severe complications after thoracic surgery are respiratory complications. Some are surgery related such as hemorrhage, bronchopleural fistula, and atelectasis. Other respiratory complications are pneumonia, acute lung injury, and acute respiratory distress syndrome (ARDS). Hypoventilation and ineffective cough caused by several mechanisms such as inappropriate pain management increase the risk of postoperative pneumonia. There are also cardiovascular complications including arrhythmias, pulmonary thromboembolism, and cardiac failure.

The incidence of pneumonia after thoracic surgery is approximately 5.3–22 % [1, 2]. Factors that influence the incidence of pneumonia include patient population, type of surgery, antibiotic prophylaxis, and diagnostic criteria for pneumonia. The incidence of pneumonia is higher when using clinical criteria compared with objective criteria.

The mortality rate of postoperative pneumonia is approximately 17 %; after thoracic surgery the rate rises to 19–40 % [1, 3]. Due to the high risk for mortality in this patient population, risk prediction is also crucial for surgical decision-making and informed patient consent. Pneumonia after thoracic surgery causes longer stays in intensive care units (ICU) and hospitals, which in turn increases the costs.

P.E. Özcan (✉) • E. Şentürk
Department of Anesthesiology and Intensive Care Medicine,
Istanbul University, Istanbul Faculty of Medicine, Istanbul, Turkey
e-mail: pergin@istanbul.edu.tr

© Springer International Publishing Switzerland 2017

M. Şentürk, M.O. Sungur (eds.), *Postoperative Care in Thoracic Surgery*,
DOI 10.1007/978-3-319-19908-5_14

Table 14.1 Risk factors for postoperative pneumonia after thoracic surgery

Age ≥ 75
Male
Smoking history
FEV_1 < 70 %
Induction therapy
Pathologic stages III–IV
Duration of operation > 3 h
COPD
Histopathologic type (squamous cell carcinoma)

FEV1 forced expiratory volume in one second, *COPD* chronic obstructive pulmonary disease

14.2 Risk Factors

During the perioperative period, many risk factors play a role in the development of postoperative pneumonia. With the exception of abdominal surgery, the risk of pneumonia after thoracic surgery is 38 times greater than other type of surgery [4]. Deterioration in pulmonary function after abdominal and thoracic surgery has previously been evidenced through pulmonary function tests, imaging methods, and physiologic measurements [5, 6].

The risk factors for postoperative pneumonia after thoracic surgery can be separated into three phases as the preoperative, intraoperative, and postoperative periods.

Risk factors related with postoperative pneumonia in thoracic surgery are listed in Table 14.1 [7, 8].

Arozullah et al. used a combination of risk factors to create a risk index for predicting pneumonia after noncardiac surgery [9]. The authors developed the risk index from the data obtained from preoperative patient-specific and operation-specific risk factors. They found that abdominal aortic aneurysm repair and thoracic surgery had the highest risk for postoperative pneumonia. The risk index may be useful for high-risk patients; therefore giving these patient groups more attention in the perioperative period and taking preventive measures may reduce the incidence of pneumonia.

Predictors of postoperative pneumonia are explained in some other chapters of this book; there we are going to focus on approach during postoperative period.

14.3 The Postoperative Period

Secretions cause atelectasis and pneumonia during the postoperative period, especially in patients with a smoking history, pain, and inefficient cough. Secretion retention in airways may cause obstruction of broncopulmonary units and atelectasis, and this is even more pronounced in smokers and in patients with chronic lung disease. The diagnosis of sputum retention can be clinical and it is characterized by respiratory distress with rapid, shallow, and bubbly breaths. There was a strong association between sputum retention and postoperative pneumonia in patients with chronic obstructive pulmonary disease (COPD), smoking history, and poor analgesia [10]. There is a great importance for physiotherapy in this situation. At least two daily visits should be performed; some patients need more. Another noteworthy point is the hydration of patients for secretion mobilization. Oxygen therapy via a facemask inevitably dries secretions when non-humidified oxygen is used. This causes mucociliary dysfunction and a decreased ability to clear secretions, so humidified oxygen should be used. Sometimes mucolytic agents can be helpful. Chest physiotherapy is a therapeutic modality that should be kept in mind. Postural drainage, percussion, and vibration are applied to the affected lung opening and promote coughing during which physicians should provide adequate analgesia. Despite these interventions, tracheal suctioning can be used in patients who cannot remove secretions. Before suctioning, high oxygen fraction should be used in patients at risk for hypoxemia.

Fiberoptic bronchoscopy may be used for clearance of secretions which has the advantage of direct visualization of the tracheobronchial tree and the ability to take sputum samples for culture when a clinically infection is suspected. Sedation is required for this procedure in nonintubated patients; noninvasive ventilation may be used during the intervention to avoid hypoxemia.

14.4 Pulmonary Rehabilitation

Many comorbid conditions accompany lung cancer surgery. Approximately 50 % of patients with lung cancer also have COPD [11]. Patients with COPD may have ineffective cough, increased secretions, and impaired gas exchange after lung resections, especially hypercapnia secondary to hypoventilation. Some patients may need re-intubation and mechanical ventilation. Pulmonary rehabilitation includes breathing exercise, cough training, and self-management education; psychosocial support has been shown to decrease complications [12, 13]. Preoperative assessment of these patients for targeting reduces postoperative complications and improves survival. Pneumonia is the most significant postoperative complication that increases morbidity and mortality. These interventions may help reduce the incidence, severity, and risks of pneumonia. Smoking cessation and pharmacological therapies such as bronchodilators, mucolytics, and antibiotics if necessary are useful for patients preparing for lung resection and also those with chronic lung disease.

Pulmonary rehabilitation programs can be preoperatively and postoperatively conducted at certain time periods. These programs include breathing and coughing techniques, inspiratory muscle strength, home-based aerobic exercise, and incentive spirometry [14–16]. Spruit et al. showed that patients with poor functional status after lung cancer treatment improved their exercise capacity using a pulmonary rehabilitation program with a 6-min walk [17]. However, after patients are diagnosed as having lung cancer, they often feel that surgery must be planned as soon as possible and thus may refuse a pulmonary rehabilitation program.

14.5 Analgesia

The thoracic analgesia is crucial to keep the patient comfortable for reducing postoperative pulmonary complications after surgery. Surgical incision, intercostal nerve injury, and inflammation are major causes of pain after thoracic surgery. Thoracic epidural analgesia is still considered the gold standard for pain relief after thoracotomies, but recently some evidence showed that a paravertebral block had a similar analgesic effect with fewer adverse effects than thoracic epidural analgesia [18]. For reduced complications after thoracic surgery, patients should be able to breathe deeply, cough, and remove secretions and should be mobilized early. Postoperative ineffective pain relief associates with worsened pulmonary complications. Belda reported that a higher postoperative pain score was an independent predictor of postoperative respiratory infections [19]. Recently, multimodal analgesia has been preferred for post thoracotomy pain. In this regimen, regional blocks are combined with opioids, nonsteroidal anti-inflammatory drugs, acetaminophen, selective cyclooxygenase −2 inhibitors, and α2 agonists. Multimodal analgesia is more effective and has fewer adverse effects. When the age and comorbid conditions of these patients are considered, more attention must be paid to the drugs used for analgesia in this population.

14.6 Does Bronchial Colonization-Airway Colonization Play a Role in Postoperative Pneumonia After Thoracic Surgery?

In normal conditions, the lower respiratory tract is sterile. Most patients who undergo surgery have a history of smoking with subsequent impairment of mucociliary function and accumulation of secretions in the lung; therefore these patients have facilitating factors for the development of infection.

The source of pathogenic microorganisms responsible for pneumonia in this patient population is not yet clear. Preoperative colonization, colonization during intubation or mechanical ventilation, and aspiration during the perioperative period can cause pneumonia after thoracic surgery [20]. The incidence of airway colonization in patients with lung cancer varied between 10 and 83 % [1, 19, 21]. Taking samples using different methods (bronchoalveolar lavage (BAL), protected specimen brush (PSB), endotracheal aspiration (ETA), spontaneous sputum) and at different times (preoperative, perioperative, or postoperative period) may account for this wide range.

Some studies have been shown that healthy, nonsmoking patients have no airway colonization [22, 23]. Healthy smokers and patients with COPD had bacterial colonization at 29 % and 66 %, respectively [24, 25]. Monso showed that 25 % of 40 stable patients with COPD had airway colonization; the most commonly isolated microorganisms were *Haemophilus influenzae* and *Streptococcus pneumonia* [26].

Patients who undergo thoracic surgery have similar colonization patterns to patients with COPD. Although the relationship between airway colonization and ventilator-associated pneumonia has been proven, bronchial colonization and pneumonia in patients after lung cancer surgery are unclear. Several studies investigated this issue. Hirakata et al. investigated the airway colonization patterns in patients with primary lung cancer and nonmalignant lung disease and healthy volunteers [27]. The rate of bacterial colonization was significantly higher in patients with lung cancer (51.9 %) than in those with nonmalignant lung disease (37.3 %) and healthy volunteers (37.8 %), and the Gram-negative colonization was higher in this cancer group than in other patient populations. The pathogenesis of airway colonization in patients with lung cancer is not clear, but centrally located tumors and high body mass index were found to be risk factors for colonization [28]. Smoking and poor pulmonary functions also add risk for colonization in patients with COPD. Furthermore, sampling methods that evaluate the incidence of airway colonization are imperative in this patient population.

Which time period is important to the development of pneumonia with respect to colonization? Sok et al. performed a study to verify the origin of microorganisms that caused pulmonary infections after lung cancer surgery [29]. They obtained samples of sputum 3 days before surgery, during surgery, and 3 days after surgery. The microorganisms that caused infections were isolated as preoperative 18 %, intraoperative 13 %, and postoperative 63 %. They found that the microorganisms which caused pneumonia were the same with microorganisms which were isolated in sputum at the 3rd postoperative day. The authors concluded that the colonization of the airway usually occurs during the postoperative period; the oral cavity and pharynx were the source of pathogens.

Cabello et al. investigated distal airway colonization in patients with pulmonary carcinoma and obtained samples from proximal to the endobronchial lesion using a PSB [22]. They used $\geq 10^2$ cfu/mL as a cutoff value for colonization and found that 42 % of patients had bronchial colonization. Sixteen of 25 isolated microorganisms were non-potential pathogenic microorganism, and the most isolated potential pathogen microorganism was *H. influenza*. Similarly, Ionas et al. found 41 % bronchial colonization in patients with resectable lung cancer [28].

Rather than the colonization of the airway, the similarity of microorganisms that colonize the airway and cause pneumonia is a more relevant issue. The correlation between these pathogens is controversial. Ionas reported that there was no relationship between postoperative infectious pulmonary complications and bronchial colonization [28]. Sok demonstrated that postoperative infective complications were caused by Gram-negative bacteria, whereas most of the positive cultures obtained preoperatively were Gram positive [29]. The change in the pattern suggests that the colonization of microorganisms in the early postoperative period may be caused by the aspiration of gastric contents and frequent interventions to the airway in the operating room and ICU. In contrast to these studies, some authors reported a good correlation between microorganisms isolated from patients who developed postoperative pneumonia with the same agents identified preoperatively [1, 19, 21, 30]. Appropriate prophylactic antibiotics and optimal duration of prophylaxis are the most imperative considerations for the prevention of postoperative pneumonia in patients who are colonized with potentially pathogenic microorganisms (PPMs) preoperatively.

The most common preoperatively isolated microorganisms from the airway are *H. influenzae*, *S. pneumonia*, and *Staphylococcus aureus*. Although approximately 50 % of postoperative pulmonary pathogens are not documented, some of the isolated pathogens have been different in various studies. In pneumonia developed during late postoperative period, resistant strains of gram-negative bacteria should be considered as potential pathogens. In the early postoperative period (first week), *H. influenzae* and *S. pneumonia* are the most common pathogens, but more resistant microorganisms such as *Pseudomonas aeruginosa*, *Acinetobacter baumannii*, and *Klebsiella pneumonia* cause pneumonia in the late postoperative period. Cytomegalovirus (CMV) infection in patients with hematologic malignancies, patients who are human immunodeficiency virus positive, and lung transplant recipients is common, but the incidence of CMV infection in other types of cancer patients is not well known. A study performed in a surgical ICU showed that the incidence of CMV infections was around 35.6 % [31]. The essential thing here is to suspect a CMV and make the correct diagnosis, especially in patients under treatment with steroids. Preemptive antiviral therapy is administered in selected patient populations but not in thoracic surgery. Antiviral therapy should be considered for patients with severe pneumonia, ARDS, and resistant to classical antibacterial therapy in postoperative period especially for patients who underwent induction therapy. The widespread use of antibiotics also affects the type of microorganisms that colonize.

14.7 Antibiotic Prophylaxis

Antibiotic prophylaxis should be used for thoracic surgery because of the clean contaminated nature of these operations. The relationship between airway colonization during the perioperative period and postoperative pneumonia after thoracic surgery enhances the significance of antibiotic prophylaxis in this field. Despite the routine use of antibiotic prophylaxis, the incidence of postoperative pneumonia is also high (24 %) [1, 2]. In several studies the onset of postoperative pneumonia developed in the first week.

Which type of prophylactic antibiotics is recommended in this type of surgery? First- and second-generation cephalosporins such as cefazolin, cefamandole, cefuroxime, and cefepime are the most frequently used agents for prophylaxis in pulmonary resections in many countries. These agents are highly successful in preventing surgical wound infections but their effectiveness in pneumonia should be questioned [32]. In a study that investigated the efficacy of prophylaxis, it was shown that the microorganisms that caused pneumonia were not sensitive to prophylactic antibiotics [32].

Most of the microorganisms responsible for postoperative pneumonia are Gram negative and are resistant to first- and second-generation cephalosporins.

Preoperative microbiologic examination of the tracheobronchial tree may be helpful to select effective antibiotic prophylaxis. Several studies investigated the effect of different prophylactic agents on postoperative pneumonia (1, 33). Schussler compared cefamandole (3 g/24 h) with amoxicillin-clavulanate (6 g/24 h) and found a significant decrease in the incidence of postoperative pneumonia in the second group and concluded that antibiotic prophylaxis may decrease the rate of pneumonia after surgery. Another study compared cefuroxime and cefepime and found that cefuroxime was more effective than cefepime as a prophylactic agent [33]. Most of the microorganisms responsible for postoperative pneumonia are Gram-negative bacteria, and 50 % of them are *Enterobacteriaceae* spp., which are resistant to these antibiotics [32].

The dose and duration of antibiotics used for prophylaxis are another major challenge. The first dose is usually administered after the induction of anesthesia. Some protocols only use a single dose, whereas other protocols use antibiotics for 24 or 48 h for prophylaxis [34].

Skin and oropharyngeal flora can be the source of microorganisms that cause postoperative pneumonia after thoracic surgery. Therefore antibiotic prophylaxis should be considered before surgery and in cases of pneumonia microorganisms from the skin, and oropharyngeal flora must be covered.

Microorganisms that colonize the bronchial tree are usually responsible for postoperative pneumonia. In addition to antibiotic prophylaxis, surveillance results and antibiotic sensitivity patterns should be considered.

Using classical criteria for diagnosis of pneumonia after lung resection is more difficult than other types of surgery because fever, hypoxemia, and abnormal chest X-ray findings are commonly seen after lung resections.

14.8 Diagnosis

The actual incidence of postoperative pneumonia after thoracic surgery is unknown. There is no gold standard for the diagnosis of postoperative pneumonia so the incidence of pneumonia varies in the literature. Many centers use only clinical criteria, whereas others use invasive diagnostic techniques. Fever > 38 °C, leukocytosis (white blood cell count ≥12000cells/μL) or leukopenia (white blood cell count ≤4000 cells/μL), purulent secretion, and new or progressive consolidation on chest X-ray are parameters used when pneumonia is suspected (Fig. 14.1). In addition to these criteria, dyspnea, worsening oxygenation, and changes in the amount or character of sputum support the diagnosis of pneumonia. Radiologic signs of pneumonia may be difficult to differentiate pneumonia from pulmonary embolism or atelectasis, especially in the immediate postoperative period. Chest X-rays are taken in the ICU with portable machines, which also add difficulty resulting in suboptimal quality images. The evaluation of chest X-rays is more difficult in patients who undergo lung surgery, and for these reasons, chest X-rays are only used to support the diagnosis; therefore thorax CT may be useful for definitive diagnosis in this situation (Figs. 14.2 and 14.3).

Endotracheal aspiration cultures are mostly used for the diagnosis of pneumonia. This is an inexpensive, easy, and quick method when compared with bronchoscopic cultures. However, its accuracy is questionable in many respects; distinguishing between infection and colonization is very difficult. If ETA samples are quantitatively analyzed, the accuracy of the results is close to bronchoscopic results.

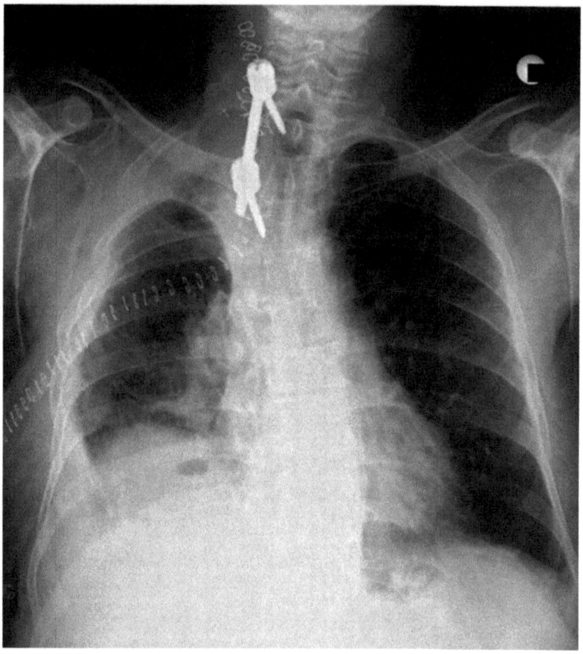

Fig. 14.1 Chest X-ray showing pneumonia after the right pulmonary resection

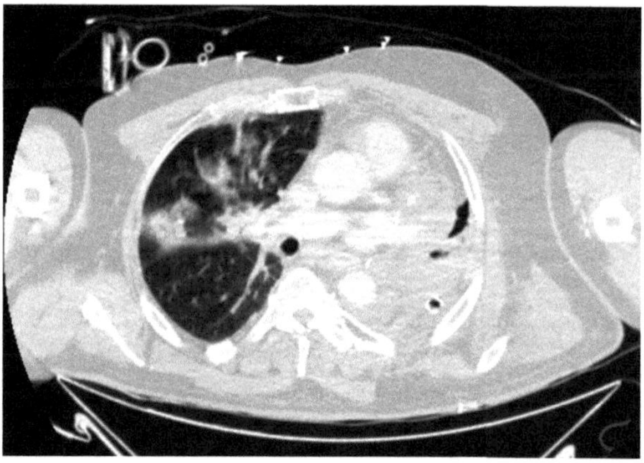

Fig. 14.2 CT image of right pneumonia after the left pneumonectomy

Differential diagnosis in this period is quite difficult. Sputum samples should be obtained if patients can cough effectively. For patients being treated in the ICU and being mechanically ventilated, fiberoptic bronchoscopy is very convenient. Bronchoscopic sampling should especially be performed in patients who fail to respond to antibiotic treatment. Bronchoscopic sampling is appropriate for rare microorganisms such as viral, fungal, and atypical etiologic agents in patients who had induction therapy before surgery. Microorganisms isolated from airways during the perioperative period may help to initiate empiric antibiotic treatment.

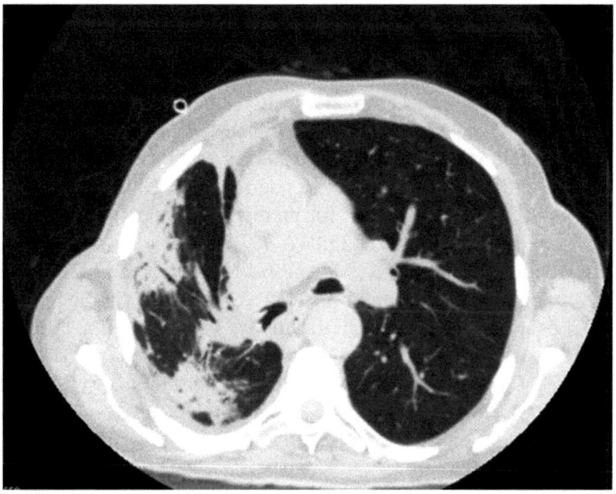

Fig. 14.3 CT image of right pneumonia after the right pulmonary resection

14.9 Treatment

The empirical antibiotic treatment should be started based on patient factors, local infection, and susceptibility patterns. If patients have no risk factors for multidrug-resistant microorganisms (MDR) such as neoadjuvant therapy, longer entubation time, and steroid therapy aminopenicillin (sulbactam/ampicillin or amoxicillin/clavulanic acid), third-generation cephalosporin (cefotaxime) or narrow-spectrum carbapenem (ertapenem) can be used. If patients have risk factors for MDR, antipseudomonal cephalosporin (cefepime, ceftazidime), or antipseudomonal carbapenem (meropenem, imipenem), β-lactam/β-lactamase inhibitor (piperacillin/tazobactam) + antipseudomonal fluoroquinolone (ciprofloxacin) or aminoglycoside (amikacin, gentamicin) can be used, and if MRSA is suspected, vancomycin or linezolid should be used. Antibiotic therapy is arranged according to culture results and patient clinical status. In recent years there has been an increased incidence of resistance to *Acinetobacter* spp., which should be taken into account because this bacteria is only susceptible to colimycin.

References

1. Schussler O, Alifano M, Dermine H et al (2006) Postoperative pneumonia after major lung resection. Am J Respir Crit Care Med 173:1161–1169
2. Bernard A, Ferrand L, Hagry O, Benoit L, Cheynel N, Favre JP (2000) Identification of prognostic factor determining risk groups for lung resection. Ann Thorac Surg 70:1161–1167
3. Nagasaki F, Flehinger BJ, Martini N (1982) Complications of surgery in the treatment of carcinoma of the lung. Chest 82:25–29
4. Torres A (2006) Respiratory infections after lung cancer resection. Expert Rev Anti Infect Ther 4(5):717–720
5. Hedenstierna G, Rothen HU (2000) Atelectasis formation during anesthesia:causes and measures to prevent it. J Clin Monit Comput 16(5–6):329–335

6. Hedenstierna G, Edmark L (2005) The effects of anesthesia and muscle paralysis on the respiratory system. Intensive Care Med 31(10):1327–1335
7. Shiono S, Yoshida J, Nishimura M et al (2007) Risk factors of postoperative respiratory infections in lung cancer surgery. J Thorac Oncol 2:34–38
8. Wang Z, Cai XJ, Shi L, Li FY, Lin NM (2014) Risk factors of postoperative nosocomial pneumonia in stage I-IIIa cancer patients. Asian Pac J Cancer Prev 15:3071–3074
9. Arozullah AM, Khuri SF, Henderson WG, Daley J (2001) Development and validation of a multifactorial risk index for predicting postoperative pneumonia after major noncardiac surgery. Ann Intern Med 135:847–857
10. Bonde P, McManus K, McAnespie M, McGuigan J (2002) Lung surgery: identifying the subgroup at risk for sputum retention. Eur J Cardiothorac Surg 22(1):18–22
11. Loganathan RS, Stover DE, Shi W, Venkatraman E (2006) Prevalence of COPD in women compared to men around the time of diagnosis of primary lung cancer. Chest 129:1305–1312
12. Nici L, Donner C, Wouters E, ATS/ERS Pulmonary Rehabilitation Writing Committee et al (2006) American Thoracic Society/European Respiratory Society statement on pulmonary rehabilitation. Am J Respir Crit Care Med 173:1390–1413
13. Ries AL, Bauldoff GS, Carlin BW et al (2007) Pulmonary rehabilitation: joint ACCP/AACVPR evidence-based clinical practice guidelines. Chest 131(5 Suppl):4S–42S
14. Bobbio A, Chetta A, Ampollini L et al (2008) Preoperative pulmonary rehabilitation in patients undergoing lung resection for non-small cell lung cancer. Eur J Cardiothorac Surg 33:95–98
15. Weiner P, Man A, Weiner M et al (1997) The effect of incentive spirometry and inspiratory muscle training on pulmonary function after lung resection. J Thorac Cardiovasc Surg 113:552–557
16. Wilson DJ (1997) Pulmonary rehabilitation exercise program for high-risk thoracic surgical patients. Chest Surg Clin N Am 7:697–706
17. Spruit MA, Janssen PP, Willemsen SC, Hochstenbag MM, Wouters EF (2006) Exercise capacity before and after an 8-week multidisciplinary inpatient rehabilitation program in lung cancer patients: a pilot study. Lung Cancer 52:257–260
18. Grider JS, Mullet TW, Saha SP, Harned ME, Sloan PA (2012) A randomized, double-blind trial comparing continuous thoracic epidural bupivacaine with and without opioid in contrast to a continuous paravertebral infusion of bupivacaine for post-thoracotomy pain. J Cardiothorac Vasc Anesth 26(1):83–89
19. Belda J, Cavalcanti M, Ferrer M et al (2005) Bronchial colonization and postoperative respiratory infections in patients undergoing lung cancer surgery. Chest 128:1571–1579
20. Morran GG, McNaught W, McArdle CS (1995) The relationship between intraoperative contamination of the lower respiratory tract and post- operative chest infection. J Hosp Infect 30:31–37
21. Yamada Y, Sekine J, Suzuki H et al (2010) Trends of bacterial colonization and the risk of postoperative pneumonia in lung cancer patients with chronic obstructive lung disease. Eur J Cardiothorac Surg 37:752–757
22. Cabello H, Torres A, Celis R et al (1997) Bacterial colonization of distal airways in healthy subjects and chronic lung disease: a bronchoscopic study. Eur Respir J 10:1137–1144
23. Kirkpatrick MB, Bass JB (1989) Quantitative bacterial cultures of bronchoalveolar lavage fluids and protected specimens from normal subjects. Am Rev Respir Dis 139:546–548
24. Soler N, Ewig S, Torres A, Filella X, Gonzalez J, Zaubet A (1999) Airway inflammation and bronchial microbial patterns in patients with stable chronic obstructive pulmonary disease. Eur Respir J 14:1015–1022
25. Riise GC, Larsson S, Larsson P, Jeansson S, Andersson BA (1994) The intrabronchial microbial flora in chronic bronchitis patients: a target for N-acetylcysteine therapy? Eur Respir J 7:94–101
26. Monsó E, Ruiz J, Rosell A et al (1995) Bacterial infection in chronic obstructive pulmonary disease. A study of stable and exacerbated outpatients using the protected specimen brush. Am J Respir Crit Care Med 152:1316–1320

27. Hirakata Y, Katoh T, Tsukagoshi M, Hayashi M, Sugiyama Y, Kitamura S (1997) Bacterial colonization of the upper respiratory tract of patients with primary lung cancer and nonmalignant lung disease. Chemotherapy 43:400–405
28. Ioanas M, Angrill J, Baldo X et al (2002) Bronchial bacterial colonization in patients with resectable lung carcinoma. Eur Respir J 19:326–332
29. Sok M, Dragas AZ, Erzˇen J, Jerman J (2002) Sources of pathogens causing pleuropulmonary infections after lung cancer resection. Eur J Cardiothorac Surg 22:23–29
30. Wansbrough-Jones MH, Nelson A, New L, Wilson A, Wright N, Pepper JR (1991) Bronchoalveolar lavage in the prediction of post-thoracotomy chest infection. Eur J Cardiothorac Surg 5:433–434
31. Heininger A, Jahn G, Engel C, Notheisen T, Unertl K, Hamprecht K (2001) Human cytomegalovirus infections in nonimmunosuppressed critically ill patients. Crit Care Med 29(3):541–547
32. Radu DM, Jauréguy F, Seguin AM et al (2007) Postoperative pneumonia after major pulmonary resections: an unsolved problem in thoracic surgery. Ann Thorac Surg 84:1669–1674
33. Turna A, Kutlu CA, Ozalp T, Karamustafaoglu A, Mulazimoğlu L, Bedirhan MA (2003) Antibiotic prophylaxis in elective thoracic surgery: cefuroxime versus cefepime. Thorac Cardiovasc Surg 51:84–88
34. Olak J, Jeyasingham K, Forrester-Wood C, Hutter J, al- Zeerah M, Brown E (1991) Randomized trial of one-dose versus six-dose cefazolin prophylaxis in elective general thoracic surgery. Ann Thorac Surg 51:956–958

When and How Do I Have to Treat the Arrhythmias After Thoracic Surgery?

15

Wilhelm Haverkamp and Thomas Hachenberg

15.1 Introduction

Cardiac arrhythmias are a common phenomenon affecting millions of people worldwide. In more than 60 % of healthy adults, atrial and ventricular premature beats can be detected on 24-h Holter monitoring [1]. In Europe, atrial fibrillation is present in about 2–3 % of the population, and its prevalence is likely to increase owing to widespread population aging [2]. Symptomatic bradycardia is a frequent reason for permanent pacemaker implantation. Ventricular extrasystoles are the most common type of arrhythmia that occurs after myocardial infarction. Arrhythmias may occur at any age but are more common among older people.

Since arrhythmias are common in the general population, it is not surprising that they are also frequently observed in patients undergoing surgery, particularly postoperatively. Some patients have a history of arrhythmias; in others, they occur for the first time. New arrhythmias are a well-known complication after surgery and may impact perioperative morbidity and mortality. This paper summarizes the pathophysiology, risk factors, and the management of arrhythmias in patients undergoing noncardiac thoracic surgery. Table 15.1 lists the negative implications these arrhythmias have.

Table 15.1 Negative implications of postoperative atrial fibrillation

Increased mortality
Increased pulmonary complications
Hemodynamic deterioration and instability
Induction or exacerbation of heart failure
Increased mean lengths of intensive care unit and hospital stay
Increased mean hospital charges

W. Haverkamp
Department of Cardiology, Charite University Medicine, Berlin, Germany

T. Hachenberg (✉)
Department of Anaesthesiology and Intensive Care Medicine, Otto-von-Guericke University, Magdeburg, Germany
e-mail: Thomas.Hachenberg@med.ovgu.de

© Springer International Publishing Switzerland 2017

M. Şentürk, M.O. Sungur (eds.), *Postoperative Care in Thoracic Surgery*,
DOI 10.1007/978-3-319-19908-5_15

Table 15.2 Risk factors for perioperative arrhythmias, particularly postoperative atrial fibrillation

Patient-related risk factors
Increasing age
Male sex
Structural heart disease (coronary artery disease, valve disease, left ventricular hypertrophy, systolic and diastolic left ventricular dysfunction)
Extracardiac risk factors (obesity, previous stroke, and concomitant lung disease)
Surgery-related risk factors
Surgical trauma (type of procedure/operation, magnitude of lung resection, dissection around the atria, mechanical factors such as instrumentation)
Hemodynamic stress (volume overload or depletion, hypertension, endogenous catecholamines)
Metabolic changes (hypoxemia, hypercarbia, acid-base imbalances)
Electrolyte disturbances (particularly hypokalemia)
Drug effects (beta-blocker withdrawal, digoxin, exogenous catecholamines, phosphodiesterase inhibitors (milrinone), levosimendan)

15.2 Pathophysiology

The clinical manifestation of arrhythmias requires both the presence of a vulnerable cardiac substrate and a trigger that initiates the arrhythmia. Changes in myocardial structure and electrical function constitute the substrate for arrhythmias. Examples for typical arrhythmia substrates are atrial fibroses (favoring atrial fibrillation) and a post-myocardial infarction scar (promoting ventricular tachycardia). The substrate is patient specific but may be modified by the below discussed risk factors. The arrhythmia trigger is defined as a single incident that may set off an arrhythmia. The trigger often takes the form of a premature beat, but may also consist of acceleration or slowing of the heart beat or myocardial stretch [3].

Many perioperative factors can be considered to affect both the arrhythmia substrate and trigger, thereby increasing atrial and ventricular susceptibility to arrhythmias. Risk factors can be classified into patient and surgery related (Table 15.2).

15.2.1 Patient-Related Risk Factors

Various patient-related clinical and nonclinical risk factors for postoperative arrhythmias have been described. One of the most relevant patient-specific risk factor is age. Increasing age has been demonstrated to be correlated with the development of arrhythmias in the general population as well as in the postoperative setting. Age-related structural and/or electrophysiological changes appear to lower the threshold for atrial and ventricular arrhythmias in the elderly. Since patients undergoing thoracic surgery present with a mean age of 67 years, the risk for the development of arrhythmias is inherently increased [4]. Arrhythmias are most likely to occur in patients with structural heart disease. Patients undergoing noncardiac thoracic surgery often have the substrate of atrial enlargement or elevation in atrial pressures, which predispose to atrial tachyarrhythmias. A history of arrhythmias predisposes to postoperative events. Reported extracardiac risk factors for postoperative atrial tachyarrhythmias include obesity, previous stroke, and history of chronic obstructive pulmonary disease [5]. These risk factors are identical to those known to increase the propensity to the development of atrial fibrillation in the nonsurgical setting.

15.2.2 Surgery-Related Risk Factors

Postoperative arrhythmias are a well-known problem during and after cardiothoracic surgery; however they may also complicate major abdominal surgery. The prevalence depends on the type of operation and the extent of cardiac monitoring after surgery. The prevalence of postoperative arrhythmias may range from 4 % of patients undergoing major general surgery, vascular, and orthopedic surgery to 20 % in patients having elective colorectal surgery [6].

The trauma associated with surgical procedures predisposes patients to atrial and ventricular arrhythmias. Inflammatory mechanisms have been proposed in the development of postoperative arrhythmias since their incidence peaks at 2 to3 days after surgery [5]. Hemodynamic stress favoring arrhythmias may result from surgical trauma, volume overload or depletion, hypertension, and increased levels of endogenous catecholamines. Hypoxemia, hypercarbia, acid-base imbalances, as well as mechanical factors such as instrumentation often predispose to electrophysiological changes favoring the occurrence of arrhythmias. Hypokalemia may provoke postoperative atrial and ventricular arrhythmias [7].

Beta-blocker withdrawal has been associated with an increased rate of postoperative supraventricular tachyarrhythmias. A state of heightened catecholamine effect occurs because chronic beta-blocker use leads to a higher density of beta-adrenergic receptors. Digoxin use has been described as a risk factor for paroxysms of atrial fibrillation after surgery. The intravenous administration of catecholamines and phosphodiesterase inhibitors such as milrinone or enoximone and levosimendan has been reported to cause ventricular premature beats, short runs of ventricular tachycardia, and atrial fibrillation [5].

It is worth noting that the pathogenesis of postoperatively occurring atrial and ventricular arrhythmias is often multifactorial; it involves some or all of the mentioned mechanisms.

15.3 Atrial Fibrillation and Other Supraventricular Arrhythmias

Isolated atrial premature beats are very common after thoracic surgery and are often related to electrolyte or other metabolic imbalances. Atrial premature beats are usually readily identified by surface ECG or continuous telemetric monitoring. Paroxysmal supraventricular tachycardia develops in about 3 % of patients undergoing general surgery. The most frequent sustained arrhythmia is atrial fibrillation. The incidence varies widely (from 12 to 44 %) depending on the type of surgery and patient characteristics. In an analysis of 2588 patients undergoing noncardiac thoracic surgery, the incidence of postoperative atrial fibrillation was 12.3 % [8]. In a multivariate analysis, significant risk factors for the occurrence of atrial fibrillation were male sex (relative risk (RR) 1.72), advanced age (RR in patients with age 70 or grater 5.3), a history of congestive heart failure (RR 2.51), a history of arrhythmias (RR 1.92), a history of peripheral vascular disease (RR 1.65), resection of mediastinal tumor or thymectomy (RR 2.36), lobectomy (8.91), bilobectomy (7.16), pneumonectomy (8.91), esophagoectomy (2.95), and intraoperative transfusions (1.39) [9].

Patients with atrial fibrillation have longer mean intensive care unit and hospital stays. Mean hospital charges are more than 30 % higher when compared with patients without atrial fibrillation. Importantly, an increased mortality in patients with postoperative atrial fibrillation has been demonstrated [10]. However, since many patients with postoperative atrial fibrillation have complex comorbidities, it is not clear to what extent the arrhythmia itself contributes to this increase in mortality [4].

With the aim to facilitate preoperative risk stratification, thoracic surgical procedures were recently divided into low- (<5 %), moderate- (5–10 %), and high- (>15 %) risk groups based on their expected incidence of postoperative atrial fibrillation (Table 15.3). In moderate- and high-risk patients, extended ECG monitoring is recommended (e.g., postoperative telemetry for 48–72 h) [11, 12].

Table 15.3 Risk stratification of thoracic surgery procedures for their risk of postoperative atrial fibrillation

Low-risk procedures (<5 % incidence)	Intermediate-risk procedures (5–15 % incidence)	High-risk procedures (>15 % incidence)
Flexible bronchoscopy with and without biopsy Photodynamic therapy Tracheal stenting Placement of thoracostomy tube or PleurX catheter (CareFusion Corporation, San Diego, California) Pleuroscopy, pleurodesis, decortication Tracheostomy Rigid bronchoscopy Mediastinoscopy Thoracoscopic wedge resection Bronchoscopic laser surgery Esophagoscopy/PEG/esophageal dilation and/or stenting	Thoracoscopic sympathectomy Segmentectomy Laparoscopic Nissen fundoplication/myotomy Zenker diverticulectomy	Resection of anterior mediastinal mass Thoracoscopic lobectomy Open thoracotomy for lobectomy Tracheal resection and reconstruction/carinal resection Pneumonectomy Pleurectomy Volume reduction/ bullectomy Bronchopleural fistula repair Clagett window Lung transplantation Esophagectomy Pericardial window

Atrial premature beats usually do not need specific treatment. Paroxysmal supraventricular tachycardia occurs from time to time and treatment is often simple. If vagal maneuvers are not successful, adenosine can be used in increasing doses (Table 15.4). Success rates exceed 95 %. Electrical cardioversion is rarely needed. The management of atrial fibrillation is much more complex.

15.3.1 Treatment of Atrial Fibrillation

Given the often transient nature of new-onset postoperative atrial fibrillation (the arrhythmia frequently resolves within 4–6 weeks), the control of the ventricular response rate is usually the initial therapy. Conventionally, nondihydropyridine calcium channel antagonists (verapamil and diltiazem) and digitalis have been used for treating postoperative atrial fibrillation (Table 15.4) [11, 12]. However, since calcium antagonists may be associated with hypotension and are contraindicated in patients with heart failure, they may not be the ideal drugs in patients with compromised heart function. The same is true for digitalis, which acts primarily by increasing vagal tone.

Table 15.4 Drugs used for postoperative arrhythmias

Drug	Dosing	Indication	Side effects
Adenosine	6 or 12 mg, the 18 mg as an iv bolus	Paroxysmal SVT	Transient heart block, flushing, chest pain, induction of AF (rare)
Atropine	0.4–1 mg iv	Bradycardia or AV block	Excessive tachycardia
Verapamil	5–10 mg iv	Rate control of AF, paroxysmal SVT	Hypotension, exacerbation of CHF, AV block
Diltiazem	10–20 mg iv bolus, then infusion at 5–15 mg/h	Rate control of AF, paroxysmal SVT	Hypotension, exacerbation of CHF, AV block
Esmolol	0.5 mg/kg bolus and infusion at 0.05 mg/kg/h; increase by 0.05 mg/kg/h every 5 min	Rate control of AF	Hypotension, bronchospasm, exacerbation of CHF
Metoprolol	5 mg iv every 5 min × 3	Rate control of AF	Hypotension
Digoxin	0.25 mg iv every 4–6 h up to 1 mg	Rate control of persisting AF	Delayed onset, nausea, vomiting
Amiodarone	Prophylaxis, 300 mg iv, then 600 mg orally for 3–5 days; treatment, 150 mg iv over 10 min, then 1 mg/min × 6 h, then 0.5 mg/min	Rate control and conversion of AF, frequent non-sustained/sustained VT, VF	Hypotension, bradycardia abnormal QTc prolongation with torsade de pointes (rare), acute respiratory distress syndrome (rare, after supra-therapeutic doses)

AF atrial fibrillation, *CHF* congestive heart failure, *SVT* supraventricular tachycardia, *VT* ventricular tachycardia, *VF* ventricular fibrillation

The effects of digitalis are attenuated postoperatively when sympathetic tome is markedly increased. Beta-blockers have been shown to be effective when atrial fibrillation occurs after surgery. Patients taking beta-blockers before surgery should have beta-blockade continued; abrupt withdrawal is associated with an increased risk of complications and should be avoided. Amiodarone iv should be preferred in patients with known severe systolic dysfunction. The drug also exerts antiarrhythmic effects, which may lead to the termination of the arrhythmias. A prospective, randomized, controlled, double-blinded study included 254 patients undergoing thoracic surgery for lung cancer. The patients received either 300 mg of amiodarone or placebo intravenously after surgery and an oral dose of 600 mg or placebo twice a day for 5 postoperative days. Amiodarone significantly decreased the prevalence of atrial fibrillation (38 patients (placebo group) vs. 11 patients (amiodarone group)). A number needed to treat of 4.4 (3.1–7.8) was calculated and adverse events occurred equally in both study arms (total of ten patients) [13].

Acute pulmonary toxicity has been reported with amiodarone in patients undergoing lung resection. Amiodarone or at least high amiodarone doses (>1000 mg/day) should be avoided in these patients. Preexisting pulmonary disease is associated with an increased risk of amiodarone pulmonary toxicity [14].

Class I antiarrhythmic drugs (sodium channel blockers like flecainide and propafenone) may be used in patients without structural heart disease. However, even in those patients, these agents may exert proarrhythmic effects (e.g., convert well-tolerated atrial fibrillation compromising atrial flutter).

Immediate electrical cardioversion is indicated in patients who demonstrate severe hemodynamic deterioration in response to new-onset atrial fibrillation. It is highly effective (>90 % conversion rate). However, early recurrences are frequent. Cardioversion from well-tolerated postoperative atrial fibrillation is usually not necessary because of a frequent self-limited course. New atrial fibrillation after thoracic surgery often resolves within 4–6 weeks, regardless of treatment.

Patients who develop atrial fibrillation after surgery are at risk of thromboembolic events, including stroke. In the individual postsurgical patient with an embolic event, the cause may be unclear, as underlying comorbidities are often responsible for such strokes, rather than the arrhythmia itself. However, based on evidence that anticoagulant therapy prevents episodes of systemic embolization in the broad population of patients with atrial fibrillation, anticoagulation seems reasonable in patients with postoperative AF who have stroke risk factors (age > 65, female gender, prior stroke, hypertension, congestive heart failure diabetes). However, a reduction of events with anticoagulant therapy in this population has never been well studied.

15.3.2 Prevention of Atrial Fibrillation

Several strategies to prevent postoperative atrial fibrillation have been studied. In daily practice, the most widely used prophylactic therapy seems to be the administration of beta-blockers. Prophylactic beta-blocker administration reduces the incidence of postoperative atrial fibrillation by about 50 % [15]. The greatest benefits are seen when beta-blockers are initiated some time prior to surgery. Contraindications need to be carefully considered. Amiodarone significantly lowers the incidence of postoperative atrial fibrillation. The prophylactic potency seems to be comparable with that of beta-blockers. It is worth reminding the rare complication of intravenous amiodarone, the onset of acute respiratory distress syndrome in the postoperative period in patients undergoing lung resection. In one randomized study, magnesium iv was effective in reducing the incidence of postoperative atrial fibrillation. However, these results have never been confirmed by other studies.

Thoracic epidural analgesia (TEA) with bupivacaine has been shown to decrease the prevalence of atrial fibrillation after lung resection surgery [16]. However, a retrospective matched pair analysis could not confirm these results. A cohort of 1,236 patients undergoing resections was included into the study: 937 received a combination of general anesthesia and TEA (TEA) and 299 received general anesthesia only (non-TEA). After matching 311 TEA patients and 132 non-TEA patients, no differences on the occurrence of postoperative atrial arrhythmia could be demonstrated [17]. Thus, the role of central neuraxial analgesia for the prevention of postoperative atrial fibrillation is unclear.

To the knowledge of the authors, no systematic data are available that have evaluated how different institutions use prophylactic drug administration for the prevention of postoperative atrial fibrillation. The own experience suggests that atrial fibrillation prophylaxis is not a routine. Most institution try to optimize all aspects of perioperative care thereby minimizing the arrhythmia risk [18].

15.4 Ventricular Arrhythmia

Isolated ventricular premature betas documented postoperatively do not indicate an increased risk for the development of malignant ventricular tachyarrhythmias (i.e., sustained ventricular tachycardia, ventricular fibrillation), and, therefore, there is no need for treatment. Non-sustained and sustained ventricular tachyarrhythmias are rare. Reported incidences after surgery range from 0.5 to 1.5 %. Ten most patients developing theses arrhythmias have severe heart disease with depressed left ventricular function or suffer from severe acute postoperative complications (e.g., hemodynamic instability, myocardial ischemia, septic shock, major surgical complications).

When frequent and complex premature beats and non-sustained ventricular tachycardia occur, the correction of any reversible cause of arrhythmias (see above) should be pursued. Antiarrhythmic drugs may be indicated when longer repeated episodes of non-sustained or sustained ventricular tachycardia develop. The preferred antiarrhythmic drug is amiodarone administered intravenously [14]. Class I antiarrhythmic drugs have also been used successfully (e.g., lidocaine); however, in this setting, they are also associated with an increased risk for ventricular proarrhythmia. In the case of hemodynamic deterioration due to sustained ventricular tachyarrhythmias, either R-wave triggered DC cardioversion (in the case of hemodynamically well-tolerated ventricular tachycardia) or, after hemodynamic collapse due to unstable ventricular tachycardia or ventricular fibrillation, immediate defibrillation and cardiopulmonary resuscitation may become necessary [10].

Most patients with known, previously documented ventricular tachyarrhythmias do have an implanted cardioverter/defibrillator. These devices are effective in terminating spontaneous arrhythmia, even in the postoperative setting. All devices should be thoroughly evaluated before and after surgery to make sure that its function has not been damaged or changed. If electrocautery is to be used, pacemakers should be placed in a triggered or asynchronous mode; implantable cardioverters should have arrhythmia detection suspended before surgery.

15.5 Bradyarrhythmias

Bradyarrhythmias are common after cardiac surgery (particularly after valve surgery), but are relatively rare after noncardiac thoracic surgery [19]. In the majority of cases, they consist of transitory episodes of low ventricular heart rate resulting from (usually preexisting) sick sinus syndrome or various degrees of atrioventricular blocks. They often result from increased vagal tone caused by an intervention, such as spinal or epidural anesthesia, laryngoscopy, or surgical intervention. Bradyarrhythmias may gain hemodynamic relevance because of a decrease in cardiac output [19]. Atropine can reverse symptomatic bradycardia. It is prudent to stop all unnecessary medications that can cause increased AV block like beta-blockers or calcium channel blockers. Temporary electrical pacing may be required in symptomatic bradycardias not responding to atropine. In some cases, when the conduction defect does not revert, permanent pacing may be necessary.

References

1. Rasmussen V, Jensen G, Schnohr P, Hansen JF (1985) Premature ventricular beats in healthy adult subjects 20 to 79 years of age. Eur Heart J 6:335–341
2. Rahman F, Kwan GF, Benjamin EJ (2014) Global epidemiology of atrial fibrillation. Nat Rev Cardiol 11:639–654
3. Iwasaki YK, Nishida K, Kato T, Nattel S (2011) Atrial fibrillation pathophysiology: implications for management. Circulation 124:2264–2274
4. Rosen JE, Hancock JG, Kim AW, Detterbeck FC, Boffa DJ (2014) Predictors of mortality after surgical management of lung cancer in the National Cancer Database. Ann Thorac Surg 98:1953–1960
5. Elrakhawy HM, Alassal MA, Elsadeck N, Shaalan A, Ezeldin TH, Shalabi A (2014) Predictive factors of supraventricular arrhythmias after noncardiac thoracic surgery: a multicenter study. Heart Surg Forum 17:E308–E312
6. Walsh SR, Tang T, Gaunt ME, Schneider HJ (2006) New arrhythmias after non-cardiothoracic surgery. BMJ 333:715
7. Fernando HC, Jaklitsch MT, Walsh GL, Tisdale JE, Bridges CD, Mitchell JD, Shrager JB (2011) The Society of Thoracic Surgeons practice guideline on the prophylaxis and management of atrial fibrillation associated with general thoracic surgery: executive summary. Ann Thorac Surg 92:1144–1152

8. Vaporciyan AA, Correa AM, Rice DC, Roth JA, Smythe WR, Swisher SG, Walsh GL, Putnam JB Jr (2004) Risk factors associated with atrial fibrillation after noncardiac thoracic surgery: analysis of 2588 patients. J Thorac Cardiovasc Surg 127:779–786
9. Riber LP, Larsen TB, Christensen TD (2014) Postoperative atrial fibrillation prophylaxis after lung surgery: systematic review and meta-analysis. Ann Thorac Surg 98:1989–1997
10. Heintz KM, Hollenberg SM (2005) Perioperative cardiac issues: postoperative arrhythmias. Surg Clin North Am 85:1103–1114, viii
11. Frendl G, Sodickson AC, Chung MK, Waldo AL, Gersh BJ, Tisdale JE, Calkins H, Aranki S, Kaneko T, Cassivi S, Smith SC Jr, Darbar D, Wee JO, Waddell TK, Amar D, Adler D, American Association for Thoracic S (2014) 2014 AATS guidelines for the prevention and management of perioperative atrial fibrillation and flutter for thoracic surgical procedures. J Thorac Cardiovasc Surg 148:e153–e193
12. Frendl G, Sodickson AC, Chung MK, Waldo AL, Gersh BJ, Tisdale JE, Calkins H, Aranki S, Kaneko T, Cassivi S, Smith SC Jr, Darbar D, Wee JO, Waddell TK, Amar D, Adler D, American Association of Thoracic S (2014) 2014 AATS guidelines for the prevention and management of perioperative atrial fibrillation and flutter for thoracic surgical procedures. Executive summary. J Thorac Cardiovasc Surg 148:772–791
13. Riber LP, Christensen TD, Jensen HK, Hoejsgaard A, Pilegaard HK (2012) Amiodarone significantly decreases atrial fibrillation in patients undergoing surgery for lung cancer. Ann Thorac Surg 94:339–344; discussion 345–6
14. Gill J, Heel RC, Fitton A (1992) Amiodarone. An overview of its pharmacological properties, and review of its therapeutic use in cardiac arrhythmias. Drugs 43:69–110
15. Sedrakyan A, Treasure T, Browne J, Krumholz H, Sharpin C, van der Meulen J (2005) Pharmacologic prophylaxis for postoperative atrial tachyarrhythmia in general thoracic surgery: evidence from randomized clinical trials. J Thorac Cardiovasc Surg 129(5):997–1005
16. Oka T, Ozawa Y, Ohkubo Y (2001) Thoracic epidural bupivacaine attenuates supraventricular tachyarrhythmias after pulmonary resection. Anesth Analg 93:253–259, 1st contents page
17. Komatsu R, Makarova N, Dalton JE, Sun Z, Chang D, Grandhe R, Sreedharan R, De Oliveira DK, Pal R, Bashour A, Murthy SC, Turan A (2015) Association of thoracic epidural analgesia with risk of atrial arrhythmias after pulmonary resection: a retrospective cohort study. J Anesth 29:47–55
18. Patel AJ, Hunt I (2014) Review of the evidence supports role for routine prophylaxis against postoperative supraventricular arrhythmia in patients undergoing pulmonary resection. Interact Cardiovasc Thorac Surg 19:111–116
19. Peretto G, Durante A, Limite LR, Cianflone D (2014) Postoperative arrhythmias after cardiac surgery: incidence, risk factors, and therapeutic management. Cardiol Res Pract 2014:615987

Management of Antiaggregated and Anticoagulated Patients Scheduled for Thoracic Surgery: Recommendations for Venous Thromboprophylaxis

16

Juan V. Llau, Manuel Granell, and Mª José Jiménez

16.1 Introduction

Thoracic surgery is performed in many cases in patients that are under the effect of some drugs. Most common drugs are, probably, antiplatelet (APA) and anticoagulant (AC) agents. The management of these patients is a common challenging problem and a cause of frequent assessment from thoracic surgeons. These patients could require temporary interruption of the administration of the antiplatelet or anticoagulant drug or could need to receive a new anticoagulant for thromboprophylaxis in the perioperative period. So, it is necessary to balance the risk of a thromboembolic event during the possible interruption of the therapy with the risk for bleeding if the antithrombotic drug is administered close to surgery.

In this chapter, current guidelines for the management of these patients are revised.

J.V. Llau
Department of Anaesthesia and Critical Care, Hospital Clínic, Valencia. University of Valencia, Valencia, Spain

University of Valencia, Valencia, Spain

M. Granell (✉)
Department of Anaesthesiology, Critical Care and Pain Relief, General University Hospital of Valencia, Valencia, Spain

University of Valencia, Valencia, Spain

Catholic University of Valencia, Valencia, Spain
e-mail: mgranellg@hotmail.com

Mª.J. Jiménez
Department of Anaesthesiology, Critical Care and Pain Relief, Hospital Clinic of Barcelona, Barcelona, Spain

© Springer International Publishing Switzerland 2017
M. Şentürk, M.O. Sungur (eds.), *Postoperative Care in Thoracic Surgery*,
DOI 10.1007/978-3-319-19908-5_16

16.2 Antiplatelet Agents and Thoracic Surgery

It is very common that patients who are scheduled for thoracic surgery are treated with APA due to their wide indications and the characteristics of these patients. They are drugs of diverse origin, whose prophylactic and therapeutic effects are especially important in the prevention and treatment of the arterial thrombosis. The most common APAs used as chronic treatment are cyclooxygenase inhibitors such as aspirin and adenosine diphosphate receptor P2Y12 antagonists such as clopidogrel or prasugrel; new antiplatelet agents include ticagrelor and cilostazol. Their main characteristics are shown in Table 16.1 [1–4].

Although the management of the APA in the perioperative period is not easy, the main challenge for the anaesthesiologist and the thoracic surgeon is those patients receiving an APA with a coronary stent (mainly, drug-eluting coronary stents).

16.2.1 Rationale for the Recommendations

Some years ago, the most common practice with the APA was their withdrawal between 7 and 10 days before thoracic surgery. But, in the last years, several general documents recommending the maintenance of the APA have been published, whenever the haemorrhagic risk allows this continuation [1–7].

Table 16.1 Main characteristics of some current antiplatelet agents

Drug	Mode of action	Half-life	Onset of action	Duration of action
Aspirin	Irreversible inhibition of the enzyme COX-1	15–20 min	Few minutes	Platelet lifespan[a]
Clopidogrel	Irreversible binding to the ADP P2Y12 receptor of the platelets	About 8 h (active metabolites after liver action)	2 h if given loading dose	Platelet lifespan[a]
Prasugrel	Irreversible binding to the ADP P2Y12 receptor of the platelets	Fast conversion in active metabolites	About 30 min	Platelet lifespan[a]
Ticagrelor	Reversible P2Y12 antagonist	Approximately 12 h	About 30 min after a loading dose	4–5 days
Cilostazol	Selective inhibition of phosphodiesterase IIIA (reversible inhibition of platelet aggregation)	Around 21 h	2–3 h	12–48 h

[a]For the recovery of haemostatic competence, the recovery of the function of all platelets could not be necessary. So, 5 days after the last administration of the majority of these antiplatelet agents could be enough

The perioperative management of APA must be based on the optimal assessment of benefit/risk relationship. This includes the stratification of the perioperative haemorrhagic risk associated with the continuation of antiplatelet agents throughout surgery and the stratification of the thrombotic risk associated with their discontinuation. In order to summarise all the information, you can find a summary in Table 16.2 [2, 4–8].

16.2.2 General Recommendations for Patients Scheduled for Thoracic Surgery

The practical guidelines for the management of APA on patients scheduled for elective thoracic surgery need the local agreement of a multidisciplinary team that includes anaesthesiologists and thoracic surgeons, with the participation and acceptance by haematologists, cardiologists and neurologists.

The decision to discontinue the antiplatelet therapy prior to surgery should be based on careful cardiovascular and thrombotic risk assessment of the patient and on the type of surgery and of bleeding risk. The recommendations about the perioperative management of antiplatelet therapy in these patients are not fully agreed, but they can be summarised as follows [1–8]:

Table 16.2 Proposed stratification of the haemorrhagic risk related with the continuation of antiplatelet agents through the perioperative period and the thrombotic risk associated with their discontinuation

Haemorrhagic risk	Minor	Moderate	Major
	Transfusion usually not needed Minor plastic/general/OS surgery Biopsies, tooth extraction, surgery of the anterior segment of eye	*Transfusion usually needed* Cardiac surgery Major OS/visceral/ENT/urology or reconstructive surgery	*Possible bleeding in an enclosed space* Cranial surgery, spinal surgery, surgery of the posterior segment of eye. Transurethral prostatectomy
Thrombotic risk	Minor	Moderate	Major
	>6 months after AMI, CABG, percutaneous coronarography, BMS, coronary surgery, CVS *(>12 months if high-risk patient or associated complications)*	>12 months after DES 6–24 weeks after AMI, CABG, BMS, CVS *(6–12 months if high-risk patient or associated complications)*	<12 months after DES <6 weeks after AMI, CABG, BMS, CVS *(<6 months if high-risk patient or associated complications)*

OS orthopaedic surgery, *ENT* ear-nose-throat surgery, *AMI* acute myocardial infarction, *CABG* coronary artery bypass grafting, *BMS* bare-metal stent, *DES* drug-eluting stent, *CVS* cerebrovascular stroke

- In all cases, it is recommended that a low dose of aspirin (75–100 mg) be maintained throughout the perioperative period, unless the risk of bleeding clearly outweighs thrombotic risk.
- In order to reduce the potential risk of bleeding, aspirin dose higher than 200 mg should be replaced by 75 or 100 mg.
- The treatment should be substituted by low-dose aspirin in the case of patients treated with clopidogrel as monotherapy and where discontinuation is mandatory (unless contraindicated).
- If antiplatelet therapy must be discontinued, it should be stopped the shortest time possible: 2 days for aspirin and 5 days for clopidogrel. Thereafter, treatment should be restarted as soon as possible following surgery after ensuring haemostasis, between 6 and 48 h during the postoperative period. Depending on the withdrawal time and in order to accelerate antiplatelet response, loading dose administration may be indicated as follows: aspirin 250 mg and clopidogrel 300 mg.

16.2.3 Current Antiplatelet Protocols in Patients with Drug-Eluting Stents

APAs are recommended in the treatment of patients who had undergone percutaneous coronary interventions (PCI) and have a coronary stent in place. After this, the current protocols of administration of APA could be summarised as follows [9]:

- After stent implantation, the use of aspirin should be continued indefinitely. It is reasonable to use aspirin around 100 mg per day in preference to higher maintenance doses.
- The duration of the therapy with a thienopyridine after stent implantation should generally be given for at least 12 months. Options could include clopidogrel 75 mg daily, prasugrel 10 mg daily and ticagrelor 90 mg twice daily.
- If the risk of morbidity from bleeding outweighs the anticipated benefit afforded by a recommended duration of thienopyridine therapy after stent implantation, earlier discontinuation (e.g. <12 months) of thienopyridine therapy is reasonable.
- Continuation of clopidogrel, prasugrel or ticagrelor beyond 12 months may be considered in patients undergoing placement of drug-eluting stent.

From this protocol in the treatment of patients with a coronary stent in place, the recommendations for their management have some special considerations [1–4, 7–10]:

- Although there is not a valid algorithm for all situations, current trend is to delay all surgery that is not life threatening if the stent has high thrombotic risk. So, elective noncardiac surgery should not be performed in the 4–6 weeks after a bare-metal stent implantation or the 12 months after drug-eluting stent implantation in patients in whom the thienopyridine will need to be discontinued perioperatively. In spite of this recommendation, the evidence supporting this practice is scarce and limited, and major adverse cardiac events (MACE) in this kind of patients undergoing surgery could be related more with emergency surgery and advanced cardiac disease but not with stent type or timing of surgery beyond 6 months after stent implantation [11].

- If surgery can't be delayed, the continuation of the antiaggregation is essential to minimise the thrombotic risk of the stent. If it is not possible to maintain the APA due to a high bleeding risk, it is necessary to know that the withdrawal of the thienopyridine and the maintenance of the aspirin alone do not assure the elimination of the thrombotic risk. So the final decision in cases of surgeries that it is not possible to be delayed should be multidisciplinary and made individually.
- In all cases, the administration of the APA treatment after surgery should be done as soon as possible. Main recommendation is to give it in the first 24 h after the end of surgery if the haemostatic competence of the patient is assured.
- After the high-risk period, if the surgery is likely to cause little or no risk of bleeding, it is recommended not to stop antiplatelet therapy. Moreover, in general, the maintenance of the treatment with aspirin in patients with a coronary stent in place is the first option.
- For patients with a coronary stent who must undergo urgent surgical procedures that mandate the discontinuation of dual antiplatelet therapy, it is reasonable to continue aspirin if possible and restart the thienopyridine as soon as possible in the immediate postoperative period.

16.3 Management of Anticoagulated Patients Scheduled for Thoracic Surgery

Many patients receive oral and chronic anticoagulation due to atrial fibrillation or a mechanical heart valve, although other indications for it include cerebrovascular pathology (repeated strokes) or prevention of recurrences of previous thromboembolic events. Nowadays, the anticoagulant therapy could be made by vitamin K antagonists (VKAs) or by any of new direct oral anticoagulants (DOACs), such as dabigatran, rivaroxaban, apixaban or edoxaban, which are recently accepted or waiting their approval for these indications.

16.3.1 Management of Patients Under Vitamin K Antagonists

The perioperative management of VKAs is well established, and nearly no change has been done in the lately recommendations [2, 12–15]. Rational decisions are made depending on the risks of thrombosis and bleeding associated with the different alternatives. In general the interruption of VKAs is required to achieve normal or near-normal haemostasis at the time of surgery (INR 1.5 or below). After stopping VKAs, between 3 and at least 5 days will be required for most anticoagulant effect to be eliminated (with acenocoumarol 3 days seem to be enough, and with warfarin the delay should be up to 5 days). So, the main recommendation in patients scheduled for thoracic surgery that require temporary interruption of a VKA before the operation is to stop VKAs approximately 5 days before surgery in the case of warfarin [2], although with acenocoumarol, the recommended time could be shorter (3 days). After surgery, it is recommended resuming VKA 12–24 h postoperative, when oral intake is permitted and there is adequate haemostasis.

The temporary discontinuation of VKAs could expose patients to a risk of thromboembolism, although some controversies have been published for this topic [14–18], mainly for a possible tendency to increase bleeding with the bridging therapy without any decrease of thrombotic events. In general, current protocols recommend:

- For patients with a mechanical heart valve, atrial fibrillation or VTE at high risk for thromboembolism, there is a need of bridging anticoagulation (administration of a short-acting anticoagulant) during the interruption of VKA therapy.
- For patients at low risk for thromboembolism, the bridging can be avoided.
- When there is a moderate risk for thromboembolism, the bridging or no-bridging approach chosen should be based on an assessment of individual patient- and surgery-related factors. If the surgery or procedure is a low risk for bleeding, the bridging may be considered, but if it is of high bleeding risk (major thoracic surgery), no bridging therapy may be better.

The best option for bridging therapy is, probably, the administration of sc LMWH. Again, the dose of the LMWH in this scenario is controversial, and the proposals go from prophylactic doses to therapeutic ones (high doses reserved only for patients at high thrombotic risk). In any case, the last dose should be given before surgery time, ensuring normal haemostasis (around 24 h for LMWH). After surgery, therapeutic-dose LMWH should be resumed 24 h postoperatively in non-high-bleeding-risk surgery. In patients who are undergoing high-bleeding-risk surgery, the resumption of therapeutic-dose LMWH should be delayed 48–72 h after surgery.

16.3.2 Management of Patients Under Direct Oral Anticoagulant

DOACs have in common that they are given orally and they do not need antithrombin for their action, but they are different drugs acting in different targets of the coagulation cascade: rivaroxaban, apixaban and edoxaban directly inhibit factor Xa; dabigatran is a direct inhibitor of factor IIa.

They can be used for thromboprophylaxis in patients scheduled for major orthopaedic surgery (total hip or knee arthroplasties), for the prevention of a stroke in patients with atrial fibrillation and for the treatment and secondary prevention in patients with venous thromboembolism [19].

As there is no experience enough about the perioperative management of DOACs, it is necessary to highlight some points:

- Some antidotes have been developed for their reversal: idarucizumab for the reversal of dabigatran [20] and andexanet for the antagonization of xabans [21]. If the antidotes are not availables, some papers propose the adminsitration of PCC for the first line control of severe bleeding related with the administration of DOACs [19].
- The dosage used for the chronic anticoagulation is quite different and higher than the dosage used for thromboprophylaxis.
- The safety objective to be reached in patients receiving DOAC for "full" anticoagulation is, in these days, unknown. The safe preoperative objective has been defined for <30 ng/ml in any DOAC [22], but it is very difficult to control plasma levels in current practice. Moreover, there is a lack of relation between this plasma level and the results of standard coagulation tests.
- Main objective for their management in patients scheduled for thoracic surgery must be the safety, considered as haemorrhage associated to the procedure. Of course, the necessary antithrombotic protection should be in mind.

With these highlighted points, main recommendations for the management of DOAC in the perioperative period of a thoracic surgery could be divided in [23]:

- Bridging strategy. Stop the anticoagulant 4–5 days before surgery and make the bridging with LMWH, as if it was AVK. This possibility has been proposed by the French [24] and the Spanish anaesthesiology societies [25]. It could be the best one (the most safe one) to manage the three DOACs as one, mainly for selected patients at high thrombotic risk (defined as a CHA2DS2-VASc score more than 4 [26] or CHADS2 more than 2 [27]). In a similar way it occurs with VKAs, the dosage of the LMWH will be based on the thrombotic risk of the patient. Nevertheless, this strategy has been abandonned by most groups.
- No bridging strategy. Stop the drug before surgery without the administration of LMWH during the window period. Based on DOAC rapid onset of action and short half-life, it has been proposed their withdrawal some days before surgery [28]. As DOACs have different half-lives and different renal clearance rates, this proposal should be adapted to each drug, to the patient, to the creatinine clearance and to the procedure's bleeding risk. Nevertheless, there is no consensus on the "exact" time for this management. Moreover, the lack of experience and data in patients undergoing high-bleeding-risk procedures (complex thoracic procedures with lung resection) demands to be extremely careful in these scenarios.

The Spanish forum, after recent article revisions and large discussions, has proposed an easy and practical protocol, summarised in Table 16.3 [8, 25–27, 29–31]. The bridging therapy is also reflected as an option in this decision algorithm, only for patients at high thrombotic risk.

Table 16.3 Proposed preoperative discontinuation time of direct oral anticoagulants based on renal function and bleeding risk

Suggested minimal time from last intake before surgery				
Drug	Apixaban Rivaroxaban		Dabigatran	
CrCl (ml/min)	>50	30–50	>50	30–50
Low bleeding risk[a]	1 d	2 d	2 d	3 d
Moderate to severe bleeding risk	2 d	3 d	3 d	4 d
High thrombotic risk	Bridging therapy with LMWH is suggested			

[a]In patients with normal renal function undergoing "very low bleeding risk" procedures, the direct oral anticoagulant may not be interrupted. In the case of apixaban and dabigatran (both given twice per day), last dose before surgery should be skipped

16.4 Thromboprophylaxis in Thoracic Surgery

Pulmonary embolism (PE) and deep vein thrombosis (DVT) are two clinical presentations of venous thromboembolism (VTE) and share the same predisposing factors, being PE in most cases a consequence of DVT. VTE is currently regarded as the result of the interaction between patient-related and setting-related risk factors. Patient-related predisposing factors are usually permanent, whereas setting-related predisposing factors are more often temporary. Patient-related predisposing factors include age, history of previous VTE, active cancer, neurological disease with extremity paresis, medical disorders causing prolonged bed rest (such as heart or acute respiratory failure) and congenital or acquired thrombophilia, hormone replacement therapy and oral contraceptive therapy [32–36].

During the perioperative period, VTE is a frequent and yet relatively preventable cause of postoperative morbidity and mortality. Although the benefits of thromboprophylaxis are broadly recognised in this context, the recently proposed objective is to offer a tailored, procedure-specific, patient-specific regimen, case-per-case decided.

16.4.1 Methods for Thromboprophylaxis

Methods used for thromboprophylaxis in surgical patients include general measures and mechanical and pharmacological methods.

- General measures include mobilisation and leg exercises. Adequate hydration should be ensured in immobilised patients.
- Mechanical methods increase mean flow velocity in leg veins and reduce venous stasis. They include graduated compression stockings (GCS), intermittent pneumatic compression (IPC) devices and pneumatic foot pumps (PFP).
- Pharmacological methods are necessary when the thrombotic risk is moderate to high. They include low-molecular-weight heparins (LMWHs) that are the most

extended drugs used for thromboprophylaxis. Other drugs available for thoracic surgical patients when indicated are fondaparinux, unfractionated heparin (UFH) and antivitamin K drugs (VKAs) (warfarin/acenocoumarol).

16.4.2 Rationale for Thromboprophylaxis in Thoracic Surgery

The rationale for the use of thromboprophylaxis in patients admitted to a hospital is based on solid principles and scientific evidence, including [34, 35, 37]:

- High prevalence of VTE among hospitalised patients, because almost all of them have one or more risk factors for VTE. If no prophylaxis is given, the risk to develop any kind of VTE is highly variable, in dependence of the medical/surgical condition of the patient.
- Adverse consequences of unprevented VTE, mainly symptomatic DVT or PE, fatal PE and post-thrombotic syndrome.
- Efficacy of thromboprophylaxis, with a good cost-effectiveness relation of pharmacological and mechanical methods.

Based on these points, it is recommended that all patients are assessed on their thrombotic risk, balanced against their bleeding risk. The final decision about the optimal thromboprophylaxis protocol to be administrated should be made after the consideration of both risk factors. In general, patients at moderate or high VTE risk with low to moderate bleeding risk should receive pharmacological thromboprophylaxis. When such patients have a high bleeding risk, they should receive mechanical thromboprophylaxis (preferably with IPC), beginning with the administration of an antithrombotic drug when the bleeding risk decreases [34, 35, 37, 38].

This rationale can be applied to patients scheduled for thoracic surgery, having in mind that:

- Many patients scheduled for thoracic surgery have a high risk for perioperative VTE because of active cancer, age, preoperative chemotherapy, complex major surgery, long surgical time, etc. Active cancer is not uncommon between patients scheduled for thoracic surgery. Only this condition must move to the clinician to consider the application of the high-risk protocol for thromboprophylaxis during the perioperative period, although the bleeding risk should be also considered.
- It is suitable to stratify the VTE risk in each patient using a validated model such as the Caprini score [39] which includes measures such as age, type/duration of surgery, obesity, history of VTE or thrombophilia, presence of a central venous catheter and malignancy. Between non-oncologic patients, the risk stratification of thoracic surgical ones based on the Caprini score classifies them in low-/intermediate-risk patients, so in most cases the use of only mechanical prophylaxis methods is enough.

Most protocols include as the first option for pharmacological thromboprophylaxis the LMWH [34–37], but some controversies have been issued related with the moment of its initiation. There are no differences reported in the literature in efficacy and safety between pre- or postoperative administration of the first dose of LMWH, and the guidelines leave each one to do their preference [40–42]. Nevertheless, the current tendency is to begin the thromboprophylaxis in the postoperative period (most drugs can be given only after surgery), and if the chosen drug is an LMWH administrated once daily, the agreement is to start between 6 and 12 h after the end of surgery.

From this basis and the recent recommendations published in some guidelines [34–37], we can summarise some suggestions for thromboprophylaxis in thoracic patients (Table 16.4).

16.4.3 Thromboprophylaxis in the Perioperative Period: Implications for the Anaesthesiologist

The performance of regional anaesthesia, particularly epidural technique that is specially indicated in this kind of surgery for postoperative analgesia, seems safe in patients receiving anticoagulant drugs for thromboprophylaxis if there is an appropriate management based on safety intervals suited to the type of anaesthetic-analgesic technique to be carried out and particularly to the characteristics of the drug [42, 43]. Nevertheless, the final decision to perform regional anaesthesia in patients receiving drugs that affect haemostasis has to be taken after careful assessment of individual risks and benefits, mainly in patients receiving one anticlotting drug for thromboprophylaxis plus one antiplatelet drug for any other medical indication [42, 43].

Table 16.4 Suggested thromboprophylaxis in thoracic surgical patients

Patient group	Suggested thromboprophylaxis options	Suggested duration
Low risk for VTE (Caprini score 0–1)	Early deambulation	–
Moderate risk for VTE (Caprini score: 2–3) and not at high risk for bleeding	LMWH or UFH or IPC/GCS (preferably IPC)	7–10 days (if pharmacological prophylaxis) or until discharge
High risk for VTE (Caprini score: 4 or more) and not at high risk for bleeding	LMWH or UFH IPC/GCS (preferably IPC) should be added to pharmacologic prophylaxis	7–10 days (in cancer patients, consider prolongation up to 4 weeks)
Moderate or high risk for VTE and high risk for bleeding	IPC/GCS (preferably IPC) Initiate LMWH or UFH when bleeding risk diminishes	7–10 days (if pharmacological prophylaxis) or until discharge (in cancer patients, consider prolongation up to 4 weeks)

VTE venous thromboembolism, *LMWH* low-molecular-weight heparin, *UFH* unfractioned heparin, *IPC* intermittent pneumatic compression, *GCS* graduated compression stockings

Main recommendations for the performance of neuraxial anaesthesia from the last guideline of the European Society of Anaesthesiology [42] can be summarised as follows:

- Low-dose aspirin does not need to be stopped.
- If clopidogrel cannot be stopped at least 5 days before surgery (ideally, 7 days), the performance of an epidural technique is not recommended.
- Prophylactic doses of an LMWH are safe if the delay between its administration and the performance of the neuraxial block is, at least, 10–12 h. If the first dose of LMWH is administrated after surgery, the delay between the epidural block and the LMWH administration should be at least 6–8 h. Finally, the epidural catheter should not be removed till 12 h has passed since the last dose of LMWH.

References

1. Llau JV, Ferrandis R, Sierra P, Gomez Luque A (2010) Prevention of renarrowing of coronary arteries using drug-eluting stents in the perioperative period: an update. Vasc Health Risk Mang 6:1–13
2. Douketis JD, Spyropoulos AC, Spencer FA, Mayr M, Jaffer AK, Eckman MH et al (2012) Perioperative management of antithrombotic therapy. Chest 141((2 Suppl)):e326S–e350S
3. Sierra P, Gómez-Luque A, Castillo J, Llau JV (2011) Guía de práctica clínica sobre el manejo perioperatorio de antiagregantes plaquetarios en cirugía no cardiaca (Sociedad Española de Anestesiología y Reanimación) (Spanish). Rev Esp Anestesiol Reanim 58(Supl 1):1–16
4. Oprea AD, Popescu WM (2013) Perioperative management of antiplatelet agents. Br J Anaesth 11(S1):i3–i17
5. Llau JV, López-Forte C, Sapena L, Ferrandis R (2009) Perioperative management of antiplatelet agents in noncardiac surgery. Eur J Anesthesiol 26:181–187
6. Korte W, Cattaneo M, Chassot PG, Elchinger S, Von Heymann C, Hofmann N et al (2011) Peri-operative management of antiplatelet therapy in patients with coronary artery disease. Thromb Haemost 105:743–749
7. Kozek-Langenecker SA, Afshari A, Albaladejo P, Aldecoa C, De Robertis E, Filipescu DC et al (2013) Management of severe perioperative bleeding – guidelines from the European Society of Anaesthesiology. Eur J Anesthesiol 30:1–112
8. Baron TH, Kamath PS, McBane RD (2013) Management of antithrombotic therapy in patients undergoing invasive procedures. N Engl J Med 368:2113–2124
9. Levine GN, Bates ER, Blankenship JC, Bailey SR, Bittl JA, Cercek B et al (2011) ACCF/AHA/SCAI guideline for percutaneous coronary intervention. J Am Coll Cardiol 2011:e44–e122
10. Howard-Alpe GM, de Bono J, Hudsmith L et al (2007) Coronary artery stents and non-cardiac surgery. Br J Anaesth 98:560–574
11. Hawn MT, Graham LA, Richman JS, Itani KM, Henderson WG, Maddox TM (2013) Risk of major adverse cardiac events following noncardiac surgery in patients with coronary stents. JAMA 310:1462–1472
12. Kearon C, Hirsh J (1997) Management of anticoagulation before and after elective surgery. N Engl J Med 336:1506–1511
13. Douketis JD, Berger PB, Dunn AS, Jaffer AK, Spyropoulos AC, Becker RC et al (2008) The perioperative management of antithrombotic therapy. Chest 133:299S–339S
14. Spyropoulos AC (2005) Bridging of oral anticoagulation therapy for invasive procedures. Curr Hematol Rep 4:405–413

15. Dunn A (2006) Perioperative management of oral anticoagulation: when and how to bridge. J Thromb Thrombolysis 21:85–89
16. Wysokinski WE, Mc Bane IIRD (2012) Periprocedural bridging management on anticoagulation. Circulation 126:486–490
17. Van Veen JJ, Makris M (2015) Management of perioperative antithrombotic therapy. Anaesthesia 70(Suppl 1):58–67
18. Siegal D, Yudin J, Kaatz S, Douketis JD, Lim W, Spyropoulos AC (2012) Periprocedural heparin bridging in patients receiving vitamin K antagonists: systematic review and meta-analysis of bleeding and thromboembolic rates. Circulation 126:1630–1639
19. Fenger-Eriksen C, Munster AM, Grove EL (2014) New oral anticoagulants: clinical indications, monitoring and treatment of acute bleeding complications. Acta Anesthesiol Scand 58:651–659
20. Pollack CV Jr, Reilly PA, Eikelboom J, Glund S, Verhamme P, Berstein RA et al (2015) Idarucizumab for Dabigatran Reversal. N Engl J Med 373:511–520
21. Connolly SJ, Milling TJ, Eikelboom JW, Gibson CM, Curnutte JT, Gold A et al (2016) Andexanet Alfa for acute major bleeding associated with Factor Xa inhibitors. N Engl J Med 375:1131–1141
22. Pernod G, Albaladejo P, Godier A, Samama CM, Susen S, Gruel Y et al (2013) Management of major bleeding complications and emergency surgery in patients on long-term treatment with direct oral anticoagulants, thrombin or factor-Xa inhibitors: proposals of the working group on perioperative haemostasis (GIHP) – March 2013. Arch Cardiovasc Dis 106(6–7):382–393
23. Ferrandis Comes R, Llau Pitarch JV (2014) Old and new anticoagulants: what are the guidelines saying? Reg Anesth Pain Med 39(Suppl 1):e63–e65
24. Sié P, Samama CM, Godier A, Rosencher N, Steib A, Llau J, et al; Working Group on Perioperative Haemostasis; French Study Group on Trombosis and Haemostasis (2011) Surgery and invasive prodecures in patients on long-term treatment with direct oral anticosgulants: thrombin or factor-Xa inhibitors. Recommendations of the Working Group on Perioperative Haemostasis and the French Study Group on Trombosis and Haemostasis. Arch Cardiovasc Dis 104:669–676
25. Llau JV, Ferrandis R, Castillo J, De Andrés J, Gomar C, Gomez-Luque A et al (2012) en representación de los participantes en el Foro de Consenso de la ESRA-España de fármacos que alteran la hemostasia. Manejo de los anticoagulantes orales de acción directa en el periodo perioperatorio y técnicas invasivas. Rev Esp Anestesiol 59:321–330
26. Ferrandis R, Castillo J, De Andrés J, Gomar C, Gomez-Luque A, Hidalgo F et al (2013) The perioperative management of new direct oral anticoagulants: a question without answers. Thromb Haemost 110:515–522
27. Kozek-Langenecker SA, Afshari A, Albaladejo P, Aldecoa Alvarez Santullano C, De Robertis E, Filipescu DC et al (2013) Management of severe perioperative bleeding. Guidelines from the European Society of Anaesthesiology. Eur J Anaesthesiol 30:270–382
28. Miesbach W, Seifried E (2012) New direct oral anticoagulants: current therapeutic options and treatment recommendations for bleeding complications. Thromb Haemost 108:625–632
29. Levy JH, Faraoni D, Spring JL, Douketis JD, Samama C (2013) Managing new oral anticoagulants in the perioperative and intensive care unit setting. Anesthesiology 118:1466–1474
30. Ortel TL (2012) Perioperative management of patients on chronic antithrombotic therapy. Blood 120:4699–4705
31. Faraoni D, Samama CM, Ranucci M, Dietrich W, Levy JH (2014) Perioperative management of patients receiving new oral anticoagulants. Clin Lab Med 34:637–654
32. Samama MM (1999) Applying risk assessment models in general surgery: effective risk stratification. Blood Coag Fibrinolysis 10(suppl 2):S79–S84
33. Samama MM, Dahl OE, Quinlan DJ, Mismetti P, Rosencher N (2003) Quantification of risk factors for venous thromboembolism: a preliminary study for the development of a risk assessment tool. Haematologica 88:1410–1421

34. Scottish Intercollegiate Guidelines Network (SIGN) (2010) Prevention and management of venous thromboembolism. SIGN, Edinburgh
35. The Royal College of Surgeons of England. Venous thromboembolism: reducing the risks. Guía NICE updated January 2010
36. Nicolaides AN, Fareed J, Kakkar AK, Comerota AJ, Goldhaber SZ, Hull R, et al (2013) Prevention and treatment of venous thromboembolism. International consensus statement (Guidelines according to scientific evidence). Int Angiol 32:111–252
37. Gould MK, García DA, Wren SN, Karanicolas PJ, Arcelus JI, Heit JA, Samama CM (2012) Prevention of VTE in non-orthopedic surgical patients. Chest 141((2 Suppl)):227–277
38. Samama CM, Gafsou B, Jeandel T, Laporte S, Steib A, Marrte E et al (2011) Guidelines on perioperative venous thromboembolism prophylaxis. Update 2011. Ann Fr Anesth Reanim 30:947–951
39. Caprini JA (2005) Thrombosis risk assessment as a guide to quality patient care. Dis Mon 51:70–78
40. Samama CM, Godier A (2011) Perioperative deep vein thrombosis prevention: what works, what does not work and does it improve outcome? Curr Opin Anesthesiol 24:166–170
41. Della Rocca G, Biggi F, Grossi P, Imberti D, Landolfi R, Palareti G et al (2011) Italian intersociety consensus statement on antithrombotic prophylaxis in hip and knee replacement and in femoral neck fracture surgery. Minerva Anestesiol 77:1003–1010
42. Gogarten W, Vandermeulen E, Van Aken H, Kozek S, Llau JV, Samama CM (2010) Regional anaesthesia and antithrombotic agents: recommendations of the European Society of Anaesthesiology. Eur J Anaesthesiol 27:999–1015
43. Llau JV, De Andrés J, Gomar C, Gómez-Luque A, Hidalgo F, Torres LM (2007) Anticlotting drugs and regional anaesthetic and analgesic techniques: comparative update of the safety recommendations. Eur J Anaestesiol 24:387–398

Pain Management Following Thoracic Surgery

17

Mukadder Orhan Sungur and Mert Şentürk

17.1 Introduction

There are numerous articles with the keywords "pain after thoracotomy" or "post-thoracotomy analgesia" emphasizing the fact that this is one of most attractive and challenging topics of anesthesiology even after decades and thousands of studies.

Several reasons contribute to this "ongoing challenge":

1. Thoracotomies (with posterolateral and posterior incisions) are one of the most painful operations. Physiopathology of postthoracotomy pain is very complicated and still not totally explained.
2. The main target organ of the complications of postoperative pain and the operation is the same: the lung. Therefore, there is a strong relationship between appropriate postoperative pain therapy and pulmonary complications like atelectasis and pneumonia [1].
3. Pain following thoracic surgery is triggered by breathing cycle constantly and exacerbated by movements such as coughing or deep breathing which can also determine efficacy of analgesic therapy [2]. Although a patient can sleep without pain (i.e., "low VAS-rest"), optimal pain therapy targets analgesia of a patient who can cough effectively (i.e., "low VAS-cough"). However, achieving such a target with high doses of opioids can also worsen the postoperative respiratory functions.
4. Last, but not least, thoracotomy is the second (after amputation) operation which is most commonly associated with a "chronic postoperative pain syndrome" [3, 4].

M.O. Sungur • M. Şentürk (✉)
Department of Anesthesiology and Intensive Care Medicine,
Istanbul University, Istanbul Faculty of Medicine, Istanbul, Turkey
e-mail: senturkm@istanbul.edu.tr

© Springer International Publishing Switzerland 2017

M. Şentürk, M.O. Sungur (eds.), *Postoperative Care in Thoracic Surgery*,
DOI 10.1007/978-3-319-19908-5_17

17.2 Physiology of Pain

Before discussing management of pain, a thorough understanding of pain physiology and surgical trauma is a must. Acute pain after thoracotomy can be due to direct or indirect trauma. Surgical dissection of tissues including skin, muscles, ribs, pulmonary parenchyma, pleura, and nerves (acute intercostal neuralgia) constitutes direct trauma. Stretching of ligaments (acute costochondritis, posterior costochondral ligament damage, costochondral dislocation), pressure exerted by rib retractors, and irritation or inflammation as a result of surgery can cause indirect trauma [5, 6]. Trauma can continue even after surgery due to drainage tubes, residual blood, sutures, or wires adjacent to neurovascular bundle [7].

Nociceptive stimuli following trauma are transmitted to the central nervous system via intercostal, thoracodorsal, long thoracic, vagus, or phrenic nerves.

- Intercostal nerves usually carry somatic nociceptive stimuli to the dorsal horn of the spinal cord by both fast-conducting, myelinated A delta and slower, unmyelinated C-fibers [8].
- Thoracodorsal and long thoracic nerves which arise from C5–C7 roots carry nociceptive stimuli due to injury of latissimus dorsi and serratus anterior muscles [9].
- Surgical manipulation of the pleura/pericardium, diaphragm, or bronchi can also result in a visceral stimuli transmitted by vagus and phrenic nerves. Diaphragmatic irritation results in phrenic nerve stimulation that is usually referred to ipsilateral shoulder pain (also known as postthoracotomy shoulder pain, PTSP) [10]. Musculoskeletal components due to distraction of posterior thoracic ligaments and brachial plexus stretching [11] also contribute to PTSP development.
- Chronic postthoracotomy pain syndrome (CPTP) is defined as "pain that recurs or persists along a thoracotomy scar at least 2 months following the surgical procedure" [4] and is thought to have neuropathic, myofascial, and visceral components. CPTP is strongly related with acute postoperative pain [12]. Other risk factors identified for CPTP besides acute neuropathic pain are female gender, radiation therapy, presence of preoperative pain, and extensive surgical trauma including pleurectomy.

Surgical technique plays an important role in both acute and chronic pain. Thoracotomy for open lung resection usually involves a posterolateral incision below the scapula tip (mostly at fifth intercostal space) and dissection of latissimus dorsi and serratus anterior muscles [13]. Limiting incision size, appropriate closing of the muscles, or avoiding splitting the latissimus dorsi can decrease surgical trauma. In recent years, surgery is modified to completely or partially preserve muscles (also called muscle-sparing thoracotomy), though their effectiveness in reducing postoperative pain is controversial [14–16]. Anterolateral incision in which surgical exposure may be limited causes less pain than posterolateral approach [17]. Acute pain due to classical techniques is more severe than thoracoscopic procedures (i.e., video-assisted thoracoscopic surgery or VATS). However, chronic pain can still be encountered in VATS (albeit at a lower incidence) [18, 19] possibly due to trocar insertion trauma [20].

17.3 Consequences of Untreated Pain

Main clinical consequence of inadequate pain relief in thoracotomy patients is altered pulmonary mechanics. Postoperative pulmonary dysfunction in thoracotomy patients is a common result of a combination of multiple factors such as preexisting lung disease, loss of parenchyma due to surgery, positioning, single-lung ventilation, and pain [21]. Surgery is known to decrease vital capacity as far as 15 % in lobectomy and 35–40 % in pneumonectomy [22]. Furthermore, general anesthesia itself may cause a functional residual capacity (FRC) reduction up to 20 % [23], and this is increased in lateral position [24]. Lastly, the patient needs to breathe to avoid postoperative deeply pulmonary complications. Thoracotomy patients often avoid deep breathing as it causes further stretching of incision, and instead "splinting," i.e., expiratory muscle contraction, is observed. Thus, uncontrolled postoperative pain results in decreased lung compliance, reduced functional residual capacity, ventilation/perfusion mismatch, splinting, atelectasis, hypoventilation, hypoxia, and hypercarbia [25].

Acute pain can also cause an increase in sympathetic flow, heart rate, preload, and postload resulting in increased myocardial oxygen consumption which may be deleterious in a patient with ischemic heart disease. For endocrine consequences, pain is associated with catecholamine, ACTH, aldosterone, cortisol, ADH, angiotensin, and glucagon increase which produces a catabolic state with hyperglycemia and free water retention. Other repercussions of untreated acute pain can be listed as altered coagulation, fibrinolysis, cytokine production, and gastrointestinal motility and CPTP.

17.4 Treatment of Pain

A wide variety of techniques and analgesics can each target different points in acute pain transmission. In the past, most authors agreed that optimal strategy should be preemptive and multimodal, and hence a preoperatively placed thoracic epidural catheter should be a standard in all patients undergoing major open thoracic surgical procedures as stated by Gottschalk et al. [20]. In less than 10 years, all three standards (preemptive, multimodal, and thoracic epidural) in this review, though still relevant, became somehow controversial.

17.5 Multimodal Analgesia

Postthoracotomy pain has complex mechanisms involving both incisional (nociceptive) pain due to the damage of myofascial structures and neuropathic component in transition from acute to chronic pain. To expect one method of analgesia to be omnipotent is to set oneself for failure. For example, as explained above, PTSP accompanying thoracic procedures is caused by afferent impulses conducted with phrenic nerves and can be treated with a phrenic nerve blockade [26], but not with thoracic epidural or paravertebral analgesia. To cover all the components and the whole pathway of thoracotomy pain, using systemic application of opioids would require very high doses with side effects and/or remain inadequate. Therefore, systemic use of opioids is not a first-choice treatment and should be considered at most as a "rescue" analgesic of other methods.

Combining strategies acting on different sites of central and peripheral nervous system is attractive as side effects of high-dose opioids can be avoided with better analgesia. A commonly used strategy is to combine local anesthetics (regional analgesia or infiltration), opioids, and non-opioid analgesics with regional anesthesia as mainstay of pain relief. This strategy theoretically may also aid in decreasing humoral inflammatory factors in circulation and hence decrease central sensitization. Role of multimodal analgesia in prevention of transition from acute to chronic pain is yet unknown [5].

17.6 Preemptive Analgesia

"Preemptive analgesia" concept, i.e., providing analgesia to prevent the establishment of central sensitization caused by incisional injury – before the noxious stimulus – had been initially advocated by experimental studies. However, the promising results of experimental studies could not be confirmed by following clinical studies [27]. Probably, this controversy was due to an incorrect definition of the concept. As a matter of fact, it is not rational to expect that only a preoperative peri-incisional injection of lidocaine would cause a change in postthoracotomy pain [28]. In a new definition, "preventive analgesia" should prevent the establishment of central sensitization caused not only by incisional but also by inflammatory injuries, covering the whole preoperative and early postoperative periods [29]. This should lead to an equal effective analgesia with lower doses of analgesics. In a prospective randomized trial comparing the effects of preoperative- or postoperative-initiated thoracic epidural anesthesia (TEA) versus intravenous opioids, it has been found that the preoperative initiation of TEA was associated with a significant improvement in both acute and chronic postthoracotomy pain [3]. A meta-analysis on timing of analgesia for postthoracotomy pain also showed that preoperative thoracic epidural analgesia is associated with a better control of acute pain [30].

17.7 Regional Analgesia

17.7.1 Thoracic Epidural Analgesia/Anesthesia

Thoracic epidural analgesia (TEA) has been traditionally regarded to be the gold standard in the treatment of postthoracotomy pain [31, 32]. TEA provides better analgesia, better quality of life [33, 34], and better preservation of FRC [34] compared to parenteral opioids. TEA is associated with a significant decrease in postoperative pulmonary complications such as pneumonia and atelectasis [35, 36]. There is also evidence that TEA may prevent chronic postthoracotomy pain [3] and provide beneficial anti-ischemic [37] and anti-arrhythmic effects [38].

One should also be aware of possible complications of epidural analgesia such as failure to place the catheter, hypotension due to bilateral sympathetic blockade, urinary retention, nausea, and rarely nerve damage, hematoma, infection, and accidental intrathecal or intravascular spread with resulting local anesthetic toxicity [39]. Therefore successful implementation of TEA depends on provider's attitude and conduct as with any anesthetic procedure. The concept is linked to several questions concerning:

17.7.1.1 How to Do It?

As thoracic epidural catheterization requires a manipulation above the conus medullaris (usually at T3–T9 level), there is possibility of medulla spinalis injury. This procedure, combined with the fact that thoracic epidural catheter is considered to be technically more difficult than the lumbar one, should be performed "awake" (or "lightly sedated") to warn the anesthetist of any possible neurological injury. Placement of thoracic epidural catheters in anesthetized patients has resulted in serious neurological damage [40]. Another advantage of placing epidural catheters prior to anesthesia would be testing of sensory block extension.

Epidural catheter is often advised to place between T3–T6 levels via a paramedian approach. There are two main reasons for such a recommendation: one is the extreme upward angulation of the processus spinosus at the mid-thoracic region, and the other is possible ligamentum flavum midline gaps in cervical and thoracic regions. With the same rationale, it is also recommended to use "hanging drop" technique instead of "loss of resistance." However, the authors' experience is that the more common approach of "loss of resistance" via the median approach is still appropriate (and easy to perform) especially in low thoracic levels. Furthermore needle for skin local anesthetic infiltration can also be used as a "relatively noninvasive" guide to locate optimum insertion angle.

The line connecting the inferior angles of the scapula is the landmark of T8; however this landmark should also be checked by counting up from the iliac crest specifically in obese patients [41]. Of note, the catheter and solution delivered should target dermatomes where nociceptive input originates to provide better analgesia with minimal side effects (right place, right drug, and right dose). Considering that the catheter would be inserted some 2–4 cm within the epidural space, the optimal level for best epidural drug spread can be adjusted. After high-thoracic epidurals, spread occurs markedly more caudal than cranial. Conversely, low-thoracic epidurals have more cranial spread, while at the mid-thoracic level, there is a homogenous spread in both directions [42].

17.7.1.2 Should It Be Mid-thoracic, or Is Low Thoracic or Lumbar Also Possible?

The "congruence" of the catheter and the incision appears to be crucial. Placing a catheter that does not coincidence with incision can result in lower pain relief [43] and possible early removal of the epidural catheter because of ineffective analgesia.

Moreover, the advantages associated with the attenuation of the stress response because of sympathetic blockade have been shown to be effective only with extensive blockade [44]. On the other hand, many anesthetists (especially the ones working in low-volume centers for thoracotomies and hence less experience with TEA) tend to prefer lumbar epidural analgesia (LEA). This approach can be advocated with a less possibility of neurologic injury and may be performed also after anesthesia induction. However the success of such approach depends on the use of opioids, specifically hydrophilic opioid morphine which tends to spread to thoracic regions [45, 46]. Similarly, single-shot intrathecal morphine may provide adequate pain relief for 12–24 h [47] with doses ranging from 15 to 20 μg/kg [48].

17.7.1.3 What and How Much to Inject?

A combination of local anesthetic and opioids has apparent benefits over the solo use of both drugs. The combination makes it possible to decrease the doses of both drugs, leading to a decreased frequency and intensity of unwarranted effects (e.g., less pruritus because of opioids and less motor blockade because of local anesthetics). Furthermore local anesthetics have been shown to facilitate the entry of opioid from the epidural space into the cerebrospinal fluid [49]. The only possible drawback of adding opioid is the possibility of a late onset of respiratory depression, but this can be minimized by using appropriate doses of appropriate opioids.

Regarding local anesthetics, bupivacaine, levobupivacaine, and ropivacaine are popular choices in differing concentrations. Application of the same amount (=dose) of the epidural cocktail in different concentrations/volumes mostly depends on "individual" choices. Although a case can be made to avoid "intense" analgesia (even "anesthesia") in a limited region for high concentration in low-volume solutions in the postoperative period, this has not shown clinically [50]. Regarding the choice of the opioid, epidural lipophilic opioids such as fentanyl or sufentanil prefer to stay in epidural fat and have low spinal bioavailability resulting in rather "narrow" but rapid-onset analgesia, whereas hydrophilic opioids such as morphine can reach cerebrospinal fluid in higher ratio and can achieve a "wider" analgesia despite increased nausea/vomiting and late onset of action. The optimal concentration of epidural fentanyl for bupivacaine 0.1 % was found to be 5 μg/ml [51]. Our center also uses patient-controlled epidural analgesia with bupivacaine 0.1 % and morphine 0.05–0.1 mg/mL solution successfully [52].

Several adjuvants have been studied regarding their effectiveness in TEA. Among them, magnesium [53], ketamine [54], clonidine [55], dexmedetomidine [56], and neostigmine [57] appear to be promising. They all are reported to be associated with a reduction in postoperative analgesic requirement; the effects on chronic pain are rather controversial. Unfortunately, almost all of these drugs are to be used "off-label" via the epidural route; this is maybe the most important reason why their use is limited to scientific trials.

17.7.1.4 When to Start?

As explained above, preoperative insertion and dosing of epidural catheter and onset of analgesia prior to incision while continuing analgesics in the postoperative

48–72 h can provide "preventive analgesia." In our institution, a loading dose of 10 mL of aforementioned epidural solution is applied before the surgery, and a constant infusion rate of 7–10 mL/h is continued throughout the surgery. However, one should be aware of possibility of hypotension at the start of surgery and be ready to counter this either by decreasing the general anesthetic levels with the depth of anesthesia monitoring or if necessary low doses of vasopressors. Obviously, loading the patient with fluids should be avoided in these cases, as long as the reason of hypotension is not hypovolemia. Second concern to preoperative or intraoperative use of TEA is that it may lead to pulmonary vasodilation. It can be assumed that the hypoxic pulmonary vasoconstriction would be inhibited, with a consequent increase in pulmonary shunt and decrease in oxygenation. Although there are some studies supporting this assumption, the increase in shunt and decrease in oxygenation appear to be statistically insignificant and clinically irrelevant with both isoflurane and propofol [52]. During the postoperative period, PCEA protocol with no loading dose, basal infusion of 5 mL/h, 3 mL bolus dose, and 30-min lockout period is used in our institution. However, this regimen is also tailored in each patient individually.

17.7.2 Paravertebral Block

Paravertebral block (PVB) with its fast-growing popularity is now considered as a serious and in some cases an even more appropriate alternative of TEA [58]. Unnecessary bilateral sympathetic blockade resulting in hypotension and urinary retention encountered in TEA can be avoided with PVB, and possibility of neurological injury, hematoma, epidural abscess, accidental intrathecal injection, and systemic local anesthetic injection, although theoretically possible, is lower in PVB than TEA. Specific complications listed for PVB include ipsilateral Horner syndrome and pneumothorax. As with TEA, infection at injection site, severe coagulopathy, and deformities of the spine resulting in technical difficulty to perform the block are the main limitations to the use of PVB. Furthermore, PVB should not be performed in patients depending on intercostal muscles for ventilation or in patients with ipsilateral diaphragmatic paresis.

In terms of outcomes, although its effect on preventing chronic postthoracotomy pain is unknown, recent reviews have stated that PVB is a safe and superior alternative to TEA for dynamic analgesia [59] and has comparable efficacy to TEA in static analgesia [60]. PVB is also successful in preserving pulmonary function and preventing complications such as failure of technique, hypotension, need for vasopressors, urinary retention, nausea and vomiting, need for ventilator support, need for reoperation, arrhythmia, anastomosis leak, and sepsis [5, 11]. Of note, most studies reporting better or comparable analgesia with TEA have been placed by the surgeon under direct vision. Also one should keep in mind that its efficacy would be limited following single-shot injection. Furthermore, according to a systematic review and metaregression study by Kotze et al., the effectiveness of PVB is increased with continuous infusion techniques when compared to intermittent boli [61]. This study also reported that higher doses of bupivacaine provided better analgesia when compared to lower doses. When using high doses, albeit infrequently, local anesthetic toxicity is possible especially if the pleural integrity is not preserved as absorption of the local anesthetic is faster from the pleural space compared to the paravertebral space [62].

The anatomy of the thoracic paravertebral space plays an important role in the application of PVB. This is a wedge-shaped space bounded medially by the bodies of the vertebrae, intervertebral discs, and intervertebral foramina, anterolaterally by the parietal pleura and the innermost intercostal membrane, and posteriorly by the transverse processes of the thoracic vertebrae, heads of the ribs, and the superior costotransverse ligament.

In the classical technique, needle is inserted 25 mm lateral to the spinous processes of the targeted vertebrae and directed posteroanterior till pars intervertebralis, articular column, or transverse process is encountered. Once the bone is met, needle is advanced in an inferior (caudal) and lateral direction while testing for a change in resistance. Change in resistance indicates penetration of the costotransverse ligament and identification of paravertebral space. We will not explain the technique of PVB in details, but one important point is that there should be a feeling of "change in resistance" as the needle is advanced caudally beyond the costotransverse ligament and needle insertion depth should be predefined (i.e., no more than 10–15 mm) [63]. This means a "click" and a "loss of resistance" similar to the ones in TEA should be avoided, for they may indicate a pleural puncture. Another important point to remember is cranial advancement can increase the risk of pleural puncture, whereas medial angulation can cause epidural, intrathecal, or spinal injection.

Although technically easy, an unacceptable high rate of misplacement is shown with classical landmark technique radiologically [64]. The advance of ultrasound technology has enabled us to visualize the transverse process, costotransverse ligament, and paravertebral space and pleura. The use of ultrasound, albeit time costly, can reduce misplacement and/or complications either with assistance as distance to paravertebral or pleural space can be measured prior to block or with direct needle visualization and guidance in real time during the block [65, 66]. Furthermore, anterior displacement of parietal pleura with injection of local anesthetic can be observed.

Interestingly, in magnetic resonance imaging studies, a discrepancy can be observed between spread of local anesthetic and somatic analgesia (i.e., although the injected local anesthetic only encompassed four vertebral levels, sensory block levels were more extensive and showed high variability) which is explained by some via a possible secondary epidural spread [67].

17.7.3 Intercostal and Interpleural Block

For intercostal block, each intercostal nerve is targeted at inferior rib margin in intercostal space. In these blocks, local anesthetic spread is mostly distal, and proximal spread is relatively limited unlike PVB requiring multiple injections and high amount of local anesthetics with possible systemic toxicity side effects for effective analgesia. However, these blocks provide fast, easy, and valuable alternative in patients when TEA and PVB cannot be used. Although intercostal nerve blocks have been shown to be effective especially in multiple injections and continuous infusions in a meta-analysis [31], this has not been the case for single-shot block [68]. Yet, there is recent interest in these blocks with the use of long-acting bupivacaine liposome [69].

Interpleural analgesia targets the spread of local anesthetic from interpleural space in a retrograde manner to intercostal and paravertebral space. However, this technique is not recommended due to possibility of air entrapment (pneumothorax) during needle pass through the pleura, large doses of local anesthetic requirement (systemic toxicity), and loss of drug via chest tubes [31].

17.7.4 Continuous Wound Catheter Analgesia

Continuous wound analgesia via ON-Q infiltration catheter had been advocated as an easy and cheaper route to administer local anesthetics compared to TEA while providing efficient analgesia for open thoracotomies [70]. However, analgesic efficacy was not confirmed in a study comparing wound analgesia with TEA and PVB [71]. Recently, a study comparing wound catheter analgesia with placebo has demonstrated better analgesia, accelerated recovery of respiratory dynamics, and suppressed postoperative inflammation markers in wound analgesia group [72].

17.7.5 Other Techniques

Cryoanalgesia which involves neurolysis by freezing intercostal nerves is nowadays an abandoned technique as its use is associated with chronic postthoracotomy pain [73]. Neuromodulation via transcutaneous electrical nerve stimulation (TENS) is a frequently underutilized technique that can complement regional or systemic analgesia and has been shown to be effective together with pharmacological analgesia when compared to TENS alone [11, 74].

17.8 Systemic Analgesia

17.8.1 Opioids

Intrathecal and epidural routes for opioid administration have been discussed above. Parenteral opioid administration is not preferred as a first choice in thoracotomy patients due to a high rate of unwarranted/warranted effects such as nausea and vomiting, constipation, altered mental status, and respiratory depression. However, in patients where regional blocks are not applicable, they can be used.

17.8.2 Acetaminophen and Nonsteroidal Anti-inflammatory Drugs (NSAID)

Acetaminophen, a weak prostaglandin and cyclooxygenase (COX)-II and COX-III inhibitor, has been shown to decrease ipsilateral shoulder pain in thoracotomy patients when given preemptively [75]. This drug can be administered via oral, rectal, and intravenous route and is a relatively safe drug in doses less than 4000 mg/day in adult patients. However, one should be cautious in higher doses or in patients with hepatic diseases. Classical NSAIDs such as ketorolac can decrease opioid requirements but are associated with gastrointestinal, renal, and cardiovascular side effects and may impair coagulation. More studies are needed to elucidate if new formulations of old drugs enabling parenteral use (such has ibuprofen) can achieve similar or yet better analgesia. COX-II selective inhibitors (such as parecoxib, celecoxib, nimesulide) can also reduce opioid consumption in an equally effective manner but do not impair coagulation. Several studies have reported successful use of NSAIDs and COX-II inhibitors for thoracotomy patients [76–78]. These drugs may also be important in suppressing postoperative inflammatory response [79], but studies are needed to investigate their effects on transition from acute to chronic pain.

17.8.3 Ketamine

Ketamine, a noncompetitive antagonist of N-methyl-D-aspartate (NMDA) receptor, has unique analgesic effects in patients with opioid tolerance, pain with neuropathic component, and acute hyperalgesia. Ketamine may be associated with an increase in neuropsychiatric disturbances but may decrease side effects of opioids such as nausea and vomiting or respiratory depression. Analgesic-sparing effects of intravenous subanesthetic doses of ketamine have been demonstrated for parenteral and paravertebral analgesia [78, 80], but not for TEA [81]. Similarly, ketamine was not shown to be effective in preventing CPTP [11].

17.8.4 Gabapentin and Pregabalin

Gabapentinoids, presynaptic calcium channel agonists, are effective in treating neuropathic pain. Common side effects of these drugs are visual disturbances, drowsiness, and vertigo which at times cannot be tolerated. Gabapentin has not been effective in preventing acute pain [82], and evidence on chronic postthoracotomy pain is conflicting [83, 84]. Interestingly, pregabalin has been shown to be effective in acute pain, CPTP, and PTSP [85–88].

17.8.5 Other Agents

Postoperative intravenous infusion of selective alpha-2-adrenergic receptor agonist dexmedetomidine has been shown to decrease opioid requirements [89, 90].

Conclusion

The effective treatment of postthoracotomy pain is one of the most important tools of thoracic anesthesia, playing an essential role in the outcome of thoracic surgery. However, neither has the exact pathogenesis been explained nor has the "best" analgesic method been defined. Proper patient preparation followed by comprehensive teamwork to apply the analgesic regimen, to monitor its effects, and to treat its side effects and complications should not be underestimated.

References

1. Belda J, Cavalcanti M, Ferrer M, Serra M, Puig de la Bellacasa J, Canalis E, Torres A (2005) Bronchial colonization and postoperative respiratory infections in patients undergoing lung cancer surgery. Chest 128:1571–1579
2. Harris DJ, Hilliard PE, Jewell ES, Brummett CM (2015) The association between incentive spirometry performance and pain in postoperative thoracic epidural analgesia. Reg Anesth Pain Med 40:232–238
3. Sentürk M, Ozcan PE, Talu GK, Kiyan E, Camci E, Ozyalçin S, Dilege S, Pembeci K (2002) The effects of three different analgesia techniques on long-term postthoracotomy pain. Anesth Analg 94:11–15
4. Classification of chronic pain. Descriptions of chronic pain syndromes and definitions of pain terms. Prepared by the International Association for the Study of Pain, Subcommittee on Taxonomy (1986) Pain Suppl 3:S1–226
5. Maxwell C, Nicoara A (2014) New developments in the treatment of acute pain after thoracic surgery. Curr Opin Anaesthesiol 27:6–11
6. De Cosmo G, Aceto P, Gualtieri E, Congedo E (2009) Analgesia in thoracic surgery: review. Minerva Anestesiol 75:393–400
7. Kolettas A, Lazaridis G, Baka S, Mpoukovinas I, Karavasilis V, Pitsiou G, Papaiwannou A, Lampaki S, Karavergou A, Machairiotis N, Katsikogiannis N, Mpakas A, Tsakiridis K, Fassiadis N, Zarogoulidis K, Zarogoulidis P (2015) Postoperative pain management. J Thorac Dis 7:62–72
8. Koehler RP, Keenan RJ (2006) Management of postthoracotomy pain: acute and chronic. Thorac Surg Clin 16:287–297
9. Bottiger BA, Esper SA, Stafford-Smith M (2014) Pain management strategies for thoracotomy and thoracic pain syndromes. Semin Cardiothorac Vasc Anesth 18:45–56
10. Doan LV, Augustus J, Androphy R, Schechter D, Gharibo C (2014) Mitigating the impact of acute and chronic post-thoracotomy pain. J Cardiothorac Vasc Anesth 28:1048–1056
11. Rodriguez-Aldrete D, Candiotti KA, Janakiraman R, Rodriguez-Blanco YF (2016) Trends and new evidence in the management of acute and chronic post-thoracotomy pain – an overview of the literature from 2005 to 2015. J Cardiothorac Vasc Anesth 30:762–772
12. Katz J, Jackson M, Kavanagh BP, Sandler AN (1996) Acute pain after thoracic surgery predicts long-term post-thoracotomy pain. Clin J Pain 12:50–55
13. Dürrleman N, Massard G (2006) Posterolateral thoracotomy. Multimed Man Cardiothorac Surg MMCTS/Eur Assoc Cardio-Thoracic Surg 2006:mmcts.2005.001453
14. Hazelrigg SR, Cetindag IB, Fullerton J (2002) Acute and chronic pain syndromes after thoracic surgery. Surg Clin North Am 82:849–865
15. Li S (2014) Analysis of 11 trials comparing muscle-sparing with posterolateral thoracotomy. Thorac Cardiovasc Surg 62:344–354
16. Elshiekh MAF, Lo TTH, Shipolini AR, Mccormack DJ (2013) Does muscle-sparing thoracotomy as opposed to posterolateral thoracotomy result in better recovery ? Interact Cardiovasc Thorac Surg 16:60–67

17. Hazelrigg SR, Landreneau RJ, Boley TM, Priesmeyer M, Schmaltz RA, Nawarawong W, Johnson JA, Walls JT, Curtis JJ (1991) The effect of muscle-sparing versus standard posterolateral thoracotomy on pulmonary function, muscle strength, and postoperative pain. J Thorac Cardiovasc Surg 101:394–400; discussion 400–1
18. Landreneau RJ, Mack MJ, Hazelrigg SR, Naunheim K, Dowling RD, Ritter P, Magee MJ, Nunchuck S, Keenan RJ, Ferson PF (1994) Prevalence of chronic pain after pulmonary resection by thoracotomy or video-assisted thoracic surgery. J Thorac Cardiovasc Surg 107:1079–1085; discussion 1085–6
19. Bertrand PC, Regnard JF, Spaggiari L, Levi JF, Magdeleinat P, Guibert L, Levasseur P (1996) Immediate and long-term results after surgical treatment of primary spontaneous pneumothorax by VATS. Ann Thorac Surg 61:1641–1645
20. Gottschalk A, Cohen SP, Yang S, Ochroch EA (2006) Preventing and treating pain after thoracic surgery. Anesthesiology 104:594–600
21. Sabanathan S, Eng J, Mearns AJ (1990) Alterations in respiratory mechanics following thoracotomy. J R Coll Surg Edinb 35:144–150
22. Van Mieghem W, Demedts M (1989) Cardiopulmonary function after lobectomy or pneumonectomy for pulmonary neoplasm. Respir Med 83:199–206
23. Hedenstierna G, Strandberg A, Brismar B, Lundquist H, Svensson L, Tokics L (1985) Functional residual capacity, thoracoabdominal dimensions, and central blood volume during general anesthesia with muscle paralysis and mechanical ventilation. Anesthesiology 62:247–254
24. Hatch D (1966) Ventilation and arterial oxygenation during thoracic surgery. Thorax 21: 310–314
25. Richardson J, Sabanathan S, Shah R (1999) Post-thoracotomy spirometric lung function: the effect of analgesia. A review. J Cardiovasc Surg (Torino) 40:445–456
26. Scawn ND, Pennefather SH, Soorae A, Wang JY, Russell GN (2001) Ipsilateral shoulder pain after thoracotomy with epidural analgesia: the influence of phrenic nerve infiltration with lidocaine. Anesth Analg 93:260–264
27. Møiniche S, Kehlet H, Dahl JB (2002) A qualitative and quantitative systematic review of preemptive analgesia for postoperative pain relief. Anesthesiology 96:725–741
28. Cerfolio RJ, Bryant AS, Bass CS, Bartolucci AA (2003) A prospective, double-blinded, randomized trial evaluating the use of preemptive analgesia of the skin before thoracotomy. Ann Thorac Surg 76:1055–1058
29. Katz J, Clarke H, Seltzer Z (2011) Preventive analgesia: quo vadimus? Anesth Analg 113:1242–1253
30. Bong CL, Samuel M, Ng JM, Ip-Yam C (2005) Effects of preemptive epidural analgesia on post-thoracotomy pain. J Cardiothorac Vasc Anesth 19:786–793
31. Joshi GP, Bonnet F, Shah R, Wilkinson RC, Camu F, Fischer B, Neugebauer EAM, Rawal N, Schug SA, Simanski C, Kehlet H (2008) A systematic review of randomized trials evaluating regional techniques for postthoracotomy analgesia. Anesth Analg 107:1026–1040
32. Procedure specific postoperative pain management. http://www.postoppain.org
33. Ali M, Winter DC, Hanly AM, O'Hagan C, Keaveny J, Broe P (2010) Prospective, randomized, controlled trial of thoracic epidural or patient-controlled opiate analgesia on perioperative quality of life. Br J Anaesth 104:292–297
34. Bauer C, Hentz J-G, Ducrocq X, Meyer N, Nicolas M, Oswald-Mammosser M, Steib A, Dupeyron J-P (2007) Lung function after lobectomy: a randomized, double-blinded trial comparing thoracic epidural ropivacaine/sufentanil and intravenous morphine for patient-controlled analgesia. Anesth Analg 105:238–244
35. Ballantyne JC, Carr DB, DeFerranti S, Suarez T, Lau J, Chalmers TC, Angelillo IF, Mosteller F (1998) The comparative effects of postoperative analgesic therapies on pulmonary outcome: cumulative meta-analyses of randomized, controlled trials. Anesth Analg 86:598–612
36. Pöpping DM, Elia N, Marret E, Remy C, Tramèr MR (2008) Protective effects of epidural analgesia on pulmonary complications after abdominal and thoracic surgery: a meta-analysis. Arch Surg 143:990–999; discussion 1000

37. Freise H, Van Aken HK (2011) Risks and benefits of thoracic epidural anaesthesia. Br J Anaesth 107:859–868
38. Oka T, Ozawa Y, Ohkubo Y (2001) Thoracic epidural bupivacaine attenuates supraventricular tachyarrhythmias after pulmonary resection. Anesth Analg 93:253–259, 1st contents page
39. Ng A, Swanevelder J (2007) Pain relief after thoracotomy: is epidural analgesia the optimal technique? Br J Anaesth 98:159–162
40. Drasner K (2004) Thoracic epidural anesthesia: asleep at the wheal? Anesth Analg 99:578–579
41. Manion SC, Brennan TJ (2011) Thoracic epidural analgesia and acute pain management. Anesthesiology 115:181–188
42. Visser WA, Lee RA, Gielen MJM (2008) Factors affecting the distribution of neural blockade by local anesthetics in epidural anesthesia and a comparison of lumbar versus thoracic epidural anesthesia. Anesth Analg 107:708–721
43. Sagiroglu G, Meydan B, Copuroglu E, Baysal A, Yoruk Y, Altemur Karamustafaoglu Y, Huseyin S (2014) A comparison of thoracic or lumbar patient-controlled epidural analgesia methods after thoracic surgery. World J Surg Oncol 12:96
44. Engquist A, Brandt MR, Fernandes A, Kehlet H (1977) The blocking effect of epidural analgesia on the adrenocortical and hyperglycemic responses to surgery. Acta Anaesthesiol Scand 21:330–335
45. Bouchard F, Drolet P (1995) Thoracic versus lumbar administration of fentanyl using patient-controlled epidural after thoracotomy. Reg Anesth 20:385–388
46. Grant GJ, Zakowski M, Ramanathan S, Boyd A, Turndorf H (1993) Thoracic versus lumbar administration of epidural morphine for postoperative analgesia after thoracotomy. Reg Anesth 18:351–355
47. Liu N, Kuhlman G, Dalibon N, Moutafis M, Levron JC, Fischler M (2001) A randomized, double-blinded comparison of intrathecal morphine, sufentanil and their combination versus IV morphine patient-controlled analgesia for postthoracotomy pain. Anesth Analg 92:31–36
48. Senturk M (2005) Acute and chronic pain after thoracotomies. Curr Opin Anaesthesiol 18:1–4
49. Hansdottir V, Woestenborghs R, Nordberg G (1995) The cerebrospinal fluid and plasma pharmacokinetics of sufentanil after thoracic or lumbar epidural administration. Anesth Analg 80:724–729
50. Dernedde M, Stadler M, Bardiau F, Seidel L, Boogaerts JG (2006) Low vs. high concentration of levobupivacaine for post-operative epidural analgesia: Influence of mode of delivery. Acta Anaesthesiol Scand 50:613–621
51. Tan CNH, Guha A, Scawn NDA, Pennefather SH, Russell GN (2004) Optimal concentration of epidural fentanyl in bupivacaine 0.1% after thoracotomy. Br J Anaesth 92:670–674
52. Ozcan PE, Sentürk M, Sungur Ulke Z, Toker A, Dilege S, Ozden E, Camci E (2007) Effects of thoracic epidural anaesthesia on pulmonary venous admixture and oxygenation during one-lung ventilation. Acta Anaesthesiol Scand 51:1117–1122
53. Bilir A, Gulec S, Erkan A, Ozcelik A (2007) Epidural magnesium reduces postoperative analgesic requirement. Br J Anaesth 98:519–523
54. Ozyalcin NS, Yucel A, Camlica H, Dereli N, Andersen OK, Arendt-Nielsen L (2004) Effect of pre-emptive ketamine on sensory changes and postoperative pain after thoracotomy: comparison of epidural and intramuscular routes. Br J Anaesth 93:356–361
55. Matot I, Drenger B, Weissman C, Shauli A, Gozal Y (2004) Epidural clonidine, bupivacaine and methadone as the sole analgesic agent after thoracotomy for lung resection. Anaesthesia 59:861–866
56. Zeng XZ, Xu YM, Cui XG, Guo YP, Li WZ (2014) Low-dose epidural dexmedetomidine improves thoracic epidural anaesthesia for nephrectomy. Anaesth Intensive Care 42:185–190
57. Chia Y-Y, Chang T-H, Liu K, Chang H-C, Ko N-H, Wang Y-M (2006) The efficacy of thoracic epidural neostigmine infusion after thoracotomy. Anesth Analg 102:201–208
58. Rawal N (2015) Current issues in postoperative pain management. Eur J Anaesthesiol 33:160–171

59. Romero A, Garcia JEL, Joshi GP (2013) The state of the art in preventing postthoracotomy pain. Semin Thorac Cardiovasc Surg 25:116–124
60. Yeung JHY, Gates S, Naidu B V, Wilson MJA, Gao Smith F (2016) Paravertebral block versus thoracic epidural for patients undergoing thoracotomy. Cochrane Database Syst Rev (2):CD009121
61. Kotzé A, Scally A, Howell S (2009) Efficacy and safety of different techniques of paravertebral block for analgesia after thoracotomy: a systematic review and metaregression. Br J Anaesth 103:626–636
62. Fagenholz PJ, Bowler GMR, Carnochan FM, Walker WS (2012) Systemic local anaesthetic toxicity from continuous thoracic paravertebral block. Br J Anaesth 109:260–262
63. Tighe S (2013) The safety of paravertebral nerve block. Anaesthesia 68:783
64. Luyet C, Siegenthaler A, Szucs-Farkas Z, Hummel G, Eichenberger U, Vogt A (2012) The location of paravertebral catheters placed using the landmark technique. Anaesthesia 67:1321–1326
65. Krediet AC, Moayeri N, van Geffen G-J, Bruhn J, Renes S, Bigeleisen PE, Groen GJ (2015) Different approaches to ultrasound-guided thoracic paravertebral block: an illustrated review. Anesthesiology 123:459–474
66. Pace MM, Sharma B, Anderson-Dam J, Fleischmann K, Warren L, Stefanovich P (2016) Ultrasound-guided thoracic paravertebral blockade: a retrospective study of the incidence of complications. Anesth Analg 122:1186–1191
67. Marhofer D, Marhofer P, Kettner SC, Fleischmann E, Prayer D, Schernthaner M, Lackner E, Willschke H, Schwetz P, Zeitlinger M (2013) Magnetic resonance imaging analysis of the spread of local anesthetic solution after ultrasound-guided lateral thoracic paravertebral blockade: a volunteer study. Anesthesiology 118:1106–1112
68. Meierhenrich R, Hock D, Kühn S, Baltes E, Muehling B, Muche R, Georgieff M, Gorsewski G (2011) Analgesia and pulmonary function after lung surgery: is a single intercostal nerve block plus patient-controlled intravenous morphine as effective as patient-controlled epidural anaesthesia? A randomized non-inferiority clinical trial. Br J Anaesth 106:580–589
69. Khalil KG, Boutrous ML, Irani AD, Miller CC, Pawelek TR, Estrera AL, Safi HJ (2015) Operative intercostal nerve blocks with long-acting bupivacaine liposome for pain control after thoracotomy. Ann Thorac Surg 100:2013–2018
70. Gebhardt R, Mehran RJ, Soliz J, Cata JP, Smallwood AK, Feeley TW (2013) Epidural versus ON-Q local anesthetic-infiltrating catheter for post-thoracotomy pain control. J Cardiothorac Vasc Anesth 27:423–426
71. Fortier S, Hanna HA, Bernard A, Girard C (2012) Comparison between systemic analgesia, continuous wound catheter analgesia and continuous thoracic paravertebral block: a randomised, controlled trial of postthoracotomy pain management. Eur J Anaesthesiol 29: 524–530
72. Fiorelli A, Izzo AC, Frongillo EM, Del Prete A, Liguori G, Di Costanzo E, Vicidomini G, Santini M (2016) Efficacy of wound analgesia for controlling post-thoracotomy pain: a randomized double-blind study†. Eur J Cardiothorac Surg 49:339–347
73. Ju H, Feng Y, Yang B-X, Wang J (2008) Comparison of epidural analgesia and intercostal nerve cryoanalgesia for post-thoracotomy pain control. Eur J Pain 12:378–384
74. Sbruzzi G, Silveira SA, Silva DV, Coronel CC, Plentz RDM (2012) Transcutaneous electrical nerve stimulation after thoracic surgery: systematic review and meta-analysis of 11 randomized trials. Rev Bras Cir Cardiovasc órgão Of da Soc Bras Cir Cardiovasc 27:75–87
75. Mac TB, Girard F, Chouinard P, Boudreault D, Lafontaine ER, Ruel M, Ferraro P (2005) Acetaminophen decreases early post-thoracotomy ipsilateral shoulder pain in patients with thoracic epidural analgesia: a double-blind placebo-controlled study. J Cardiothorac Vasc Anesth 19:475–478
76. Singh H, Bossard RF, White PF, Yeatts RW (1997) Effects of ketorolac versus bupivacaine coadministration during patient-controlled hydromorphone epidural analgesia after thoracotomy procedures. Anesth Analg 84:564–569

77. Senard M, Deflandre EP, Ledoux D, Roediger L, Hubert BM, Radermecker M, Libbrecht D, Joris JL (2010) Effect of celecoxib combined with thoracic epidural analgesia on pain after thoracotomy. Br J Anaesth 105:196–200
78. Argiriadou H, Papagiannopoulou P, Foroulis CN, Anastasiadis K, Thomaidou E, Papakonstantinou C, Himmelseher S (2011) Intraoperative infusion of S(+)-ketamine enhances post-thoracotomy pain control compared with perioperative parecoxib when used in conjunction with thoracic paravertebral ropivacaine infusion. J Cardiothorac Vasc Anesth 25: 455–461
79. Esme H, Kesli R, Apiliogullari B, Duran FM, Yoldas B (2011) Effects of flurbiprofen on CRP, TNF-α, IL-6, and postoperative pain of thoracotomy. Int J Med Sci 8:216–221
80. Nesher N, Ekstein MP, Paz Y, Marouani N, Chazan S, Weinbroum AA (2009) Morphine with adjuvant ketamine vs higher dose of morphine alone for immediate postthoracotomy analgesia. Chest 136:245–252
81. Joseph C, Gaillat F, Duponq R, Lieven R, Baumstarck K, Thomas P, Penot-Ragon C, Kerbaul F (2012) Is there any benefit to adding intravenous ketamine to patient-controlled epidural analgesia after thoracic surgery? A randomized double-blind study. Eur J Cardiothorac Surg 42:e58–e65
82. Zakkar M, Frazer S, Hunt I (2013) Is there a role for gabapentin in preventing or treating pain following thoracic surgery? Interact Cardiovasc Thorac Surg 17:716–719
83. Solak O, Metin M, Esme H, Solak O, Yaman M, Pekcolaklar A, Gurses A, Kavuncu V (2007) Effectiveness of gabapentin in the treatment of chronic post-thoracotomy pain. Eur J Cardiothorac Surg 32:9–12
84. Grosen K, Drewes AM, Højsgaard A, Pfeiffer-Jensen M, Hjortdal VE, Pilegaard HK (2014) Perioperative gabapentin for the prevention of persistent pain after thoracotomy: a randomized controlled trial. Eur J Cardiothorac Surg 46:76–85
85. Yoshimura N, Iida H, Takenaka M, Tanabe K, Yamaguchi S, Kitoh K, Shirahashi K, Iwata H (2015) Effect of postoperative administration of pregabalin for post-thoracotomy pain: a randomized study. J Cardiothorac Vasc Anesth 29:1567–1572
86. Matsutani N, Dejima H, Takahashi Y, Kawamura M (2015) Pregabalin reduces post-surgical pain after thoracotomy: a prospective, randomized, controlled trial. Surg Today 45: 1411–1416
87. Imai Y, Imai K, Kimura T, Horiguchi T, Goyagi T, Saito H, Sato Y, Motoyama S, Nishikawa T, Minamiya Y (2015) Evaluation of postoperative pregabalin for attenuation of postoperative shoulder pain after thoracotomy in patients with lung cancer, a preliminary result. Gen Thorac Cardiovasc Surg 63:99–104
88. Mishra A, Nar AS, Bawa A, Kaur G, Bawa S, Mishra S (2013) Pregabalin in chronic post-thoracotomy pain. J Clin Diagn Res 7:1659–1661
89. Wahlander S, Frumento RJ, Wagener G, Saldana-Ferretti B, Joshi RR, Playford HR, Sladen RN (2005) A prospective, double-blind, randomized, placebo-controlled study of dexmedetomidine as an adjunct to epidural analgesia after thoracic surgery. J Cardiothorac Vasc Anesth 19:630–635
90. Ramsay MAE, Newman KB, Leeper B, Hamman BL, Hebeler RF, Henry AC, Kourlis H, Wood RE, Stecher JA, Hein HAT (2014) Dexmedetomidine infusion for analgesia up to 48 hours after lung surgery performed by lateral thoracotomy. Proc (Bayl Univ Med Cent) 27:3–10

Rehabilitation for Thoracic Surgical Patients: Why, When, and How

18

Grégoire Blaudszun, Frédéric Triponez, Pierre-Olivier Bridevaux, and Marc Joseph Licker

18.1 Physical Fitness: A Marker of Health

A wealth of studies has provided convincing evidence of the remarkable ability of aerobic fitness to assess general health status and to predict all-cause mortality in numerous adult populations. According to the World Health Organization (WHO), physical inactivity is highly prevalent in both Western and emerging countries (31 % in men and 34 % in women) and has become the fourth leading risk factor for global mortality – just behind hypertension, tobacco-related illnesses, and diabetes mellitus. Approximately 3.2 million deaths are attributable each year to poor physical activity (http://whqlibdoc.who.int/publications/2010/9789241599979_eng.pdf).

Likewise, assessing aerobic fitness is helpful in preoperative risk stratification as poor physical performance is considered a valuable predictor of mortality and morbidity as well as prolonged hospital stay following major surgical procedures.

Using self-report questionnaires such as the Duke Activity Status Index or simple motion detectors (accelerometer, pedometer), physical fitness can be qualitatively rated in metabolic equivalents of task (METs), one MET being equivalent to the amount of energy expanded or oxygen consumed (VO_2) at rest (0.8–1 kcal.kg-1.hour-1, resting VO_2 2.5–3.5 ml.kg-1.min-1). Physical fitness level is inversely related to mortality after adjustment for the presence of cardiopulmonary disease,

G. Blaudszun • M.J. Licker (✉)
Department of Anaesthesiology, Pharmacology, and Intensive Care,
Geneva University Hospitals, Geneva, Switzerland
e-mail: Marc-Joseph.Licker@hcuge.ch

F. Triponez
Service of Thoracic and Endocrine Surgery, Geneva University Hospitals,
Geneva, Switzerland

P.-O. Bridevaux
Division of Pulmonary Medicine, Geneva University Hospitals, Geneva, Switzerland

© Springer International Publishing Switzerland 2017

M. Şentürk, M.O. Sungur (eds.), *Postoperative Care in Thoracic Surgery*,
DOI 10.1007/978-3-319-19908-5_18

socioeconomic factors, and age, 1-year mortality increasing by 13 % for every 1 MET decrement in exercise capacity [1].

Aerobic physical fitness as assessed quantitatively by the maximal or peak oxygen consumption (VO_{2peak}, VO_{2max}) reflects the integrative functioning of the pulmonary and circulatory systems, blood oxygen-carrying content (hemoglobin), and skeletal muscle mechanical performances. Oxygen transport from the environment to the skeletal muscle mitochondria entails a series of convective and diffusive steps, the so-called oxygen cascade that represents key processes essential for oxidative metabolism implicated in cellular growth, internal enzymatic processes, and mechanical work (Fig. 18.1). As genetics accounts for only 20–30 % of VO_{2peak} values, morphometric characteristics, lifestyle, and concomitant diseases are the main contributory factors in human aerobic capacity. Compared with men, VO_{2peak} is approximately 15–25 % lower in women and decreases on average by 5–15 % per decade, the decline being sharper among sedentary persons and after the age of 60.

Considerable evidence suggests that exercise training programs may alleviate symptoms and improve long-term outcome in various diseases such as chronic obstructive pulmonary disease (COPD), diabetes, arterial hypertension, heart failure (HF), coronary artery disease, cancer, and neuropsychiatric disorders. Over the last 15 years, some clinicians have hypothesized that implementation of exercise training programs prior to and/or following surgery had the potential to "recondition" the patient by increasing aerobic fitness and thereby minimizing perioperative risk of major organ dysfunction while enhancing functional recovery soon after surgery.

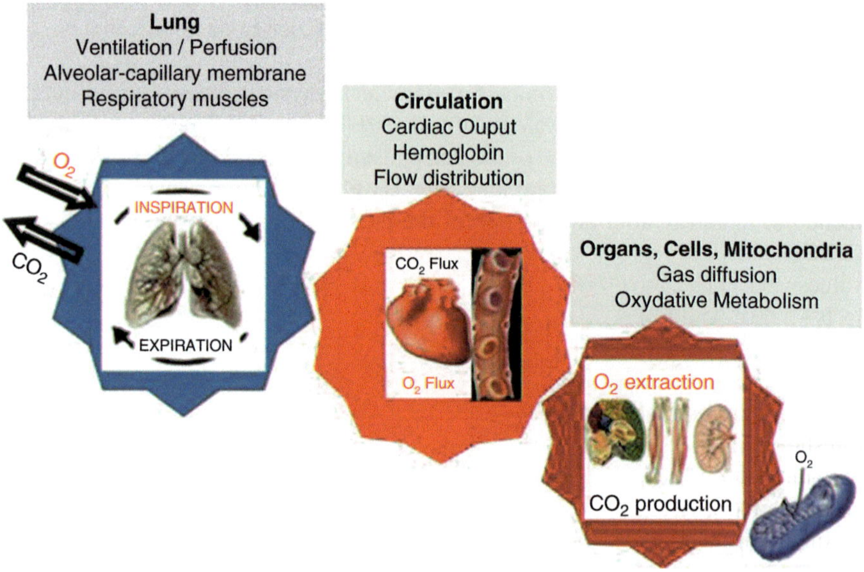

Fig. 18.1 Oxygen cascade

In this chapter, we will review the current knowledge regarding physiological impairment observed in thoracic surgical patients, the mechanisms underlying endurance and strength exercise-induced improvement in physical fitness, and the efficacy of exercise training program when prescribed prior to and/or after surgery.

18.2 Physical Fitness in Thoracic Surgical Candidates

18.2.1 Assessment of Fitness Before Surgery

Cardiopulmonary exercise testing (CPET) on a cycloergometer or a treadmill represents the gold standard to assess patient's physical fitness and the effectiveness of physical training interventions. Besides VO_{2peak} (highest value attained during CPET) and VO_{2max} (plateau level of VO_2 achieved beyond which no increase in effort can raise it further), other parameters such as peak workload or peak power (Wmax), peak heart rate (peakHR), O_2 pulse (VO_2/HR), ventilator equivalent for CO_2 (ratio of minute ventilation to the production of carbon dioxide, VE/VCO_2), anaerobic threshold (AT), and respiratory gas exchange ratio (VCO_2/VO_2) all characterize the patient's aerobic capacity. Overall, the predicted VO_{2max} of any individual takes into account age, gender, height, and lean body mass. Alternate testing modalities have also been developed and validated to provide physiological surrogates of patient's physical fitness as derived from stair climbing (speed of ascent, number of stairs) and the shuttle test or the 6-min walk test (6MWT, distance) (Table 18.1). In elderly and "frail" patients, simple tests of active mobilization such as the gait speed test (time needed to walk 5 m), maximal handgrip strength test (dynamometer), recording of all movement throughout the day (pedometer, accelerometer), the mini-mental test, and subjective performance scoring status (e.g., Karnofsky Performance Status) all complement valuable information on patient physical autonomy and bear important prognostic significance.

Guidelines issued from the American College of Chest Physicians (ACCP), from the British Thoracic Society (BTS), and jointly from the European Society of Thoracic Surgeons and the European Respiratory Society (ESTS/ERS) all recommend performing CPET whenever the diffusion capacity for carbon monoxide (DLCO) and/or forced expiratory volume in 1 s (FEV1) are below 80 % of predicted values [2–4]. The scientific rationale to perform CPET is to identify "unfit" subjects – those with low VO_{2peak} – who might not be able to sustain the postoperative physiological impairments and the increased metabolic burden consequent to the surgical-induced neuroendocrine and inflammatory responses. Cutoff values of 15–16 ml.kg-1.min-1 VO_{2max} (four METs) and 10–12 ml.kg-1.min-1 anaerobic threshold (three METs) have been shown to be helpful in discriminating patients at low–moderate risk and those at high (or very high) risk of major postoperative complications.

Importantly, patients with lung cancer awaiting surgery and particularly those receiving chemotherapeutic agents present VO_{2max} on average 25–30 % lower than age- and gender-matched individuals (sedentary, active, or trained) (Fig. 18.2).

Table 18.1 Cardiorespiratory fitness testing modalities

	Cardiopulmonary exercise testing CPET	Stair climbing or other physical stress tests	Shuttle or 6-min walk test	Age-predicted HR test
	Maximal		Submaximal	
Principle	Direct measurements of VO_2, VCO_2, HR, BP, and airflow	Estimated VO_2max from highest workload, HR achieved	Distance (m)	Workload achieved at 70–85 % $_{Pred}$HR
Equipment	Cycle ergometer/ treadmill Expired–inspired gas HR (SpO_2, BP)	Stair climbing[a] (6 floors) or cycle ergometer/treadmill (SpO_2,BP, ECG)	30-m corridor monitor HR, SpO_2, stop watch	Cycle ergometer/ treadmill monitor HR, SpO_2, BP (ECG), stop watch
Duration	8–12 min	5–20 min	4–6 min	*5–20 min*
Operative risk				
Low	$VO_{2\ max}$ > 20 ml/kg/min	>22 m altitude or 6 floors or 15 m/min	>600 m	
Moderate	$VO_{2\ max}$ 15–20 ml/kg/min	8–20 m alt. or 3–5 floors		
High	$VO_{2\ max}$ 10–15 ml/kg/min	3–7 m alt. or 1–2 floors	400 m	
Very High	$VO_{2\ max}$< 10 ml/kg/min	<2.4 m alt. or 1 floor		

BP blood pressure, *ECG* electrocardiogram, *HR* heart rate, *SpO2* pulsed oxygen saturation, *VO2max* maximal oxygen consumption
[a]Stair climbing test assumes reasonable speed of ascent

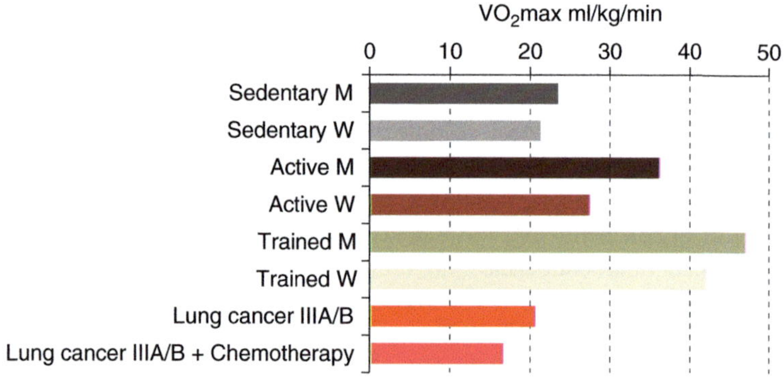

Fig. 18.2 Aerobic capacity assessed in healthy men and women (sedentary, active, and trained) and in patients with lung cancer receiving or not neoadjuvant chemotherapy

18.2.2 Causes of Poor Physical Fitness

Among thoracic surgical patients, the loss of muscular mass and aerobic physical fitness is often multifactorial as a result of aging, physical inactivity, tobacco-related illnesses, tumor burden, and chemotherapy, with no single organ or step of the oxygen cascade being identified as solely responsible.

Based on CPET, poor aerobic physical fitness is primarily linked to respiratory limitations (ventilator and gas exchange capacity), cardiovascular limitations (cardiac and vascular components, hemoglobin level), skeletal muscle limitations (muscular deconditioning, joint disorders, or neurological deficits), or a combination of these factors. The age-related decline in VO_{2max} is largely attributed to impaired peripheral oxygen utilization coupled to the loss of lean body mass and decreased HR reserve (downregulation of β-adrenergic receptor and cardiac autonomic imbalance) that limits the exercise-induced increase in cardiac output. Likewise, a sedentary lifestyle, malnutrition, and prolonged immobilization have all been associated with low VO_{2max} owing to lower heart rate response, loss of skeletal muscle mass, and impaired mitochondrial oxidative capacity.

18.2.3 Stress- and Inactivity-Induced Muscle Wasting

After surgery, afferent nerve signals from the injured tissues and pro-inflammatory cytokines released from activated leukocytes, fibroblasts, and endothelial cells all activate the sympathetic nervous system and the hypothalamic–pituitary axis. This so-called surgical stress-induced neuroendocrine and inflammatory response is proportional to the extent of tissue trauma. Concomitant to the peak release of inflammatory mediators and counter-regulatory hormones (cortisol, catecholamines, and glucagon), basal VO_2 and VCO_2 have been shown to increase by 10–25 % within the first 2 days after thoracic surgery, peaking at 30–45 % in patients with pneumonia [5, 6]. This hypermetabolic state reflects increased synthesis of acute phase proteins in the liver and enhanced tissue repair activity involving leukocytes, fibroblasts, and mesenchymal cells. The high levels of counter-regulatory hormones lead to a decrease in glucose cellular uptake/utilization (insulin resistance) and promote the breakdown of skeletal and visceral proteins into amino acids, as well as degradation of fat into glycerol and free fatty acids. Both amino acids and glycerol serve as substrates for hepatic neoglucogenesis and protein synthesis, while energy needs are predominantly met by free fatty acids in most tissues, except a few obligate glucose users (e.g., leukocytes, red blood cells, neurons).

Following major surgery, urinary nitrogen excretion increases to 40–100 g per day reflecting early muscle wasting (loss of 2–4 kg skeletal muscles) that takes several weeks for complete recovery [7]. The ensuing muscle weakness and fatigability when completing minor tasks impede early mobilization and return to functional autonomy. Frail subjects with sarcopenia and altered capacity to utilize nutrients are prone to experience postoperative multiorgan dysfunction resulting in admission to intensive care units (ICU), prolonged hospital stay, and discharge in institutional care facilities.

Besides the neuroendocrine and inflammatory components, physical inactivity associated with the intraoperative and postoperative period causes maladaptive changes in organ components of oxygen transport. Muscular disuse associated with short immobilization periods (5–10 days) has been shown to result in loss of muscle mass and strength due to an accelerated protein breakdown and in lower VO_{2max} (−10–20 %) owing to reduced cardiac output and reduced red blood cell mass [8]. Interestingly, among all skeletal muscles, the diaphragm is most prone to inactivity-induced proteolysis leading to the so-called ventilation-induced diaphragmatic dysfunction. Unlike nonrespiratory muscles in the limbs or thoracoabdominal wall, the functioning and morphology of the diaphragm have been shown to be sensitive to ventilation-induced muscle loading conditions. In brain-dead patients, Levine et al. reported severe diaphragm muscle fiber atrophy after 18–69 h of mechanical ventilation, whereas pectoralis muscle fibers were entirely preserved [9]. An average 30% loss of the force-generating capacity of the diaphragm has been observed following thoracic surgery with short mechanical ventilation periods (less than 2 h), whereas the contractile performance of latissimus dorsi muscle was preserved [10].

18.3 Exercise-Induced Muscular and Cardiopulmonary Function

Compared with pharmacological interventions, exercise training is currently recognized as one of the most efficient interventions to improve physical and psychological health in patients with cardiovascular, pulmonary, and rheumatic diseases as well as with cancer, obesity, or mental disorders.

18.3.1 Type of Exercise

Physical training programs encompass resistance or strength-type exercises and endurance or aerobic-type exercises. Increasing muscular mass is usually achieved by "resistive work" or static (isometric) contraction without any change in muscle length. In contrast, dynamic (isotonic) muscle actions entail concentric and eccentric contractions leading to muscle shortening and lengthening, respectively.

18.3.2 Mechanism of Exercise-Induced Improvement in Physical Fitness (Fig. 18.3)

In "frail" sarcopenic subjects, resistance exercises (isometric contractions) are particularly effective in (re)building up muscle mass (hypertrophic changes dominates hyperplasia) with significant improvement in strength and joint mobility. In

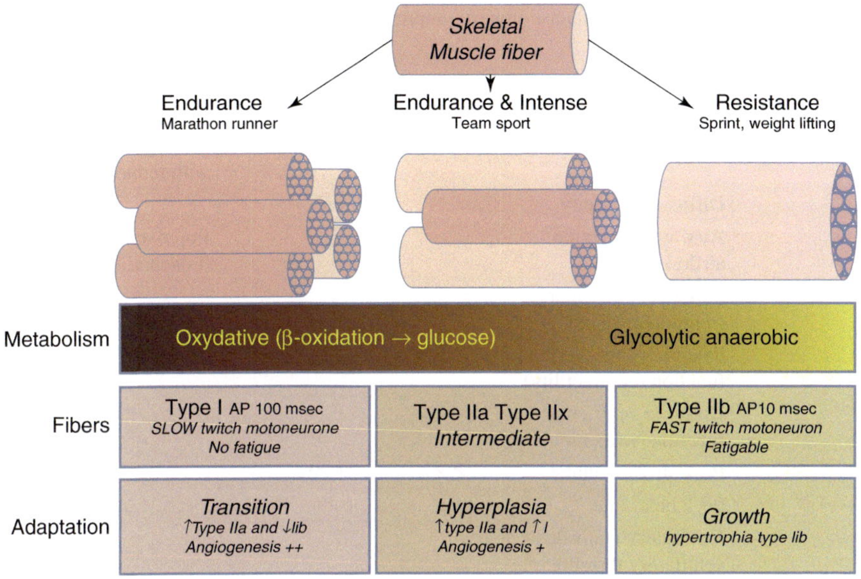

Fig. 18.3 Mechanisms of exercise-induced changes in muscle fiber phenotype

contrast, aerobic exercises lead to a minor increase in muscle mass/strength, but their beneficial health benefits are attributed to attenuation of systemic inflammation, enhanced angiogenesis, and phenotypical changes of cardiac and skeletal myocytes from type IIb into type IIa fibers with increased oxidative capacity (Fig. 18.3). The mechanisms underlying the aerobic exercise-induced increase in VO_{2max} are multifactorial involving partial reversal of endothelial dysfunction and adrenergic receptor responsiveness, higher capillary density, restoration of insulin sensitivity, and enhanced mitochondrial performances owing to tighter coupling between beta-oxidation and the tricarboxylic acid cycle. The enhanced cardiac output and facilitated tissue oxygen diffusion coupled with greater extraction of oxygen by the working muscle all contribute to increase in aerobic capacity after short training periods (Table 18.2).

18.3.2.1 Experimental Data

In several animal models, repeated bouts of intense muscular activity (equivalent to high-intensity interval training [HIIT]) to achieve 80–90 % HRmax or VO_{2max} have demonstrated cardioprotective effects quite similar to ischemic preconditioning. Protective cellular processes in the heart are mediated by sarcolemmal and mitochondrial ATP-sensitive potassium channels, generation of antioxidant molecules (superoxide dismutase, catalase), overexpression of heat shock protein (HSP70, HSP27), and upregulation of autophagic responses (Fig. 18.4). Exercise-induced cardiac mitochondrial adaptations have been shown to result in decreased reactive oxygen species production, increasing the heart's ability to tolerate high calcium levels and to sustain subsequent acute ischemic events.

Table 18.2 Mechanisms of exercise-induced improvement in oxygen transport components

Oxygen transport component		Long term (≥4 weeks)	Short term (<4 weeks)	Comment
Pulmonary	Respiratory muscles (breathing exercise)	=	=	Respiratory muscle training is associated with reduced dyspnea
	Diffusion capacity	=	=	
	Airway obstruction, airflow trapping	=	=	Improved by bronchodilators
	Pulmonary vascular (remodeling)	=	=	
Cardiac	Systolic ventricular function (contractility)	↗or =	?	
	Diastolic ventricular function (relaxation)	↗or =	?	
	Peak stroke volume	↗↗	(↗)	
	Peak heart rate	↗↗	↗	
	Ventilatory equivalents at ventilatory threshold	↙	?	
	Cardiac Output	↗↗↗ (♂>♀)	↗ (♂>♀)	
	Tolerance to myocardial ischemia	↗	↗	
Vascular	Endothelial function (NO release)	↗	↗	
	Arterial stiffness	↙	?	
	Anti-inflammatory expression	↗	?	
Blood	Hemoglobin concentration	↗	=	
All	Ventilatory (anaerobic) threshold	↗	?	
Skeletal muscle	Arteriovenous oxygen difference	= elderly ♂ ↗elderly ♀		
	Capillary density	↗	?	
	Enzymes for oxidative phosphorylation	↗↗	↗	
	Mitochondrial density	↗↗	↗	
	Myoglobin concentration	↗	?	
	Fiber transition to fatigue resistant phenotype (type I to type IIA)	Yes	?	
	Muscle mass	↗	(↗)	

↗ enhancement, ↙ decrement, = no change

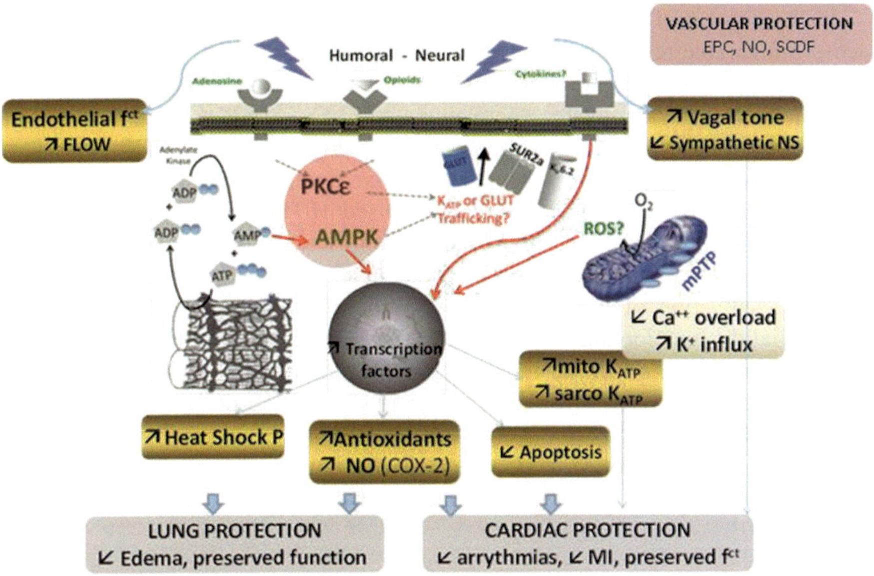

Fig. 18.4 Organ-protective mechanisms induced by aerobic high-intensity training. *EPC* endothelial progenitor cells; *NO* nitric oxide; *SCDF* stromal cell-derived factor; *COX-2* cyclooxygenase type 2; *PKC* protein kinase C; *AMPK* adenosine monophosphate kinase; *ROS* reactive oxygen species; *AMP*, *ADP*, and *ATP* adenosine mono-, di-, and triphosphate; *mPTP* mitochondrial permeability transition pore; *mito* and *sarco KATP* mitochondrial and sarcolemmal potassium ATP channel

Regarding the risk of ventilation-induced diaphragmatic dysfunction, Smuder et al. elegantly demonstrated that endurance training (10 days, 60-min treadmill at 70 % VO_{2max}) increased both antioxidant and HSP72 capacity while minimizing oxidative damage, protease activation, diaphragm myofiber atrophy, and contractile dysfunction induced by 12-h mechanical ventilation [11]. Similar short-lasting training programs in rats (running in a wheel) have been shown to protect against lung ischemia–reperfusion injuries and preserve alveolar–capillary permeability by limiting pro-inflammatory mediators (TNF-alpha and IL-1) and oxidative stress (superoxide dismutase activity) [12].

18.3.2.2 Clinical Data

Even short-term aerobic or endurance exercise programs (1–3 weeks) have been shown to improve physical fitness reflected by increases in VO_{2max}, maximal workload, ventilatory aerobic threshold, anaerobic threshold coupled with faster heart rate recovery (expressing sympatho-vagal balance), and lesser fatigue. Perceived dyspnea is often alleviated although airflow limitation and diffusion capacity remain unchanged. The increased VO_{2max} is mainly related to increase in peak stroke volume and peak HR in elderly man, whereas widening in peak arteriovenous oxygen difference predominates in elderly woman, suggesting gender differences in cardiovascular and skeletal muscle responses to exercise training.

In the context of surgery, physical training modalities need to be tailored to achieve favorable results within a short time frame (2–4 weeks). Compared with continuous low-intensity training, 8 weeks of HIIT in sedentary individuals have been shown to provide greater improvements in VO_{2max} (+22 % vs 15 %) and left ventricular mass (6 % vs 1 %) with faster post-exercise recovery of HR consistent with enhanced vagal neural tone [13]. Similar findings have been reported in patients with CHF after 4 weeks of supervised HIIT (average 7 h/week): the increased VO_{2max} (+26 %) and improved left ventricular function were associated with a reduced expression of MuRF-1 levels in skeletal muscles, reflecting lower catabolic activation of the ubiquitin–proteasome system [14, 15]. Reversal of endothelial dysfunction and improvement of oxygen delivery in the skeletal muscles have been related to the mobilization of bone marrow-derived endothelial progenitor cells (EPCs), nitric oxide (NO), and stromal cell-derived factor (SCDF) following short training period among healthy sedentary subjects, in frail elderly, and in patients with cardiovascular diseases [16]. This angiogenic response can be further amplified by performing intermittent physical training in a hypoxic environment [17].

18.4 Exercise Training in Patients Undergoing Thoracic Surgery: Prohabilitation and Rehabilitation

Currently, only 10–20 % of patients diagnosed with lung cancer are eligible for curative surgical resection. Reasons to dismiss surgical treatment are not only related to advanced disease stage (TNM stage IIIB, IV) or histological type (small cell carcinoma) but also to comorbidities and poor functional capacity that are amenable to appropriate therapeutic strategies. According to the ESTS/ERS guidelines, patients with $VO_{2max} < 10$ ml/kg/ml are declared unfit for major surgical resection, and those with $VO_{2max} < 14–16$ ml/kg/min are considered at high risk of postoperative cardiopulmonary complications [2].

Physical interventions aimed at enhancing patient's functional capacity before surgery and to improve the tolerance to postoperative surgical stress have been lumped under the concept of "prohabilitation" in contrast to "rehabilitation" that is related to physical therapy prescribed after surgery to speed up functional recovery.

The preoperative period represents a window of "therapeutic opportunity"; patients are in better physical condition than in the early postoperative period and more receptive to adopt a "healthy behavior" (tobacco and alcohol cessation, enhanced mobilization, better diet). Whether patient's poor physical fitness is "intrinsic" or "reversible" by implementing structured exercise programs associated (or not) with nutritional and psychological support remains questionable.

A growing interest is now focusing on non-pharmacological interventions such as physical exercise, smoking cessation, nutritional supplementation, and psychological support aimed to optimize patient physiological condition before and/or shortly after thoracic, cardiac, orthopedic, and abdominal procedures. Since 2000, 13 meta-analyses and systematic reviews encompassing more than 50 studies have been published in the field of preoperative preparation, aerobic exercise training, and postoperative rehabilitation [18–30]. Short-term exercise training by improving aerobic fitness could potentially increase the number of candidates for curative therapy. The interval of time from diagnosis to curative cancer surgery should not exceed 4 weeks and would be sufficient to partly reverse the poor functional capacity by improving patient's physiological reserves.

In abdominal and cardiac surgery, a systematic review including 12 RCTs reported shorter length of hospital stay and fewer postoperative pulmonary complications among patients enrolled in various forms of preoperative exercise training programs [30]. A preoperative inspiratory muscle training program (incentive spirometry; education in active cycle of breathing and forced expiration techniques) was shown to prevent postoperative pneumonia and reduce length of hospital stay [31]. In contrast, another systematic review of 8 RCTs failed to demonstrate exercise-induced physiological and clinical benefits in patients undergoing cardiac, abdominal, or orthopedic surgery [22]. Failure to achieve favorable effects could be attributed to poor adhesion and low attendance to the program as well as performance of low-intensity aerobic exercise program. More recently, among patients scheduled for colorectal surgery, Gillis et al. demonstrated the superiority of a tri-modal reconditioning program (exercise, diet, and anti-stress therapy) conducted preoperatively instead of postoperatively, as evidenced by better recovery of walking capacity 8 weeks after surgery; however, the length of hospital stay and the incidence of perioperative complications were similar regardless of the timing of the optimization strategy [32].

Regarding thoracic surgery, a literature search from 1990 to 2015 yielded 14 cohort studies (N=365: 49 prohabilitation, 316 rehabilitation) [33–46] and 8 RCTs (N=381: 196 prohabilitation, 185 rehabilitation) [47–54] focusing on different exercise training protocols and reporting objective measures of physical fitness (walking capacity, $VO_{2max,\ peak}$ work rate), pulmonary function, blood gas exchange, and/or clinical outcome along with health-related quality of life parameters (HRQL).

Altogether, these studies support the safety and feasibility of implementing physical training programs within a limited time frame before surgery (11 days to 4 weeks) that can eventually be continued postoperatively. Minor adverse effects such as transient hypotension, low back pain, or exacerbation of shoulder arthritis have been reported anecdotally. The variable eligibility rate (from 20 to 85 %) mainly depended on the existing physiological status and the inclusion/exclusion criteria, some investigators excluding patients with cardiovascular diseases, those with joint or neurological disabilities, and those with neuropsychological disorders. Among patients enrolled in the training program, the completion/retention rate was fair (60–100 %) along with variable attendance to most planned sessions (from 40 to 125 %), except in patients treated with adjuvant chemotherapy (43 % attendance).

Six of eight RCTs reported some improvement in at least one surrogate marker of physical fitness after prohabilitation intervention. In four of six studies using CPET, mean VO_{2max} or mean VO_{2peak} improved by 1.7–6.3 ml/kg/min (approximately +10–20 % of predicted $VO_{2max/peak}$) along with significant increase in peak workload (+25–35 % power). Consistent with these findings, nine of ten studies using the 6MWT reported a significant increase in walking distance (+28 m to 377 m) and reduced fatigability after prohabilitation. Unchanged walking distance at the 6MWT (one study) could be explained by therapy focusing only on muscle strength training. Regarding health quality of life (QOL), few favorable outcomes were observed that might be related to the possible ceiling effect or the use of non-validated questionnaires. Regarding clinical outcomes, despite consistent reports of improved exercise capacity, a lower rate of postoperative complications was observed in only one small RCT (N=24), and a shorter hospital stay was reported in 3 RCTs in the prohabilitation group compared with the control group.

Not surprisingly, insignificant changes in airflow limitation (forced vital capacity and forced FEV1) and in gas exchange (diffusion capacity to carbon monoxide [DLCO]) were reported after short-term prohabilitation intervention. In a small prospective study (N=22 COPD patients), Sekine et al. reported that intensive chest physiotherapy (incentive spirometry, breathing exercise) combined with walking (>5'000 steps/day), which started on average 2 weeks preoperatively and continued postoperatively, resulted in a lesser fall in FEV1, lesser requirement for oxygen therapy, and shorter length of hospital stay after lobectomy [44].

The rather low quality of these studies (selection biases, noncontrolled studies) and lack of relevant clinical endpoints (major postoperative complications) preclude any conclusions regarding the benefits of the physical interventions in the perioperative period.

The overall methodological quality was poor to moderate with an overall high to unclear risk of bias. Few RCTs have been conducted so far and include small numbers of patients. Hence, the generalizability of these preliminary positive findings is further limited due to considerable heterogeneity in therapeutic protocols and outcome measurement across studies, notwithstanding the exclusion of patients with significant comorbid diseases, a population that has the potential to benefit most from pre- and postoperative physical training.

Conclusion

The risk of developing major postoperative complications is partially related to "modifiable" factors, aerobic fitness, smoking habits, alcohol consumption, and poor nutrition. Low VO_{2max} or poor exercise tolerance has been identified as a strong predictor of perioperative complications and functional recovery. Besides lifestyle modifications and nutritional support, implementing pre- and postoperative muscle training is grounded on strong experimental data and should be considered to downgrade high-risk patient into a lower-risk profile.

In 2016, emerging data indicate that short-term physical training prescribed in patients awaiting lung cancer resection results in a consistent increase in aerobic capacity (average +10–20 % VO_{2max}, increase walking distance).

However, the current evidence for exercise-induced clinical improvement is skewed toward small RCTs or cohort studies with relatively fit patients, undergoing mostly generalized ("one size fits all") moderate-to-high-intensity exercise programs that are neither targeted to achieve significant improvement in aerobic fitness nor tailored to the patient's own abilities. Moreover, studies largely differ regarding type, dose, and timing of physical interventions.

Future research should identify which aspects of exercise training programs (strength, endurance, or functional mobility) are appropriate and tolerable for each individual and specific group of patients. Moreover, exercise training-related research should also incorporate monitoring principles to establish the optimum in training parameters. High-intensity training is likely necessary to achieve improvements given the often short time available before surgery. Fortunately, even frail and older patients can tolerate these specific programs.

References

1. Kokkinos P, Myers J, Kokkinos JP, Pittaras A, Narayan P, Manolis A, Karasik P, Greenberg M, Papademetriou V, Singh S (2008) Exercise capacity and mortality in black and white men. Circulation 117:614–622
2. Brunelli A, Charloux A, Bolliger CT, Rocco G, Sculier J-P, Varela G, Licker M, Ferguson MK, Faivre-Finn C, Huber RM, Clini EM, Win T, De Ruysscher D, Goldman L, European Respiratory Society, European Society of Thoracic Surgeons Joint Task Force on Fitness For Radical Therapy (2009) The European Respiratory Society and European Society of Thoracic Surgeons clinical guidelines for evaluating fitness for radical treatment (surgery and chemoradiotherapy) in patients with lung cancer. Eur J Cardiothorac Surg 36:181–184
3. Brunelli A, Kim AW, Berger KI, Addrizzo-Harris DJ (2013) Physiologic evaluation of the patient with lung cancer being considered for resectional surgery: diagnosis and management of lung cancer, 3rd ed: American College of Chest Physicians evidence-based clinical practice guidelines. Chest 143(5 Suppl):e166S–e190S
4. Lim E, Baldwin D, Beckles M, Duffy J, Entwisle J, Faivre-Finn C, Kerr K, Macfie A, McGuigan J, Padley S, Popat S, Screaton N, Snee M, Waller D, Warburton C, Win T, British Thoracic Society, Society for Cardiothoracic Surgery in Great Britain and Ireland (2010) Guidelines on the radical management of patients with lung cancer. Thorax 65(Suppl 3):iii1–iii27
5. Brandi LS, Bertolini R, Janni A, Gioia A, Angeletti CA (1996) Energy metabolism of thoracic surgical patients in the early postoperative period. Effect of posture. Chest 109:630–637
6. Saito H, Minamiya Y, Kawai H, Motoyama S, Katayose Y, Kimura K, Saito R, Ogawa J-I (2007) Estimation of pulmonary oxygen consumption in the early postoperative period after thoracic surgery. Anaesthesia 62:648–653
7. López Hellín J, Baena-Fustegueras JA, Sabín-Urkía P, Schwartz-Riera S, García-Arumí E (2008) Nutritional modulation of protein metabolism after gastrointestinal surgery. Eur J Clin Nutr 62:254–262
8. Convertino VA (1997) Cardiovascular consequences of bed rest: effect on maximal oxygen uptake. Med Sci Sports Exerc 29:191–196
9. Levine S, Nguyen T, Taylor N, Friscia ME, Budak MT, Rothenberg P, Zhu J, Sachdeva R, Sonnad S, Kaiser LR, Rubinstein NA, Powers SK, Shrager JB (2008) Rapid disuse atrophy of diaphragm fibers in mechanically ventilated humans. N Engl J Med 358:1327–1335
10. Welvaart WN, Paul MA, Stienen GJM, van Hees HWH, Loer SA, Bouwman R, Niessen H, de Man FS, Witt CC, Granzier H, Vonk-Noordegraaf A, Ottenheijm CAC (2011) Selective diaphragm muscle weakness after contractile inactivity during thoracic surgery. Ann Surg 254:1044–1049
11. Smuder AJ, Min K, Hudson MB, Kavazis AN, Kwon O-S, Nelson WB, Powers SK (2012) Endurance exercise attenuates ventilator-induced diaphragm dysfunction. J Appl Physiol 112:501–510

12. Mussi RK, Camargo EA, Ferreira T, De Moraes C, Delbin MA, Toro IFC, Brancher S, Landucci ECT, Zanesco A, Antunes E (2008) Exercise training reduces pulmonary ischaemia-reperfusion-induced inflammatory responses. Eur Respir J 31:645–649
13. Matsuo T, Saotome K, Seino S, Eto M, Shimojo N, Matsushita A, Iemitsu M, Ohshima H, Tanaka K, Mukai C (2014) Low-volume, high-intensity, aerobic interval exercise for sedentary adults: VO_2max, cardiac mass, and heart rate recovery. Eur J Appl Physiol 114:1963–1972
14. Gielen S, Sandri M, Kozarez I, Kratzsch J, Teupser D, Thiery J, Erbs S, Mangner N, Lenk K, Hambrecht R, Schuler G, Adams V (2012) Exercise training attenuates MuRF-1 expression in the skeletal muscle of patients with chronic heart failure independent of age: the randomized Leipzig Exercise Intervention in Chronic Heart Failure and Aging catabolism study. Circulation 125:2716–2727
15. Höllriegel R, Beck EB, Linke A, Adams V, Möbius-Winkler S, Mangner N, Sandri M, Gielen S, Gutberlet M, Hambrecht R, Schuler G, Erbs S (2013) Anabolic effects of exercise training in patients with advanced chronic heart failure (NYHA IIIb): impact on ubiquitin-protein ligases expression and skeletal muscle size. Int J Cardiol 167:975–980
16. Ross MD, Wekesa AL, Phelan JP, Harrison M (2014) Resistance exercise increases endothelial progenitor cells and angiogenic factors. Med Sci Sports Exerc 46:16–23
17. Wang J-S, Lee M-Y, Lien H-Y, Weng T-P (2014) Hypoxic exercise training improves cardiac/muscular hemodynamics and is associated with modulated circulating progenitor cells in sedentary men. Int J Cardiol 170:315–323
18. Debes C, Aissou M, Beaussier M (2014) [Prehabilitation. Preparing patients for surgery to improve functional recovery and reduce postoperative morbidity]. Ann Fr Anesth Rèanim 33:33–40
19. Egberts K, Brown WA, Brennan L, O'Brien PE (2012) Does exercise improve weight loss after bariatric surgery? a systematic review. Obes Surg 22:335–341
20. Gill SD, McBurney H (2013) Does exercise reduce pain and improve physical function before hip or knee replacement surgery? a systematic review and meta-analysis of randomized controlled trials. Arch Phys Med Rehabil 94:164–176
21. Hulzebos EHJ, Smit Y, Helders PPJM, van Meeteren NLU (2012) Preoperative physical therapy for elective cardiac surgery patients. Cochrane Database Syst Rev 11:CD010118
22. Lemanu DP, Singh PP, MacCormick AD, Arroll B, Hill AG (2013) Effect of preoperative exercise on cardiorespiratory function and recovery after surgery: a systematic review. World J Surg 37:711–720
23. Livhits M, Mercado C, Yermilov I, Parikh JA, Dutson E, Mehran A, Ko CY, Gibbons MM (2010) Exercise following bariatric surgery: systematic review. Obes Surg 20:657–665
24. Nagarajan K, Bennett A, Agostini P, Naidu B (2011) Is preoperative physiotherapy/pulmonary rehabilitation beneficial in lung resection patients? Interact Cardiovasc Thorac Surg 13:300–302
25. O'Doherty AF, West M, Jack S, Grocott MPW (2013) Preoperative aerobic exercise training in elective intra-cavity surgery: a systematic review. Br J Anaesth 110:679–689
26. Pouwels S, Stokmans RA, Willigendael EM, Nienhuijs SW, Rosman C, van Ramshorst B, Teijink JAW (2014) Preoperative exercise therapy for elective major abdominal surgery: a systematic review. Int J Surg 12:134–140
27. Singh F, Newton RU, Galvão DA, Spry N, Baker MK (2013) A systematic review of pre-surgical exercise intervention studies with cancer patients. Surg Oncol 22:92–104
28. Snowdon D, Haines TP, Skinner EH (2014) Preoperative intervention reduces postoperative pulmonary complications but not length of stay in cardiac surgical patients: a systematic review. J Physiother 60:66–77
29. Speck RM, Bond DS, Sarwer DB, Farrar JT (2014) A systematic review of musculoskeletal pain among bariatric surgery patients: implications for physical activity and exercise. Surg Obes Relat Dis 10:161–170
30. Valkenet K, van de Port IGL, Dronkers JJ, de Vries WR, Lindeman E, Backx FJG (2011) The effects of preoperative exercise therapy on postoperative outcome: a systematic review. Clin Rehabil 25:99–111

31. Hulzebos EHJ, Helders PJM, Favié NJ, De Bie RA, Brutel de la Riviere A, Van Meeteren NLU (2006) Preoperative intensive inspiratory muscle training to prevent postoperative pulmonary complications in high-risk patients undergoing CABG surgery: a randomized clinical trial. JAMA 296:1851–1857
32. Gillis C, Li C, Lee L, Awasthi R, Augustin B, Gamsa A, Liberman AS, Stein B, Charlebois P, Feldman LS, Carli F (2014) Prehabilitation versus rehabilitation: a randomized control trial in patients undergoing colorectal resection for cancer. Anesthesiology 121:937–947
33. Bobbio A, Chetta A, Ampollini L, Primomo GL, Internullo E, Carbognani P, Rusca M, Olivieri D (2008) Preoperative pulmonary rehabilitation in patients undergoing lung resection for non-small cell lung cancer. Eur J Cardiothorac Surg 33:95–98
34. Cesario A, Ferri L, Galetta D, Pasqua F, Bonassi S, Clini E, Biscione G, Cardaci V, di Toro S, Zarzana A, Margaritora S, Piraino A, Russo P, Sterzi S, Granone P (2007) Post-operative respiratory rehabilitation after lung resection for non-small cell lung cancer. Lung Cancer 57:175–180
35. Cesario A, Ferri L, Galetta D, Cardaci V, Biscione G, Pasqua F, Piraino A, Bonassi S, Russo P, Sterzi S, Margaritora S, Granone P (2007) Pre-operative pulmonary rehabilitation and surgery for lung cancer. Lung Cancer 57:118–119
36. Coats V, Maltais F, Simard S, Fréchette E, Tremblay L, Ribeiro F, Saey D (2013) Feasibility and effectiveness of a home-based exercise training program before lung resection surgery. Can Respir J 20:e10–e16
37. Divisi D, Di Francesco C, Di Leonardo G, Crisci R (2013) Preoperative pulmonary rehabilitation in patients with lung cancer and chronic obstructive pulmonary disease. Eur J Cardiothorac Surg 43:293–296
38. Hoffman AJ, Brintnall RA, Brown JK, Eye AV, Jones LW, Alderink G, Ritz-Holland D, Enter M, Patzelt LH, Vanotteren GM (2013) Too sick not to exercise: using a 6-week, home-based exercise intervention for cancer-related fatigue self-management for postsurgical non-small cell lung cancer patients. Cancer Nurs 36:175–188
39. Irie M, Nakanishi R, Hamada K, Kido M (2011) Perioperative short-term pulmonary rehabilitation for patients undergoing lung volume reduction surgery. COPD 8:444–449
40. Jones LW, Peddle CJ, Eves ND, Haykowsky MJ, Courneya KS, Mackey JR, Joy AA, Kumar V, Winton TW, Reiman T (2007) Effects of presurgical exercise training on cardiorespiratory fitness among patients undergoing thoracic surgery for malignant lung lesions. Cancer 110:590–598
41. Jones LW, Eves ND, Peterson BL, Garst J, Crawford J, West MJ, Mabe S, Harpole D, Kraus WE, Douglas PS (2008) Safety and feasibility of aerobic training on cardiopulmonary function and quality of life in postsurgical nonsmall cell lung cancer patients: a pilot study. Cancer 113:3430–3439
42. Peddle-McIntyre CJ, Bell G, Fenton D, McCargar L, Courneya KS (2012) Feasibility and preliminary efficacy of progressive resistance exercise training in lung cancer survivors. Lung Cancer 75:126–132
43. Riesenberg H, Lübbe AS (2010) In-patient rehabilitation of lung cancer patients–a prospective study. Support Care Cancer 18:877–882
44. Sekine Y, Chiyo M, Iwata T, Yasufuku K, Furukawa S, Amada Y, Iyoda A, Shibuya K, Iizasa T, Fujisawa T (2005) Perioperative rehabilitation and physiotherapy for lung cancer patients with chronic obstructive pulmonary disease. Jpn J Thorac Cardiovasc Surg Off Publ Japanese Assoc Thorac Surg = Nihon Kyōbu Geka Gakkai zasshi 53:237–243
45. Spruit MA, Janssen PP, Willemsen SCP, Hochstenbag MMH, Wouters EFM (2006) Exercise capacity before and after an 8-week multidisciplinary inpatient rehabilitation program in lung cancer patients: a pilot study. Lung Cancer 52:257–260
46. Sterzi S, Cesario A, Cusumano G, Dall'Armi V, Lapenna LM, Cardaci V, Novellis P, Lococo F, Corbo GM, Cafarotti S, Margaritora S, Granone P (2013) Post-operative rehabilitation for surgically resected non-small cell lung cancer patients: serial pulmonary functional analysis. J Rehabil Med 45:911–915
47. Arbane G, Tropman D, Jackson D, Garrod R (2011) Evaluation of an early exercise intervention after thoracotomy for non-small cell lung cancer (NSCLC), effects on quality of life,

muscle strength and exercise tolerance: randomised controlled trial. Lung Cancer 71:229–234
48. Benzo R, Wigle D, Novotny P, Wetzstein M, Nichols F, Shen RK, Cassivi S, Deschamps C (2011) Preoperative pulmonary rehabilitation before lung cancer resection: results from two randomized studies. Lung Cancer 74:441–445
49. Granger CL, Chao C, McDonald CF, Berney S, Denehy L (2013) Safety and feasibility of an exercise intervention for patients following lung resection: a pilot randomized controlled trial. Integr Cancer Ther 12:213–224
50. Morano MT, Araújo AS, Nascimento FB, da Silva GF, Mesquita R, Pinto JS, de Moraes Filho MO, Pereira ED (2013) Preoperative pulmonary rehabilitation versus chest physical therapy in patients undergoing lung cancer resection: a pilot randomized controlled trial. Arch Phys Med Rehabil 94:53–58
51. Pehlivan E, Turna A, Gurses A, Gurses HN (2011) The effects of preoperative short-term intense physical therapy in lung cancer patients: a randomized controlled trial. Ann Thorac Cardiovasc Surg 17:461–468
52. Stefanelli F, Meoli I, Cobuccio R, Curcio C, Amore D, Casazza D, Tracey M, Rocco G (2013) High-intensity training and cardiopulmonary exercise testing in patients with chronic obstructive pulmonary disease and non-small-cell lung cancer undergoing lobectomy. Eur J Cardiothorac Surg 44:e260–e265
53. Stigt JA, Uil SM, van Riesen SJH, Simons FJNA, Denekamp M, Shahin GM, Groen HJM (2013) A randomized controlled trial of postthoracotomy pulmonary rehabilitation in patients with resectable lung cancer. J Thorac Oncol 8:214–221
54. Wall LM (2000) Changes in hope and power in lung cancer patients who exercise. Nurs Sci Q 13:234–242

Perioperative Care of Thoracic Trauma Patient

19

Kemalettin Koltka

19.1 Introduction

Trauma is one of the leading causes of death in the world. Thoracic trauma accounts for 20–25 % of the trauma mortality; in these cases, cardiac trauma or the rupture of great vessels is the main reason of immediate mortality.

Penetrating and blunt traumas are the two mechanisms for thoracic trauma; the mechanism is important: if a patient has a penetrating thoracic trauma (stab wounds, gunshot wounds, etc.), searching an injury in the tracheobronchial tree is the first priority in the initial examination of the patient.

In blunt trauma, traffic road accidents and falls are the most frequent mechanisms of injury [1]. In a series of 22613 patients, Huber et al. found that nearly half of the cases had pulmonary contusion (10864, 48 %); pneumothorax (8878, 39 %), rib fractures (7794, 35 %), hemothorax (6223, 28 %), flail chest (3681, 16 %), and lung laceration (2644, 12 %) are the other common injuries following thoracic trauma [1].

Blunt or penetrating thoracic trauma can cause injury to the larynx, tracheobronchial tree, lungs, or chest wall. The incidence of extrathoracic injuries associated with major blunt trauma is high; in most cases head trauma (cerebral concussion, cerebral contusion, skull fracture, facial fractures), lower and/or upper extremity injuries, and abdominal injuries are also present [2]. This chapter will focus on blunt thoracic trauma and the common diagnosis/problems after blunt thoracic trauma. As anesthesiology contains the perioperative period, an anesthetist can meet the thoracic trauma patient in the emergency department, in the operating rooms, in the ICU, and in the algology department, and the thoracic trauma patient will be discussed according to this fact.

K. Koltka
Department of Anesthesiology and Intensive Care Medicine, Istanbul University, Istanbul Faculty of Medicine, Istanbul, Turkey
e-mail: ahmetkoltka@yahoo.com

© Springer International Publishing Switzerland 2017

M. Şentürk, M.O. Sungur (eds.), *Postoperative Care in Thoracic Surgery*,
DOI 10.1007/978-3-319-19908-5_19

19.2 Traumatic Pneumothorax

Pneumothorax is one of the most common manifestations of thoracic trauma and may be noted in 40–50 % of patients with chest trauma [3]. Unfortunately a huge number of pneumothoraces are occult and cannot be seen on an initial chest x-ray but found later by additional imaging. The high incidences of occult pneumothoraces emphasize the early routine CT in all polytrauma patients. CT scan can detect not only pneumothorax but also other complications, including lung contusion, diaphragmatic rupture, and hemothorax. Detecting pneumothorax is critical, given the likelihood of pneumothorax progression if mechanical ventilation or anesthesia is required.

The use of ultrasonography is increasing for pneumothorax evaluation.

Ultrasonography is especially important in unstable trauma patients whose transport for CT scans is not possible.

The etiology of the development of a pneumothorax in blunt chest trauma in the absence of a rib fracture lacerating the visceral pleura is not very clear. A sudden increase in alveolar pressure can lead to alveolar rupture and dissection of air into the interstitium of the lung that may then dissect to the visceral pleural surface and to the mediastinum. The rupture of the visceral pleura or mediastinal pleura may lead to a pneumothorax [3].

The treatment of choice in a traumatic pneumothorax is the placement of a chest tube. In the presence of known hemothorax or mechanical ventilation, a large-bore chest tube (28–36 F) must be used; most clinicians will recommend immediate placement of a large-bore chest tube in all patients with a traumatic pneumothorax [3].

The treatment of choice in occult pneumothoraces is less clear although most occult pneumothoraces likely do not warrant the potential risk associated with a tube thoracostomy. If there is a need of positive-pressure ventilation or there is an accompanying hemothorax, then a chest tube placement must be considered. Chest tube placement not only evacuates air and blood but also can be used as a monitor of the rate of blood loss which can be a reason for immediate operative intervention [3].

19.3 Hemothorax

Massive hemothorax is defined as a rapid accumulation of more than 1.500 ml of blood in the pleural space. Such a huge hemothorax can be due to large pulmonary lacerations and great vessel or intercostal vessel injury [4]. A hemothorax can accommodate nearly half of the total blood volume. A massive hemothorax may induce hemodynamic instability due to the loss of intravascular volume and respiratory compromise due to mass effect. A trauma patient in shock, associated with the absence of breath sounds and/or dullness on one side of the chest, should be treated for massive hemothorax until proven otherwise [4]. Volume resuscitation and placement of a large-bore chest tube are initial treatment modalities, and these will be the adequate treatment for most of the cases. Bleeding generally stops in a few minutes after lung expansion. An initial drainage of > 1.500 ml blood from the chest tube or > 250 ml/h drainage for more than 3 consecutive hours or a drainage requiring blood transfusion is the main indication for operation [4].

19.4 Pulmonary Contusion

Pulmonary contusion is a common result of major trauma [1]. Although thoracic injuries among children are uncommon, 50 % of such lesions involve pulmonary contusion [5].

The clinical manifestations of pulmonary contusion may be insidious; the initial chest x-ray may be normal, and respiratory difficulty may become evident hours after injury. Patients who sustain pulmonary contusions have higher risks of pneumonia and acute respiratory distress syndrome (ARDS) and long-term respiratory disability. The outcomes of pulmonary contusions appear to be similar for pediatric and adult age groups [6].

Patients who have experienced trauma involving high-energy transfer should be evaluated for pulmonary contusion because prompt diagnosis and intervention may improve outcome [6].

It is difficult to diagnose pulmonary contusion with chest x-ray; only half of the lesions are detected at the initial chest x-ray, whereas 92 % of pulmonary contusions can be seen 24 h after the trauma. Enlargement of lung contusions on chest x-ray during the first 24 h is generally a sign of bad prognosis. Furthermore, the degree of contusion can be hard to separate clinically from the effects of aspiration, fluid overload, transfusion-related acute lung injury (TRALI), and pulmonary embolism [6].

CT scan of the thorax is currently the standard of care for the diagnosis and risk stratification of pulmonary contusions. However, there are many patients with pulmonary contusions found at CT scans and without physiologic deterioration, and some authors have suggested that newer CT scans are overly sensitive in this situation.

19.4.1 Treatment

The treatment of pulmonary contusion is primarily supportive: supplemental oxygen and rapid assessment of airway and breathing should be done according to standard trauma protocols. Pulmonary contusions may be associated with severe hypoxemia, so patient transport can be hazardous even in the prehospital setting.

In the emergency department, patients with pulmonary contusions are examined and treated according to modern trauma care protocols. Although uncommon, in patients with unilateral pulmonary contusions and/or massive intratracheal bleeding or in patients having severe air leaks, selective intubation is useful. Endobronchial blockers are useful in controlling hemoptysis in patients with diffuse pulmonary contusions [6]. Blockers are also used to protect the uninjured lung from blood and decrease the risk of air embolization. They also avoid the changing of endotracheal tubes which can be a risky procedure due to difficult intubation and problems due to trauma. But it should be kept in mind that most of the anesthetists are more familiar with the double-lumen tubes for one-lung ventilation.

Regarding the use of the devices for one-lung ventilation, one has to be aware to differentiate "lung isolation" and "lung separation." "Lung isolation" is rather a method to prevent the non-diseased lung from the contamination (such as massive bleeding, pus, etc.) of the diseased one. Therefore, it should be underlined that in "emergency" cases, lung isolation can play a more important role than lung separation. For lung isolation, double-lumen tubes are considered to be more appropriate, while blockers are designed more for the lung separation. On the other hand, the recently introduced EZBlocker can be a rational alternative, for it is easy to manage, can be used to block both lungs consequently, and can be positioned even if no fiber-optic bronchoscopy is available.

Anesthesiologists/intensivists should be familiar with the use of fiber-optic bronchoscopy (FOB) also in the emergency units. FOB should be considered as a very important part of not only the general management of the thoracic trauma patient, such as (not exclusively):

- Diagnosis and aspiration of blood and pus in the major airways
- Diagnosis of problems in airway integrity
- Lung isolation
- Lung separation during operation

Aggressive pulmonary toilet, meticulous fluid management, and an effective pain control therapy using multimodal analgesic techniques (especially regional techniques such as epidural and paravertebral blockades) are the cornerstones of treatment.

Noninvasive positive-pressure ventilation (NPPV) may be appropriate for selected patients with pulmonary contusion and hypoxemia. In a prospective evaluation of 2.770 patients with hypoxemic acute respiratory failure, NPPV was successful in patients with cardiogenic pulmonary edema (90 %) and pulmonary contusion (82 %); the success rate for patients with acute lung injury (ALI) was only 10 % [7, 8].

If endotracheal intubation is necessary, mechanical ventilation strategies should aim the optimization of oxygenation while avoiding secondary injuries. Limiting peak and plateau pressures and the use of low tidal volumes and avoiding overdistension are the cornerstones of ventilation strategies in patients with pulmonary contusions. Pressure-controlled ventilation minimizes peak (but not plateau) airway pressures and "may" help prevent barotrauma. Lung contusions usually begin to resolve in 2–5 days after trauma if other pulmonary complications are not superimposed [4]. In some cases permissive hypercapnia or alveolar recruitment maneuvers can be necessary, but these techniques must be used cautiously in patients having head trauma.

Pulmonary parenchymal repair or resection, including thoracotomy and repair, wedge resection, lobectomy, or pneumonectomy, is required in less than 2% of blunt thoracic trauma patients [9].

Pulmonary contusion should always be considered when there is an unexpectedly high alveolar-arterial PO2 difference in the course of resuscitation from or surgical repair of any thoracic injury. Rib fractures are often associated with pulmonary contusion in the area adjacent to the fractures. Pneumonia and ARDS may occur with subsequent long-term disability [4].

With the increase of our knowledge about the pathophysiology of hemorrhagic shock, innovative resuscitative approaches have emerged. Hypertonic saline has been shown to effectively restore perfusion after hemorrhagic shock, and the volume requirement is smaller than that for traditional high-volume isotonic alternatives or blood product-based approaches [10]. This treatment modality was used by several authors for thoracic trauma, but no clinical studies have demonstrated a pulmonary physiologic benefit from the use of hypertonic saline after thoracic trauma [6].

There is not enough data about the long-term impacts of pulmonary contusion on quality of life of survivors. In a small series of patients with flail chest who had or did not have pulmonary contusion, persistent abnormalities in functional residual capacity (approaching closing volume) and oxygenation were found after lung contusion. Patients with pulmonary contusion, but not those with flail chest alone, frequently exhibited disabling dyspnea. Subsequent chest CT scans revealed fibrosis in the lungs of pulmonary contusion patients with dyspnea [11]. The authors of a long-term follow-up on 55 patients with multiple trauma associated with blunt chest trauma found out that the pulmonary function tests were impaired and physical function was decreased in 70% of patients, resulting in reduced pulmonary-specific quality of life [12].

In children the prognosis is much better; in a long follow-up investigation of pediatric patients with pulmonary contusion, the results showed unremarkable chest x-rays and normal lung function, and the authors concluded that children who recover after a pulmonary contusion-laceration trauma do not suffer from significant late respiratory problems [13].

19.5 Rib Fractures

Rib fractures are one of the most common injuries found in blunt chest trauma patients [1]. In a textbook, the incidence of rib fractures after blunt trauma is stated as 60% [14]. The ribs typically involved are IV–X. If the first two ribs are broken, the patient had suffered a high-energy trauma, and as these ribs provide protection to vital structures, lesions of the brachial plexus and vessels (subclavian artery and vein) may occur, and pulmonary contusions are likely [14]. If the lower ribs are broken, injuries to the abdominal organs such as the liver, spleen, and kidneys must be sought. The fractures of the lower ribs are generally due to direct local trauma. In the elderly population, even minor traumas often result in rib fractures due to osteoporosis and decreased bone elasticity [14].

Rib fractures cause two important problems: chest wall pain and pulmonary lacerations. Untreated or poorly treated chest wall pain leads to reduced ventilation with and subsequent complications such as pneumonia and atelectasis. Pulmonary lacerations may cause pulmonary hematoma, hemothorax, and pneumothorax.

Serial rib fractures are defined as the fracture of at least three ribs and occur in almost one third of all rib fracture cases. As the number of rib fractures increases, the risk for developing a flail chest also increases.

Flail chest is a common result of blunt chest trauma and occurs in 16% of patients with blunt chest trauma [1]. There are different definitions of flail chest: at least five contiguous single rib fractures or three adjacent segmental rib fractures or at least two adjacent ribs are broken in at least two places [14, 15]. This results in an unstable flail segment with a paradoxical respiratory motion (inward motion during inspiration and outward motion during expiration). Posterior flail segments are stabilized by overlying muscles as well as the scapula and therefore may not cause severe complications. In contrast, anterior and lateral flail segments are mobile and can seriously impair respiratory function. Additionally, a flail chest is generally associated with a lung contusion [16].

19.5.1 Acute Pain Management of Patients with Multiple Fractured Ribs

Patients with multiple fractured ribs (MFR) have severe pain that adversely affects a patient's ability to cough and breathe deeply, predisposing the patient to sputum retention and respiratory insufficiency. Effective analgesia, chest physiotherapy, and respiratory care are the cornerstones of management. Effective analgesia is vital because it allows patients to breathe deeply, cough effectively, and comply with chest physiotherapy [17].

There are many analgesic options available for pain treatment in patients with MFR. If the number of ribs fractured is low and the patient is young and without other major comorbidities, systemic analgesics may suffice. Nonsteroidal anti-inflammatory drugs (NSAID), codeine, or paracetamol can be used for effective pain treatment, and patients can be discharged from the hospital safely with these medications. Generally in the acute phase, a strong opioid such as morphine is added to the treatment. Ketamine is a good option for analgesia supplementation. Both opioids and ketamine can be given in the prehospital setting [18]. If the patient has a concomitant head trauma and the observation of his/her level of consciousness is mandatory, then strong opioids or ketamine is no longer a desired option. In such cases regional techniques can be used as the main analgesic modality.

For older patients (>65 years of age) and for patients with ≥ 4 fractured ribs, regional techniques are better choices of analgesia [18]. Furthermore, underlying lung injury may not manifest early in plain chest x-rays. As such, regional nerve block should be considered in all patients when there is significant pain and/or the respiratory status is unstable.

19.5.2 Thoracic Epidural Analgesia

Thoracic epidural analgesia (TEA) can be used in these patients because it provides good pain relief, and the improvements in respiratory functions are better than intravenous opioid patient-controlled analgesia [19, 20].

In patients with bilateral MFR, TEA is the technique of choice; thoracic epidural catheter must be inserted close to the middle level of the fractured ribs.

An example of TEA protocol in trauma patients: After a test dose of 3 ml of 2.0% lignocaine with epinephrine (1:200.000), 0.5% bupivacaine in a volume of 1 ml/segment to 1.5 ml/segment can be administered as bolus followed by an infusion of 0.125% bupivacaine at a rate of 0.1 ml/kg/h to 0.2 ml/kg/h [21]. The elderly patients are the group of patients who will benefit the most from TEA because the mortality due thoracic trauma is higher in this group of patients than their younger counterparts. Contraindications of TEA in trauma patients include vertebral fracture, hemodynamic instability, and traumatic coagulopathy. In elderly patients, to have information about previous medications is mandatory: many elderly patients are using anticoagulant or antiplatelet agents. TEA has also been associated with prolonged length of stay and increased complications in elderly patients [22].

19.5.3 Thoracic Paravertebral Block

Unilateral thoracic paravertebral block (TPVB) is a good alternative to TEA in patients with MFR or to patients undergoing thoracotomy [21, 23]. TPVB has been found to be a simple and an effective method of providing continuous pain relief in patients with unilateral MFR [17]. It is technically less complex with a few absolute contraindications [24]. Specifically, the block can be performed (and the catheter withdrawn) in the presence of even a moderate degree of coagulopathy which is frequently present in polytrauma patients. Hypovolemia and hypotension are not absolute contraindications, because TPVB is associated with minimal hemodynamic problems. Opioids are infrequently used, so risks like urinary retention and pruritus are very low. Epidural and intrathecal drug administration and pneumothorax are the complications of the technique, but the incidences are low. Local anesthetic toxicity is possible, if more than one catheter is used such as in bilateral blocks [25].

An example of TPVB: After a test dose of 3 ml of 2.0% lignocaine with epinephrine (1:200.000), a bolus dose of 0.5% bupivacaine in a volume of 0.3 ml/kg (1.5 mg/kg) was injected, and this was followed by a continuous infusion of 0.25% bupivacaine at a rate of 0.1 ml/kg/h to 0.2 ml/kg/h [21].

In their study comparing TPVB with TEA in unilateral MRF patients, Mohta et al. concluded that continuous bupivacaine infusion through TPVB is as effective as through TEA for pain management in patients with unilateral fractured ribs and the outcome after two techniques is comparable [21].

19.5.4 Intercostal Nerve Block

Intercostal nerve block (ICNB) is an effective block; the main disadvantage of this block is the necessity for multiple injections at each of the levels and one level above and one below the fractured ribs. The block is generally effective for 4–8 h when a long-acting local anesthetic or epinephrine-local anesthetic combination is used [25]. The block is technically easy and simple to perform. A major disadvantage of ICNB is the necessity for repeated multiple injections which makes this cheap, easy, and effective analgesic modality a secondary option for MFR patients. However, a higher number of injections increase the risk of pneumothorax, intravascular injection, and local anesthetic toxicity.

To increase the effectiveness and utilization of ICNB, novel techniques were investigated: Truitt et al. placed two multiport catheters in an extrathoracic paraspinous location to create a continuous intercostal nerve block and started an infusion of 0.2 % ropivacaine at a constant rate of 14 ml/h in total (7 ml in each catheter) and achieved excellent analgesia, improvements in pulmonary functions, and a decreased length of stay when compared with historic controls [26]. Moving the scapula as lateral as possible and using ultrasound or fluoroscopy may facilitate ICNB at the upper thoracic levels [25]. Depending on the location of the rib fractures, ICNB can be performed at the angle of the rib (5–8 cm from midline in adults) or at the posterior axillary line. When ICNB was performed immediately lateral to the paraspinal muscles, the epidural catheter can be send toward the midline to effect a continuous TPVB without the disadvantages of multiple and repeated injections [27].

19.5.5 Interpleural Block

Interpleural analgesia has been evaluated for multiple uses, including multiple rib fracture patients [28]. Interpleural block was compared with intercostal nerve block, and the latter technique was better [29, 30].

The block is easy to perform when clear landmarks are present and usually involves the placement of a continuous catheter for infusion. The technique can be performed percutaneously, and a posterior approach is a better choice. The amount of local anesthetic injected can vary from 10 to 30 ml, and most will select a 20 ml of 0.25%–0.5% bupivacaine with epinephrine [31]. Pneumothorax, local anesthetic toxicity, unilateral Horner's syndrome, and phrenic nerve blockade are the complications of interpleural block.

Preexisting pleural effusions or hemothorax can be accepted as relative contraindication, because the fluid will make diffusion of the local anesthetic unpredictable and diminish the efficacy of the block. Infection at the insertion site or within the pleural cavity is an absolute contraindication of interpleural block [31].

References

1. Huber S, Biberthaler P, Delhey P et al (2014) Scandinavian journal of trauma. Resusc Emerg Med 22:1–9
2. Besson A, Saegesser F (1983) Color atlas of chest trauma and associated injuries. Medical Economics Books, Oradell, pp 12–14
3. Haynes D, Baumann MH (2010) Seminars in respiratory and critical care medicine. 31:769–780
4. Gerhardt MA, Gravlee GP (2008) Anesthesia considerations for cardiothoracic trauma. In: Smith CE (ed) Trauma anesthesia. Cambridge University Press, New York, pp 279–299
5. Balcı AE, Kazez A, Eren S et al (2004) Blunt thoracic trauma in children: review of 137 cases. Eur J Cardiothorac Surg 26:387–392
6. Cohn SM, DuBose JJ (2010) Pulmonary contusion: an update on recent advances in clinical management. World J Surg 34:1959–1970
7. Antonelli M, Conti G, Moro ML et al (2001) Predictors of failure of noninvasive positive pressure ventilation in patients with acute hypoxemic respiratory failure: a multi-center study. Intensive Care Med 27:1718–1728
8. Vidhani K, Kause J, Parr M (2002) Should we follow ATLS guidelines for the management of traumatic pulmonary contusion: the role of non-invasive ventilatory support. Resuscitation 52:265–268
9. Karmy-Jones R, Jurkovich J, Shatz DV et al (2001) Management of traumatic lung injury: a western trauma association multicenter review. J Trauma 51:1049–1053
10. Velasco IT, Pontieri V, Jr Rocha e Silva M et al (1980) Hyperosmotic NaCl and severe hemorrhagic shock. Am J Physiol 239:H664–H673
11. Kishikawa M, Yoshioka T, Shimazu T et al (1991) Pulmonary contusion causes long-term respiratory dysfunction with decreased functional residual capacity. J Trauma 31:1203–1208
12. Leone M, Bregeon F, Antonini F et al (2008) Long-term outcome in chest trauma. Anesthesiology 109:864–871
13. Haxhija EQ, Nöres H, Schober P et al (2004) Lung contusion-lacerations after blunt thoracic trauma in children. Pediatr Surg Int 20:412–414
14. Mommsen P, Krettek C, Hildebrand F (2011) Chest trauma: classification and influence on the general management. In: Pape HC, Sanders R, Borrelli J Jr (eds) The poly-traumatized patient with fractures. Springer, Berlin/Heidelberg, pp 75–88
15. Lorene N, Laura MC (2005) Sheehy's manual of emergency care, 6th edn. Elsevier Mosby St Louis, St. Louis, pp 655–657
16. Trupka A, Nast-Kolb D, Schweiberer L (1998) Thoracic trauma. Unfallchirurg 101:244–258
17. Karmakar MK, Critchley LA, Ho AM et al (2003) Continuous thoracic paravertebral infusion of bupivacaine for pain management in patients with multiple fractured ribs. Chest 123: 424–431
18. Michelet P, Boussen S (2013) Case scenario – thoracic trauma. Ann Fr Anesth Reanim 32: 504–509
19. Wu CL, Jani ND, Perkins FM, Barquist E (1999) Thoracic epidural analgesia versus intravenous patient-controlled analgesia for the treatment of rib fracture pain after motor vehicle crash. J Trauma 47:564–567
20. Moon MR, Luchette FA, Gibson SW et al (1999) Prospective, randomized comparison of epidural versus parenteral opioid analgesia in thoracic trauma. Ann Surg 229:684–691
21. Mohta M, Verma P, Saxena AK et al (2009) Prospective, randomized comparison of continuous thoracic epidural and thoracic paravertebral infusion in patients with unilateral multiple fractured ribs-a pilot study. J Trauma 66:1096–1101
22. Kieninger AN, Bair HA, Bendick PJ, Howells GA (2005) Epidural versus intravenous pain control in elderly patients with rib fractures. Am J Surg 189:327–330
23. Casati A, Alessandrini P, Nuzzi M et al (2006) A prospective, randomized, blinded comparison between continuous thoracic paravertebral and epidural infusion of 0.2% ropivacaine after lung resection surgery. Eur J Anaesthesiol 23:999–1004

24. Karmakar MK, Ho AMH (2007) Thoracic and lumbar paravertebral block. In: Hadzic A (ed) The New York School of Regional Anesthesia textbook of regional anesthesia and acute pain management. McGraw-Hill, New York, pp 583–597
25. Ho AM, Karmakar MK, Critchley LA (2011) Acute pain management of patients with multiple fractured ribs: a focus on regional techniques. Curr Opin Crit Care 17:323–327
26. Truitt MS, Murry J, Amos J et al (2011) Continuous intercostal nerve blockade for rib fractures: ready for primetime? J Trauma 71:1548–1552
27. Ben-Ari A, Moreno M, Chelly JE, Bigeleisen PE (2009) Ultrasound-guided paravertebral block using an intercostal approach. Anesth Analg 109:1691–1694
28. Karmakar MK, Ho AM-H (2003) Acute pain management of patients with multiple fractured ribs. J Trauma 54:615–625
29. Blake DW, Donnan G, Novella J (1989) Interpleural administration of bupivacaine after cholecystectomy: a comparison with intercostal nerve block. Anaesth Intensive Care 17:269–274
30. Bachmann-Mennenga B, Boscoping J, Kuhn DFM et al (1993) Intercostal nerve block, interpleural analgesia, thoracic epidural block or systemic opioid application for pain relief after thoracotomy? Eur J Cardiothorac Surg 7:12–18
31. Hidalgo NRA, Ferrante FM (2007) Complications of paravertebral, intercostal nerve blocks and interpleural analgesia. In: Finucane BT (ed) Complications of regional anesthesia. Springer Science, New York, pp 102–120

Chronic Obstructive Pulmonary Disease and the Postoperative Period

20

Gary H. Mills

20.1 Introduction

Chronic obstructive pulmonary disease (COPD) is encountered during thoracic surgery in four broad circumstances: (1) during one-lung anesthesia for lobectomy or removal of a lung in a patient who is/was usually a smoker and has developed lung cancer, (2) during lung volume resection surgery in emphysema or (3) bullectomy as a treatment for large bullae which are causing dyspnea or are at risk of causing pneumothoraces, and (4) in patients with COPD who may undergo lung transplantation.

Mortality after thoracic surgery is relatively high. When considering surgery for lung cancer, the mortality rates for lobectomy are 4 and 11.5 % for pneumonectomy. Postoperative pulmonary complications include air leak, pneumonia, bronchopleural fistula, and acute respiratory failure. ARDS or barotrauma may occur, often in the nonsurgical lung. Long operating times and the need for postoperative mechanical ventilation greatly increase the likelihood of complications [1].

G.H. Mills
Sheffield Teaching Hospitals and University of Sheffield, Sheffield, UK
e-mail: g.h.mills@sheffield.ac.uk

© Springer International Publishing Switzerland 2017

M. Şentürk, M.O. Sungur (eds.), *Postoperative Care in Thoracic Surgery*,
DOI 10.1007/978-3-319-19908-5_20

20.2 Which Factors Suggest Postoperative Complications in Patients with COPD?

Although COPD is an independent risk factor for perioperative complications in major surgery, somewhat surprisingly specific lung function test values in COPD alone have not been a good predictor of postoperative complications. However, certain closely related factors are important, such as low preoperative SpO_2 or recent pulmonary infection as seen in ARISCAT [2], especially in prolonged abdominal surgery and even more so in thoracic surgery. One study suggests perioperative risk may be increased by COPD with a preoperative FEV1 <70 % predicted or FEV1/FVC ratio <65 % [3]. Diffusing capacity for carbon monoxide is also a guide to severity of emphysematous change in the lung in moderate and severe COPD. Some recent studies have also confirmed COPD as an independent risk factor. In a recent analysis of over 300,000 patients (including 1200 with COPD) in the National Surgical Quality Improvement Program database undergoing abdominal surgery, COPD was independently associated with increased postoperative morbidity and with increased length of stay and mortality in some types of surgery [4]. Postoperative respiratory failure is more common in COPD [5], as is postoperative pneumonia [6]. Surgery during an exacerbation of COPD poses high risks and should only be entertained in an emergency situation. Patients should be optimally treated, until they settle back to baseline lung function. This treatment would normally involve steroids, which – if prolonged – will necessitate additional steroids to reduce the risk of adrenal suppression when surgery is eventually undertaken.

Pulmonary risk during lung resection is associated with abnormal preoperative lung function tests including a preoperative FEV1 under 60 % of predicted in lung resection surgery. DLCO is also useful in predicting risk [7, 8]. Low-risk groups include those with a preoperative FEV1 and DLCO of over 80 % predicted. Predicting postoperative pulmonary function is also important and has involved using formulas such as below that examine the amount of the lung to be resected and its functional contribution.

Predicted postoperative FEV1 (PPOFEV1) = Preoperative FEV1 × (1-(number functional lung segments being removed/total number of functional lung segments, which may be 19)).

One study has suggested that a predicted postoperative FEV1 value and DLCO of >40 % of the predicted normal preoperative values were not associated with mortality. Guidelines from the European Respiratory Society and European Society of Thoracic Surgery use a predicted postoperative FEV1 or DLCO of >30 % as the cutoff, below which death is a likely outcome [9]. Between 60 and 30 % may suggest that exercise testing such as a stair climb or shuttle test is required to better delineate the risk. More precise assessment would involve cardiopulmonary exercise testing. VO_2 max <15 ml/kg produces a high risk of complications [10]. If the predicted postoperative (PPO) VO_2 is likely to be <10 ml/kg, then resection is likely to result in death. Traditional tests such as stair climbing are effective, but unfortunately stairs are not standardized; however, being able to climb less than 12 m increased complications including death [11].

20.3 Preoperative Physiotherapy or Cardiopulmonary Rehabilitation and Their Impact on the Postoperative Period in COPD

It is important to reduce the postoperative risks in COPD patients by whatever means have been shown to be effective, as postoperative complications are common in patients undergoing one-lung anesthesia especially for lung resection surgery [12–17]. Unfortunately most work in this area has been conducted on abdominal and cardiac surgery and generally in patients without COPD. However some evidence is available, especially prior to lung volume reduction surgery, lung transplant, and, to a lesser extent, prior to lung resection for lung cancer. Preoperative pulmonary rehabilitation improves exercise capacity and dyspnea. One study has looked at the impact on moderate to severe COPD undergoing lung resection due to cancer. Prolonged rehabilitation lasting 1 month proved very difficult to deliver, whereas a ten-session program (including lower extremity endurance training for 20 mins, upper extremity endurance training, strengthening exercises, inspiratory muscle training, and slow breathing) was much more practical and appeared to reduce length of stay and shortened chest drain duration [18].

Despite the inherent potential delay to surgery, several studies have managed to look at pulmonary rehabilitation for 4 weeks prior to lung cancer resection. They have shown a reduction in postoperative respiratory morbidity, including a study by Cesario [19] and an observational study by Bobbio [20]. Unfortunately in one study of lung resection, the patients in the pulmonary rehabilitation arm had a better baseline maximal inspiratory and expiratory pressure [21], which could have influence their future outcomes.

The ability of COPD patients to exercise may not just be related to lung and cardiovascular performance. COPD patients may be unable to exercise because of limb weakness that has occurred secondary to a lack of mobility caused by the lung disease [22, 23]. Some exercise programs can overcome this and produce an improvement in walking distance, dyspnea, pulmonary functional status scale [24], cardiovascular fitness, and leg muscle strength. This then benefits patients in the postoperative period.

20.4 Smoking, COPD, and Postoperative Recovery

COPD is most commonly caused by smoking. Therefore many patients with COPD undergoing surgery are still smokers, which is likely to increase postoperative complications [25]. Smoking cessation 8 weeks prior to surgery appears to be beneficial, improving pulmonary outcomes and wound healing [26, 27]. Frequently, patients will require surgery in less than 8 weeks. It is often thought that stopping smoking close to surgery causes a worsening of pulmonary postoperative complications; however, the evidence for this is not strong [28]. Smokers undergoing surgery will need to stop in the immediate postoperative period, because of the safety requirements of supplemental oxygen. So any concern that stopping may produce respiratory secretions and related issues should not stop a patient from trying to cut down or quit prior to surgery. Consideration of the need for nicotine patches may be important in the postoperative period.

20.5 COPD in Non-thoracic Surgery

Operations on the thorax or upper abdomen are likely to significantly reduce functional residual capacity. How can this problem be reduced? If a patient can lie flat or in a suitable position for surgery, then a peripheral nerve block (such as in ophthalmic surgery) and regional or spinal/epidural analgesia/anesthesia are likely to have a lesser impact on the lung. General anesthesia using techniques that avoid intubation will reduce related bronchospasm. Unfortunately this will not be suitable for most major surgery. Laparoscopic techniques reduce postoperative pain, which is also helpful in COPD. However insufflation of CO_2 and the compressing effect of gas passed into the abdomen or thorax will add a load onto the respiratory system and contribute to atelectasis.

Induction agents including propofol obtund laryngeal and tracheal reflexes and ketamine has bronchodilator properties. During maintenance, sevoflurane is a good bronchodilator. Desflurane has rapid emergence, which may be helpful. Opioids need to be used carefully to avoid respiratory depression, especially in patients who are already CO_2 retainers. The combination of epidural anesthesia and general anesthesia reduces the incidence of postoperative pneumonia from 16 to 11 % and mortality from 9 to 5 % [29].

20.6 Mechanical Ventilation

Air trapping is a potential major issue in one- and two-lung anesthesia, leading to dynamic hyperinflation, which produces raised intrathoracic pressure in the intraoperative period, with potential respiratory and cardiovascular consequences during and after surgery. This can be visualized as failure to complete exhalation on the monitored flow time graph. Increased expiratory time can be provided by decreasing inspiratory time, increasing I/E ratio, and slowing respiratory rate. Air trapping can become severe, producing an elevation of intrathoracic pressure, which may even require temporary disconnection from the breathing circuit to allow the trapped air to escape. Application of some PEEP may hold airways open during expiration if set to levels equivalent to intrinsic PEEP. However pressures and the tendency to air trapping may vary in different parts of the lung, so the applied PEEP may not suit all lung units and a relatively low PEEP may be more effective in patients with bronchospasm. High FiO_2 leads to absorption atelectasis [30], which appears rapidly after induction of anesthesia [31, 32], becoming exponentially more of an issue when we consider time to increase in atelectasis, especially at end-tidal oxygen levels 90 % and above [33]. This is made even worse in patients with poor V/Q mismatch [34]. However, in the postoperative period, the importance of limiting inspired oxygen concentrations to avoid atelectasis is in some doubt [35], although some have postulated this confusion in the evidence is because of the use of high FiO_2 levels earlier in the anesthesia [34]. However, there are times in COPD when administration of a high FiO_2 may cause problems in patients with a raised $PaCO_2$, which may lead them to retain even more $PaCO_2$. Lung protective ventilation during surgery is also important and is dealt with in a separate chapter.

Duration of surgery is very important with a postoperative pneumonia rate of 8 % in operations lasting under 2 h, rising to 40 % for operations over 4 h in length [36].

Complete reversal of neuromuscular blockade is essential to avoid postoperative pulmonary complications [36, 37, 38, 39].

Patients with postoperative lung injury, especially after thoracic surgery, may have a huge increase in mortality (up to 39 %) at 30 days [40]. During one-lung anesthesia, lungs are subject to deflation, atelectasis, reinflation, and the effects of released inflammatory mediators, as well as the threat to anastomoses in terms of airway pressure, vascular supply, and healing.

20.7 Postoperative Interventions

Thoracic, abdominal, and aortic aneurysm surgeries are frequently complicated by postoperative pulmonary complications. Studies have looked at techniques and exercises that can be introduced or taught to patients in the preoperative period, which can be continued after surgery. Unfortunately, most of these studies have not involved thoracic surgery patients. Despite this, there are some areas where basic principles appear to make a difference. These include mobilization and adequate pain relief. Less invasive surgery can help here. Studies on major abdominal surgery have concluded that postoperative complications including postoperative pneumonia and 30-day mortality are reduced in patients with COPD when thoracic epidural analgesia is used [29].

Early mobilization reduces postoperative pulmonary complications, whereas slow mobilization adds risk with each day of delay [41]. The greatest first day barrier to mobilization was hypotension.

Patients with malnutrition or who have a low albumin are at risk of postoperative complications, and this may require intervention both before and after surgery.

20.8 Continuous Positive Airway Pressure

Continuous positive airway pressure (CPAP) has good theoretical advantages after surgery, in that it can increase transpulmonary pressure, improve functional residual capacity, expand collapsed areas, and improve gas exchange. Most studies have looked at major abdominal and cardiac surgeries. Comparisons between very brief periods of CPAP versus 6 h continuous CPAP have shown reduced incidence of pneumonia and re-ventilation with the more sustained treatment [42]. Similarly postoperative CPAP after major abdominal surgery has been shown to reduce atelectasis, pneumonia, and reintubation [43].

20.9 Noninvasive Ventilation

Noninvasive ventilation (NIV) could theoretically be useful after thoracic surgery, especially if CO2 retention is present. One concern with both CPAP and NIV is whether there will be an increased incidence of air leaks (air leaks are relatively common after pulmonary lobectomy at around 9.7 %). Fortunately the small number of studies performed on thoracic surgery patients does not appear to have found an increase [44, 45]. NIV has been used after thoracic surgery and has been found to increase arterial oxygenation.

20.10 Simpler Techniques for Improving Oxygenation

Deep breathing exercises and incentive spirometry may be effective in the post-op care of thoracic surgery patients and have the advantage that they can be quickly taught to patients both pre- and post-op [46]. Unfortunately, clinical studies in upper abdominal surgery have not been conclusive in showing major benefits [47, 48].

20.11 Lung Volume Reduction Surgery (LVRS) in COPD

Loss of elastic tissue and alveolar walls in emphysema leads to hyperinflation. This puts the respiratory muscles at a mechanical disadvantage during inspiration, especially the diaphragm which in extreme cases becomes flattened and unable to descend effectively during inspiration [49]. Therefore if patients can be selected who will gain elastic recoil following surgery, the likely outcome is an improvement in dyspnea and exercise capacity [50]. The reduction in extreme stretch on the lung may also reduce pulmonary vascular resistance. Most LVRS is performed via thoracotomy or median sternotomy. A thoracoscopic approach is also common and more recently bronchoscopic techniques have been developed.

Perioperative mortality and morbidity in LVRS is best reduced by excluding patients from surgery in the first instance with an FEV1 and homogenous emphysema of ≤20 % predicted or a DLCO ≤20 % predicted. Perioperative complications include persistent air leak, reintubation possibly with prolonged ventilation, respiratory failure, pneumonia, arrhythmias, myocardial infarction, pulmonary embolism, and bleeding. Prior to surgery, most patients will have undergone extensive pulmonary rehabilitation, treatment of COPD, and any other underlying conditions. Postoperatively, bronchospasm will be treated and if ventilator failure occurs, NIV commenced. Most air leaks settle with pleural drainage, but around 3 % persist and re-exploration may be needed. Hemorrhage requiring re-exploration occurs in around 1 %.

20.12 Bullectomy and COPD

Giant bullae occupy more than 30 % of a hemithorax. They are most commonly caused by smoking, occasionally are associated with marijuana and intravenous drug abuse. They may also occur in association with alpha-1 antitrypsin deficiency. Rarely, they occur with Marfans and Ehlers-Danlos syndrome and sarcoidosis. They make breathing less efficient and sometimes produce a secondary spontaneous pneumothorax. Postoperatively complications are similar to LVRS.

Conclusion

Care of patients with COPD in the postoperative after lung surgery relies to some extent on evidence gathered during the study of other types of major surgery. More study specific to thoracic anesthesia is needed. However, most problems that develop in the perioperative period can most effectively be dealt with by good preoperative assessment, selection, and preparation. This preparation will involve respiratory rehabilitation. Early postoperative mobilization is important. Good pain relief is also vital. Epidural analgesia has been shown to reduce the incidence of pneumonia.

References

1. Stephan F, Boucheseiche S, Hollande J, Flahault A, Cheffi A, Bazelly B, Bonnet F (2000) Pulmonary complications following lung resection: a comprehensive analysis of incidence and possible risk factors. Chest 118(5):1263–1270
2. Canet J, Gallart L, Gomar C et al (2010) Prediction of postoperative pulmonary complications in a population-based surgical cohort. Anesthesiology 113:1338
3. Gass GD, Olsen GN (1986) Preoperative pulmonary function testing to predict postoperative morbidity and mortality. Chest 89(1):127
4. Fields AC, Divino CM (2016) Surgical outcomes in patients with chronic obstructive pulmonary disease undergoing abdominal operations: an analysis of 331,425 patients. Surgery 159(4):1210
5. Arozulla AM, Daley J, Henderson WG, Khuri SF (2000) Multifactorial risk index for predicting postoperative respiratory failure in men after major noncardiac surgery. The National Veterans Administration Surgical Quality Improvement Program. Ann Surg 232:242
6. Gupta H, Gupta PK, Schuller D, Fang X, Miller WJ, Modrykamien A, Wichman TO, Morrow LE (2013) Development and validation of a risk calculator for predicting postoperative pneumonia. Mayo Clin Proc 88(11):1241–9
7. Keagy BA, Lores ME, Starek PJ, Murray GF, Lucas CL, Wilcox BR (1985) Elective pulmonary lobectomy: factors associated with morbidity and operative mortality. Ann Thorac Surg 40(4):349
8. Zhang R, Lee SM, Wigfield C, Vigneswaran WT, Ferguson MK (2015) Lung function predicts pulmonary complications regardless of the surgical approach. Ann Thorac Surg 99(5):1761
9. Brunelli A, Charloux A, Bolliger CT, Rocco G, Sculier JP, Varela G, Licker M, Ferguson MK, Faivre-Finn C, Huber RM, Clini EM, Win T, De Ruysscher D, Goldman L, European Respiratory Society and European Society of Thoracic Surgeons joint task force on fitness for radical therapy (2009) ERS/ESTS clinical guidelines on fitness for radical therapy in lung cancer patients (surgery and chemo-radiotherapy). Eur Respir J 34(1):17
10. Smith TP, Kinasewitz GT, Tucker WY, Spillers WP, George RB (1984) Exercise capacity as a predictor of post-thoracotomy morbidity. Am Rev Respir Dis 129(5):730
11. Brunelli A, Refai M, Xiumé F, Salati M, Sciarra V, Socci L, Sabbatini A, 1 (2008) Performance at symptom-limited stair-climbing test is associated with increased cardiopulmonary complications, mortality, and costs after major lung resection. Ann Thorac Surg 86:240
12. Win T, Sharples L, Groves AM et al (2008) Predicting survival in potentially curable lung cancer patients. Lung 86:97–102
13. Damhuis RAM, Schutte PR (1996) Resection rates and postoperative mortality in 7,899 patients with lung cancer. Eur Respir J 9:7–10
14. Little AG, Rusch VW, Bonner JA et al (2005) Patterns of surgical care of lung cancer patients. Ann Thorac Surg 80:2051–6

15. Benzo R, Kelley GA, Recchi L et al (2007) Complications of lung resection and exercise capacity: a meta-analysis. Respir Med 101:1790–7
16. Bartels M, Kim H, Whiteson J et al (2006) Pulmonary rehabilitation in patients undergoing lung-volume reduction surgery. Arch Phys Med Rehabil 87:84–8
17. Takaoka ST (2005) The value of preoperative pulmonary rehabilitation. Thorac Surg Clin 15:203–11
18. Benzo R, Wigle D, Novotny P et al (2011) Preoperative pulmonary rehabilitation before lung cancer resection: results from 2 randomized studies. Lung Cancer 74(3):441–445. doi:10.1016/j.lungcan.2011.05.011
19. Cesario A, Ferri L, Galetta D et al (2007) Pre-operative pulmonary rehabilitation and surgery for lung cancer. Lung Cancer 57:118–9
20. Bobbio A, Chetta A, Ampollini L et al (2008) Preoperative pulmonary rehabilitation in patients undergoing lung resection for non-small cell lung cancer. Eur J Cardiothorac Surg 33:95–8
21. Morano MT, Arau'jo AS, Nascimento FB, da Silva GF, Mesquita R, Pinto JS, de Moraes Filho MO, Pereira ED (2013) Preoperative pulmonary rehabilitation versus chest physical therapy in patients undergoing lung cancer resection: a pilot randomized controlled trial. Arch Phys Med Rehabil 94:53–8
22. Kyroussis D, Polkey MI, Hamnegard CH, Mills GH, Green M, Moxham J (2000) Respiratory muscle activity in patients with COPD walking to exhaustion with and without pressure support. Eur Respir J 15(4):649–55
23. Polkey MI, Kyroussis D, Keilty SE, Hamnegard CH, Mills GH, Green M, Moxham J (1995) Exhaustive treadmill exercise does not reduce twitch transdiaphragmatic pressure in patients with COPD. Am J Respir Crit Care Med 152(3):959–64
24. Votto J, Bowen J, Scalise P, Wollschlager C, ZuWallack R (1996) Short-stay comprehensive inpatient pulmonary rehabilitation for advanced chronic obstructive pulmonary disease. Arch Phys Med Rehabil 77:1115–8
25. Fagevik Olsén M, Hahn I, Nordgren S, Lönroth H, Lundholm K (1997) Randomized controlled trial of prophylactic chest physiotherapy in major abdominal surgery. Br J Surg 84(11):1535
26. Thomsen T, Villebro N, Møller AM (2010) Interventions for preoperative smoking cessation. Cochrane Database Syst Rev 2010 Jul 7;(7):CD002294. doi: 10.1002/14651858.CD002294.pub3.
27. Jung KH, Kim SM, Choi MG, Lee JH, Noh JH, Sohn TS, Bae JM, Kim S (2015) Preoperative smoking cessation can reduce postoperative complications in gastric cancer surgery. Gastric Cancer 18(4):683
28. Myers K, Hajek P, Hinds C, McRobbie H (2011) Stopping smoking shortly before surgery and postoperative complications: a systematic review and meta-analysis. Arch Intern Med 171(11):983
29. van Lier F, van der Geest PJ, Hoeks SE, van Gestel YR, Hol JW, Sin DD, Stolker RJ, Poldermans D (2011) Epidural analgesia is associated with improved health outcomes of surgical patients with chronic obstructive pulmonary disease. Anesthesiology 115(2):315–21
30. Magnusson L, Spahn DR (2003) New concepts of atelectasis during general anaesthesia. Br J Anaesth 91:61–72
31. Brismar B, Hedenstierna G, Lundquist H et al (1985) Pulmonary densities during anesthesia with muscular relaxation: a proposal of atelectasis. Anesthesiology 62:422–8
32. Lundquist H, Hedenstierna G, Strandberg A et al (1995) CT assessment of dependent lung densities in man during general anaesthesia. Acta Radiol 36:626–32
33. Edmark L, Kostova-Aherdan K, Enlund M, Hedenstierna G (2003) Optimal oxygen concentration during induction of general anesthesia. Anesthesiology 98:28–33
34. Hedenstierna G, Rothen HU. (2012) Respiratory function during anesthesia: effects on gas exchange. Compr Physiol. 2012 Jan;2(1):69-96. doi: 10.1002/cphy.c080111. Review. PMID: 23728971

35. Akca O, Podolsky A, Eisenhuber E et al (1999) Comparable postoperative pulmonary atelectasis in patients given 30% or 80% oxygen during and 2 hours after colon resection. Anesthesiology 91:991–8
36. Schmid M, Sood A, Campbell L, Kapoor V, Dalela D, Klett DE, Chun FK, Kibel AS, Sammon JD, Menon M, Fisch M, Trinh QD (2015) Impact of smoking on perioperative outcomes after major surgery. Am J Surg 210(2):221–229, e6. Epub 2015 Apr 23
37. Murphy GS, Brull SJ (2010) Residual neuromuscular block: lessons unlearned. Part I: definitions, incidence, and adverse physiologic effects of residual neuromuscular block. Anesth Analg 111:120
38. Brull SJ, Murphy GS (2010) Residual neuromuscular block: lessons unlearned. Part II: methods to reduce the risk of residual weakness. Anesth Analg 111:129
39. Grosse-Sundrup M, Henneman JP, Sandberg WS et al (2012) Intermediate acting non-depolarizing neuromuscular blocking agents and risk of postoperative respiratory complications: prospective propensity score matched cohort study. BMJ 345:e6329
40. Serpa NA et al (2014) Incidence of mortality and morbidity related to postoperative lung injury in patients who have undergone abdominal or thoracic surgery: a systematic review and meta-analysis. Lancet Respir Med 2(12):1007–15
41. Haines KJ, Skinner EH, Berney S, Austin Health POST Study Investigators (2013) Association of postoperative pulmonary complications with delayed mobilisation following major abdominal surgery: an observational cohort study. Physiotherapy 99(2):119–25. Epub 2012 Sep 23
42. Zarbock A, Mueller E, Netzer S et al (2009) Prophylactic nasal continuous positive airway pressure following cardiac surgery protects from postoperative pulmonary complications: a prospective, randomized, controlled trial in 500 patients. Chest 135:1252
43. Ireland CJ, Chapman TM, Mathew SF, Herbison GP, Zacharias M. (2014) Continuous positive airway pressure (CPAP) during the postoperative period for prevention of postoperative morbidity and mortality following major abdominal surgery. Cochrane Database Syst Rev. 2014 Aug 1;(8):CD008930. doi: 10.1002/14651858.CD008930.pub2.
44. Aguilo R, Togores B, Pons S, Rubi M, Barbe F, Agusti AG (1997) Non-invasive ventilatory support after lung resectional surgery. Chest 112(1):117–121
45. Nery FP, Lopes AJ, Domingos DN, Cunha RF, Peixoto MG, Higa C et al (2011) CPAP increases 6-minute walk distance after lung resection surgery. Respir Care 57(3):363–369
46. Perrin C, Jullien V, Venissac N, Berthier F, Padovani B, Guillot F et al (2007) Prophylactic use of noninvasive ventilation in patients under-going lung resectional surgery. Respir Med 101(7):1572–1578
47. Agostini P, Naidu B, Cieslik H, Steyn R, Rajesh PB, Bishay E, Kalkat MS, Singh S (2013) Effectiveness of incentive spirometry in patients following thoracotomy and lung resection including those at high risk for developing pulmonary complications. Thorax 68(6):580–5. Epub 2013 Feb 21
48. do Nascimento Junior P, Módolo NS, Andrade S, Guimarães MM, Braz LG, El Dib R. Cochrane Database Syst Rev. 2014 Feb 8;(2):CD006058. doi: 10.1002/14651858.CD006058.pub3. Review. PMID: 24510642
49. Bloch KE, Li Y, Zhang J et al (1997) Effect of surgical lung volume reduction on breathing patterns in severe pulmonary emphysema. Am J Respir Crit Care Med 156:553
50. National Emphysema Treatment Trial Research Group (2001) Patients at high risk of death after lung-volume-reduction surgery. N Engl J Med 345:1075

Index

© Springer International Publishing Switzerland 2017

M. Şentürk, M.O. Sungur (eds.), *Postoperative Care in Thoracic Surgery*,
DOI 10.1007/978-3-319-19908-5

J

L

M

N

9783319199078